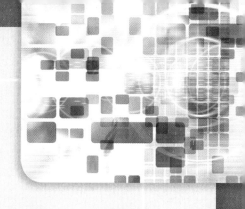

D1599590

Coding Review
for National Certification

Passing the CPC and CCS-P Exams

Mary Harmon, BS, CMA, CPC

MedTech College
Indianapolis, Indiana

Mc Graw Hill **Higher Education**

Boston   Burr Ridge, IL   Dubuque, IA   New York   San Francisco   St. Louis
Bangkok   Bogotá   Caracas   Kuala Lumpur   Lisbon   London   Madrid   Mexico City
Milan   Montreal   New Delhi   Santiago   Seoul   Singapore   Sydney   Taipei   Toronto

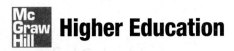

The McGraw·Hill Companies

Higher Education

CODING REVIEW FOR NATIONAL CERTIFICATION: PASSING THE CPC AND CCS-P EXAMS

Published by McGraw-Hill, a business unit of The McGraw-Hill Companies, Inc., 1221 Avenue of the Americas, New York, NY, 10020.

This book is printed on acid-free paper.

1 2 3 4 5 6 7 8 9 0 QPD/QPD 0 9

ISBN 978-0-07-337398-0
MHID 0-07-337398-2

Vice president/Editor in chief: *Elizabeth Haefele*
Vice president/Director of marketing: *John E. Biernat*
Sponsoring editor: *Natalie J. Ruffatto*
Director of development, Allied Health: *Patricia Hesse*
Executive marketing manager: *Roxan Kinsey*
Lead media producer: *Damian Moshak*
Media developmental editor: *Marc Mattson*
Director, Editing/Design/Production: *Jess Ann Kosic*
Project manager: *Christine M. Demma*
Senior production supervisor: *Janean A. Utley*
Senior designer: *Srdjan Savanovic*
Senior photo research coordinator: *John C. Leland*
Media project manager: *Mark A. S. Dierker*
Outside development house: *Barb Tucker, S4Carlisle Publishing Services*
Cover design: *Srdjan Savanovic*
Interior design: *Pam Verros*
Typeface: *10/12 Times New Roman*
Compositor: *Laserwords Private Limited*
Printer: *Quebecor World Dubuque Inc.*
Cover credit: © *GRAFIKA/Miyano Takuya/Norihiro Uehara*
Photo Credits: **Frontmatter:** © Photodisc/Punchstock/RF; © Photodisc/Getty Images/RF; © dynamicgraphics/Jupiterimages/RF; and © Veer/RF; **Unit Opener 1:** © Brand X Pictures/Punchstock/RF; **Unit Opener 2:** © Brand X Pictures/Punchstock/RF; **Unit Opener 3:** © Brand X Pictures/Punchstock/RF; **Unit Opener 4:** © Brand X Pictures/Punchstock/RF; **Chapter Opener 1:** © BananaStock/JupiterImages/RF; **Chapter Opener 2:** © Brand X Pictures/Punchstock/RF; **Chapter Opener 3:** © Getty Images/RF; **Chapter Opener 4:** © Royalty-Free/CORBIS; **Chapter Opener 5:** © Comstock Images/PictureQuest/RF; **Chapter Opener 6:** © Royalty-Free/CORBIS; **Chapter Opener 7:** © Royalty-Free/CORBIS; **Chapter Opener 8:** © JupiterImages/Dynamic/RF; **Chapter Opener 9:** © liquidlibrary/PictureQuest/RF; **Chapter Opener 10:** © Getty Images/Steve Allen/RF; **Chapter Opener 11:** © Steve Mason/Getty Images/RF; **Chapter Opener 12:** © Glowimages/RF; **Chapter Opener 13:** © David Chase/Getty Images/RF; and **Chapter Opener 14:** (c) Veer/RF.

Library of Congress Cataloging-in-Publication Data
Harmon, Mary.
 Coding review for national certification : passing the CPC and CCS-P exams / Mary Harmon.
  p. ; cm.
 Includes index.
 ISBN-13: 978-0-07-337398-0 (alk. paper)
 ISBN-10: 0-07-337398-2 (alk. paper)
 1. Nosology—Code numbers—Examinations, questions, etc. 2. Medical records—Management—Examinations, questions, etc. 3. Medicine—Code numbers—Study guides. I. Title.
 [DNLM: 1. Forms and Records Control—Examination Questions. 2. Medical Records—Examination Questions. W 18.2 H288c 2010]
 RB115.H37 2010
 616.001'2—dc22   2008050327

The Internet addresses listed in the text were accurate at the time of publication. The inclusion of a Web site does not indicate an endorsement by the authors or McGraw-Hill, and McGraw-Hill does not guarantee the accuracy of the information presented at these sites.

www.mhhe.com

Dedication

To the greatest inspirations in my life; Zakk, Jake, and Jordan. Remember, all who wander are not lost . . .

About the Author

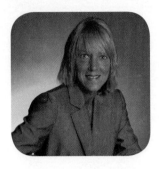

Mary Harmon is a professional, credentialed medical coder and the Executive Vice President of Academics for a chain of allied health schools based in Indianapolis, of which she is one of the owners. She started out 18 years ago as a medical coder and medical assistant. She began coding in an OB/GYN office back when it was still acceptable for insurance companies to "write in" the diagnosis and procedures instead of using codes on an insurance claim form.

As the onset of the computer age took hold, medical coding began to take on a new form. Computers processed numbers much more quickly than alpha characters and the use of medical codes became prominent. Along with that, medical reimbursement in the United States became a priority with the ever-growing deficits in the health care system. The need for medical coders was imminent as they began to take their place in the allied health care system. The need for individuals to become formally educated in the field of medical coding, insurance, and reimbursement was growing. With the early coding experience Mary obtained, coupled with the opportunities presented to her to train other medical personnel, Mary became an instructor in this field. She realized that the need for trained professional coders was not going to wane and she wanted to be instrumental in training individuals for a career in medical coding.

Mary taught for many years in medical coding and medical assisting programs and eventually began to write curriculum for many allied health programs with a focus on medical coding. She gained degrees in Adult Education and Psychology to aid in the process of understanding how adults learn. During her years of instructing, she continually encountered problems with finding textbooks written for medical coding classes. Thus began the writing of her own material for ICD-9, CPT, HCPCS, and reimbursement courses. As time went on, textbooks written for medical coding courses began to take hold; however, there was not enough material to quench the thirst her students had for more practice in medical coding. She would go home at night and on weekends to create "coding problems" for her students so that she could challenge them in every way possible to become professionals in their area and heighten their skills.

Eventually, Mary's career involved writing medical curriculum, training instructors on how to teach medical coding, and preparing students to write for a national certification to gain professional credentialing in coding. With the onset of creating a chain of allied health schools with her business partners Mary realized she could use this opportunity to offer the best, most concentrated medical coding programs possible. However, she felt that one very important aspect of her coding programs was lacking. With the demand for medical coders to become certified, Mary needed a capstone course that specifically focused on passing a national coding credential. She searched for a textbook that would accomplish this and was unsuccessful. There just was not a review text that she was comfortable with, that gave her the reassurance that her students would be provided with a comprehensive review to prepare them for certification. A moderate amount of coding practice alone was not enough. Mary needed each of her students to "think like a coder;" and her philosophy is that if you think like a coder you will become a coder.

With the demand for medical coders to become certified, Mary quickly identified the areas her students would need to work on at the end of their coding program to help them pass an examination. The need for an overall review, coding practice, in-depth knowledge, and applied understanding of coding guidelines was necessary. Each of Mary's students needed to "think like a coder" in order to pass a coding examination with relative ease. You cannot do this without applied practice and a comprehensive review that sets the stage for a real-life examination. Tips for indexing, applied coding practice, review of medical terminology, anatomy and physiology, pathophysiology, coding guidelines, modifiers, abstracting, special coding alerts, and a logical thinking process is what it takes in a review course to pass a medical coding examination. So she decided to author her own review textbook and wrote this review textbook, for you the student.

Mary is very excited about this project, and hopes that it provides students' with an overall view of medical coding and applied understanding of coding guidelines and prepares them for the challenge of professional medical coding. If you practice your skills and follow the suggestions and tips in this textbook, you will be prepared for the challenge of passing a national coding certification.

Brief Contents

Preface xiv

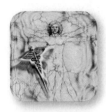

UNIT 1: Foundation for Taking the Coding Examination   1

Chapter 1: Test-Taking skills   2

Chapter 2: Anatomy and Physiology Review   12

Chapter 3: Medical Terminology and Pathophysiology Review   31

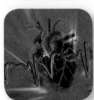

UNIT 2: Procedures Review   61

Chapter 4: CPT Guidelines Review   62

Chapter 5: Evaluation and Management Review   72

Chapter 6: Anesthesia Review   91

Chapter 7: Surgery Review   98

Chapter 8: Radiology Review   122

Chapter 9: Pathology and Laboratory Review   131

Chapter 10: Medicine Section Review   141

Chapter 11: HCPCS Level II Coding Review   157

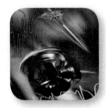

UNIT 3: Diagnoses Review   163

Chapter 12: ICD-9-CM Guidelines and Coding Conventions
Review, Part I   164

Chapter 13: ICD-9-CM Guidelines and Coding Conventions
Review, Part II   192

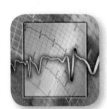

UNIT 4: Practice Coding Examination   217

Chapter 14: Practice Examination   218

Appendix A: Answers and Rationale   236

Appendix B: Abbreviations   250

Appendix C: Correlations to Certification Examinations   255

Glossary   259

Index   262

Contents

Preface   xiv

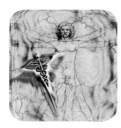

UNIT 1: Foundation for Taking the Coding Examination   1

Chapter 1:

Test-Taking Skills   2
  Recommended Time for Study   3
  Time Management   3
  Making the Most of your Time   3
  Examination Content   5
  Study Skills Strategies   6
  Focusing   6
  Pre-reading Strategies   6
  Open Book Tests   6
  Test-Taking Skills   7
  Studying/Comprehending Medical Records   8
  Multiple Choice Questions   8
  How to Overcome Text Anxiety   9
  Preparing for Your Examination   10
  The Day of the Examination   10

Chapter 2:

Anatomy and Physiology Review   12
  Directional Terms   13
  Anatomy and Physiology Overview   13
  The Integumentary System   13
  The Respiratory System   15
  The Urinary System   16
  The Male Reproductive System   16
  The Female Reproductive System   17
  The Cardiovascular and Blood Systems   18
  The Digestive System   19
  Eyes, Ears, and Nose (Senses)   20
  The Musculoskeletal System   21
  The Nervous System   23
  Parts of the Brain   24
  Spinal Cord   25
  The Endocrine System   25

Chapter 3:

Medical Terminology and Pathophysiology Review   31
  Medical Word Components   32
  Word Roots Review   32
  Combining Forms Review   32
  Prefixes Review   33
  Suffixes Review   34
  Integumentary System Terminology Review   34
  Respiratory System Terminology Review   36
  Urinary System Terminology Review   38
  Male Reproductive System Terminology Review   38
  Female Reproductive System Terminology Review   42
  Cardiovascular System Terminology Review   44
  Blood and Lymphatic System Terminology Review   46
  Digestive System Terminology Review   48
  Terminology Review of the Senses   50
  Terminology Review of the Musculoskeletal System   52
  Terminology Review of the Nervous System   54
  Endocrine System Terminology Review   57

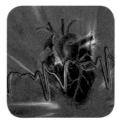

UNIT 2: Procedures Review   61

Chapter 4:

CPT Guidelines Review   62
  Introduction   63
  Section Numbers and their Sequence   63
  Review Instructions for Using the CPT Manual   64
  Format of the Terminology   65

Guidelines **65**

Add-on Codes **67**

Modifiers **67**

Unlisted Procedure of Service **69**

Special Report **69**

Code Changes **69**

Listing of CPT Appendices: A-M **69**

Chapter 5:

Evaluation and Management Review **72**

Classification of Evaluation and Management Services 73

New and Established Patients 73

Chief Complaint 73

Concurrent Care 74

Counseling 74

Family History and History of Present Illness 74

Levels of Service 74

Nature of Presenting Problem 74

Past and Social History 75

Past History 75

Social History 75

Review of Systems 75

Time 76

Face-to-Face Time 76

Non–Face-to-Face Time 76

Unit-Floor Time 76

Clinical Examples 77

Review of Instructions for Selecting a Level of Evaluation and Management Service 77

Determining Extent of History 77

Extent of Examination Performed 78

Level of Medical Decision Making 79

Appropriate Level of E&M Services 80

Office or Other Outpatient Services 80

Hospital Observation Services 81

Hospital Inpatient Services 82

Consultations 82

Emergency Department Services 83

Critical Care Services 83

Inpatient Neonatal and Pediatric Critical Care Intensive Services 84

Nursing Facility Services 84

Home Services, Prolonged Services 85

Case Management Services, Care Plan Oversight Services 85

Preventive Medicine Services and Newborn Care 85

Chapter 6:

Anesthesia Review **91**

Time Reporting 92

Physician's Services and Materials Supplied by the Physician 92

Special Report 92

Anesthesia Modifiers 92

Physical Status Modifiers 93

Qualifying Circumstances 93

Types of Anesthesia 94

How to Locate Anesthesia Codes 94

Chapter 7:

Surgery Review **98**

Surgery 99

CPT Surgical Package Definition 99

Commonly Used Modifiers in the Surgery Section 99

Separate Procedures 101

Materials Supplied by a Physician 101

Reporting More Than One Procedure/Service 101

Special Report 101

Unlisted Service or Procedure 102

Quick and Accurate Coding 102

Add-On Codes 102

Integumentary System 103

Skin, Subcutaneous, and Accessory Structures 103

Repair 103

Destruction and Excision—Breast 104

Musculoskeletal System 105

Fractures 105

Spine (Vertebral Column) 105

Arthrodesis 107

Application of Casts and Strapping 107

Respiratory System 107

Endoscopy 107

Lung Transplantation 107

Cardiovascular System   108
Pacemaker or Pacing Cardioverter-Defibrillator   108
Electrophysiological Operative Procedures   109
Venous Grafting Only for Coronary Artery Bypass   110
Combined Arterial-Venous Grafting for Coronary Bypass   110
Arterial Grafting for Coronary Artery Bypass   110
Endovascular Repair of Descending Thoracic Aorta   110
Heart/Lung Transplant   111
Vascular Injection Procedures   111
Central Venous Access Procedures   111
Digestive System   112
Endoscopy/Laparoscopy   112
Intestines   112
Repair of Hernia   112
Urinary System   113
Renal Transplantation   113
Urodynamics   113
Endoscopy: Cystoscopy, Urethrosocopy, Cystourethrosocopy   113
Male and Female Genital System   114
Female Genital System   114
Maternity Care and Delivery   114
Male Genital System   115
Nervous and Endocrine Systems   115
Surgery of Skull Base   115
Injection, Drainage, or Aspiration   116
Eye, Ocular, Adnexa, and Auditory System   117

Chapter 8:

Radiology Review   122
Supervision and Interpretation   123
Modifiers in the Radiology Section   123
Professional Versus Technical Component   124
Special Report   124
Administration of Contrast Materials   124
Radiology System Coding Notes for Review   125
Aorta and Arteries   125
Veins and Lymphatics   126
Diagnostic Ultrasound   126
Radiation Oncology   127

Clinical Treatment Planning   127
Radiation Treatment Management   127
Proton Beam Treatment Delivery   128
Clinical Brachytherapy   128

Chapter 9:

Pathology and Laboratory Review   131
Qualitative and Quantitative Tests   132
Pathology and Laboratory Notes for Review   133
Organ or Disease-Oriented Panels   133
Drug Testing   133
Evocative/Suppression Testing   134
Urinalysis   134
Chemistry   134
Hematology and Coagulation   135
Immunology   136
Microbiology   136
Cytopathology   136
Surgical Pathology   136

Chapter 10:

Medicine Section Review   141
Modifiers   142
Special Report   142
Separate Procedures   143
Add-On Codes   143
Unlisted Service or Procedures   143
Medicine Coding Notes   143
Immunization Administration for Vaccines/Toxoids   143
Hydration, Therapeutic, Prophylactic, and Diagnostic Injections and Infusions (Excludes Chemotherapy)   144
Hydration   145
Psychiatry   145
Dialysis   146
Ophthalmology   146
Special Otorhinolaryngological Services   147
Cardiovascular   148
Pulmonary   149
Neurology and Neuromuscular Procedures   149
Chemotherapy Administration   150
Acupuncture   151
Osteopathic and Chiropractic Manipulative Treatment   151
On-Line Medical Evaluation   151

Moderate Conscious Sedation 151
Category II Codes 152
Modifiers Used with Category II Codes 153
Category III Codes 153

Chapter 11:

HCPCS Level II Codes Review 157
**HCPCS Level II Codes Section
Breakdowns 158**
**General Guidelines for HCPCS Coding
Assignments 158**
HCPCS Table of Drugs 159
**Medical and Surgical Supplies
A4000-A8999 159**
Dental Procedures 160
Durable Medical Equipment 160
**Alcohol and Drug Abuse Treatment
Services 160**
Orthotic and Prosthetic Procedures 160
HCPCS Level II Modifiers 160

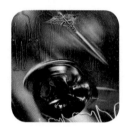

**UNIT 3: Diagnoses
Review 163**

Chapter 12:

ICD-9-CM Guidelines and Coding Conventions
Review, Part I 164
**ICD-9-CM Coding Conventions
and Guidelines 165**
Review of the ICD-9-CM Coding Manual 165
ICD-9-CM Official Coding Conventions 166
ICD-9-CM Official Coding Guidelines 168
**V Codes and E Codes: Supplementary
Classifications 169**
*Chapter 18: Classification of Factors Influencing
Health Status and Contact with Health Service
(V01-V86) 169*
*Chapter 19: Supplemental Classification
of External Causes of Injury and Poisoning
(E800-E999) 171*
Tables within the Index to Diseases 173
Table of Drugs and Chemicals 173
Neoplasm Table 173
Hypertension Table 175

ICD-9-CM Coding Notes for Review 175
*Chapter 1: Infectious and Parasitic Diseases
(001-139) 175*
Chapter 2: Neoplasms (140-239) 177
*Chapter 3: Endocrine, Nutritional, and Metabolic
Diseases and Immunity Disorders (240-279) 179*
*Chapter 4: Diseases of Blood and Blood-Forming
Organs (280-289) 180*
Chapter 5: Mental Disorders (290-319) 180
*Chapter 6: Diseases of Nervous System and Sense
Organs (320-389) 181*
*Chapter 7: Diseases of the Circulatory System
(390-459) 182*
*Chapter 8: Disease of the Respiratory System
(460-519) 185*
**Review of Health Insurance
Portability and Accountability Act
Enforcement 187**
Preventing Health Care Fraud and Abuse 187
**Review of Uniform Hospital Data
Discharge Set 188**
Procedures 188
Diagnoses 189

Chapter 13:

ICD-9-CM Guidelines and Coding Conventions
Review, Part II 192
ICD-9 CM Coding Notes for Review 193
*Chapter 9: Diseases of the Digestive System
(520-579) 193*
*Chapter 10: Diseases of the Genitourinary System
(580-629) 195*
*Chapter 11: Complications of Pregnancy,
Childbirth, and Puerperium (630-677) 196*
*Chapter 12: Diseases of Skin and Subcutaneous
Tissue (680-709) 200*
*Chapter 13: Diseases of Musculoskeletal System and
Connective Tissue (710-739) 201*
Chapter 14: Congenital Anomalies (740-759) 203
*Chapter 15: Conditions in the Perinatal Period
(760-779) 204*
*Chapter 16: Signs, Symptoms, and Ill-Defined
Conditions (780-799) 206*
Chapter 17: Injury and Poisoning (800-999) 207
**Review of Date Quality and
Management 210**
Insurance Claims 210
Diagnostic Related Groups Review 212

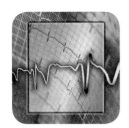

UNIT 4: Practice Coding Examination   217

Chapter 14:

Practice Examination   218
   Directions   219
   Medical Terminology   219
   Anatomy and Physiology   219
   Health Information Management   220
   Reimbursement   221
   Data Quality   222
   ICD-9-CM Coding   223

HCPCS Codes   224
Evaluation and Management Codes   224
Anesthesia   227
Surgery Section   228
Radiology   229
Pathology and Laboratory   231
Medicine   232
Miscellaneous   232

Appendix A: Answers and Rationale   236
Appendix B: Abbreviations   250
Appendix C: Correlations to Certification
Examinations   255

Glossary   259
Index   262

Preface

To the Student

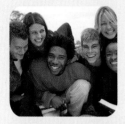

This review text was designed for you, the student, to help you successfully pass your national coding examination. It is a useful resource to review areas of medical coding that are somewhat difficult for you or are vague in your memory. I have taken a very comprehensive approach to this review, in which all content areas in both the CPC and CCS-P credentials are covered. The field of medical coding is continually expanding, and the demand for certification is greater now that it ever has been. Because of reimbursement issues and health care costs in the United States, health care systems cannot afford to hire individuals who are not educated or credentialed. The greatest value, for medical coders, is placed on the highest levels of technical specialty. Although medical coding positions can be very specialized and compartmental, the trend in this area is towards a greater degree of generalization and overall professional knowledge.

Over the years, it has been my privilege to instruct students in the field of medical coding. I have instructed students who were unsure of themselves and did not think that they could "make it" in this field. Today, many of those students are colleagues of mine. My philosophy with them was practice, practice, practice and "think like a coder." My advice to you is the same. You must have intimate knowledge of the CPT and ICD-9 manuals, including their sections, subsections, guidelines, tables, indexes, and tabular listings, in order to think like a coder. Only practice can provide you with this type of in-depth knowledge of your most useful tools. The coding manuals should be likened to shopping in your favorite store; you always know where everything is. If you know where everything is, it cannot be hard to find!

To the Medical Coding Instructor

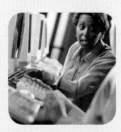

The first edition of *Coding Review for National Certification; Passing the CPC and CCS-P Exams* is addressed to the student who has completed a formal education in medical coding or an individual with at least three years full-time medical coding experience who is seeking certification. As an instructor, the goal of this textbook is three-fold.

- First, the student needs to be guided through an overall review of the CPT and ICD-9 manuals, their guidelines, modifiers, coding conventions, and specific notations to coding descriptors.

- Secondly, practice must be facilitated by you, the instructor. Statistics in learning have shown that repeated practice of a skill objective by an adult learner increases performance that leads to the mastery of the skill. This textbook includes many practice problems throughout the body of the text, coding problems at the end of each chapter, and a mock examination at the end of the textbook. Lastly, as an instructor using this textbook, you want to help each student to "think like a coder." This concept is very important in order to set the stage for success for the student. Learning to think through every coding problem or question in an analytical, organized, sequential approach teaches the student to attack the "problem" in a consistent manner, which in turn, provides consistent accuracy in coding.

- Features such as "Think Like a Coder," "Indexing Tips," and "Coding Alert" are all mechanisms used to expound on the importance of ideas or concepts that help the student to relate to medical coding in a logical manner. Reinforcers are used consistently throughout the textbook in the form of questions, coding problems/scenarios, examples, tables, and illustrations. The textbook follows all of the ICD-9, CPT, and HCPCS guidelines and coding conventions that are up to date; these guidelines and conventions are applied in the textbook in a logical and sequential manner.

About the Textbook

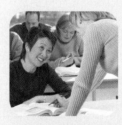

Coding Review for National Certification; Passing the CPC and CCS-P Exams, first edition, represents a comprehensive approach to mastering concepts needed for obtaining a professional credential in medical coding.

- This first edition review textbook can be used in a vocational academic setting, in the work environment, and for home study by individuals choosing to obtain credentialing in the coding field.

- It is designed for individuals who have had a formal education in medical coding or for individuals who have at least 3 years of full-time coding experience in both ICD-9-CM and CPT coding.

- The review is targeted for the CPC credential offered by the American Academy of Professional Coders

(AAPC) and the CCS-P credential offered by the American Health Information Management Association (AHIMA) through the Commission on Accreditation for Health Informatics and Information Management Education (CAHIIM).

- Both examinations are geared toward physician-based coding and are similar, yet different in various ways. Both examinations include content for ICD-9 and CPT guidelines, abstracting, HCPCS, diagnosis code linking to CPT, and modifier concepts.
- The CPC examination includes medical terminology, anatomy and physiology, and ICD-9 coding with a concentration in CPT coding and their appropriate modifiers.
- The CCS-P examination includes content for health information documentation, reimbursement methods and regulatory guidelines, and data quality.

Approach to the Coding Review Text

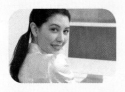 The foundation of this textbook is the preparation of you, the student, on writing for a national coding certification with a successful outcome. Each chapter contains the following elements:

- Chapter Objectives
- *From the Author*
- Indexing Tips
- Coding Alerts!
- Think Like a Coder
- Examples
- Tables
- Applying Coding Theory to Practice

Chapter one begins the textbook with Test-Taking Skills.

This chapter provides you with sound test-taking techniques, tips on how to manage study time through scheduling for weekly and daily planning, study skill strategies, and focus on examination content.

Chapter two is an anatomy and physiology review.

This review includes directional terms relevant to organ structures and body systems in tandem with their relevance to coding practices. Through the use of "Coding Alerts," students will review the most common procedures relevant to the body system begin reviewed.

Chapter three consists of the medical terminology and pathophysiology review.

More than 200 prefixes, suffixes, and word roots are reviewed and examined. You will review the four medical word components and the most commonly used medical terms in each of the body systems. Also presented is the review of the most common diseases encountered in each of the body systems.

Chapter four begins the CPT guidelines review.

Included in this chapter is the review of CPT as a set of codes, these codes' descriptors and guidelines, instructions for the use of the CPT manual, applying section numbers and their sequences, and explanations of coding symbols used throughout the coding manual.

Chapter five is focused on the comprehensive review of the assignment of Evaluation and Management codes.

Included in this comprehensive chapter is the review of all of the standards and guidelines, subsections, subheadings, and descriptors relevant the E&M codes. You will review and apply all levels of service as they relate to each E&M category by using clinical examples and working through problems.

Chapter six reviews the Anesthesia Section of the CPT manual.

Focused in this chapter are standards and guidelines, physical status modifiers, qualifying circumstances, and applicable modifiers.

Chapter seven introduces the review of the largest section of the CPT manual, the Surgery Section.

Focused in this chapter are the review of the standards and guidelines, modifiers that are appropriate to the Surgery Section, subsection information breakdown and application. The chapter is laid out in accordance with the CPT manual itself. It begins with a review of the standards and guidelines, then is broken down into the body systems beginning with the Integumentary System through to the Sense Organs; Auditory System. Notes, coding descriptors and exercises accompany this chapter.

Chapter eight reintroduces and reviews the Radiology Section of the CPT manual.

The focus begins with how the Radiology Section is arranged and lays out indexing tips that aid you in quickly and accurately finding codes in this section. Also reviewed are the interpretation of the radiology notes and modifiers pertinent to this section. An emphasis is placed on the difference between technical components and supervision and interpretation as it relates to radiology.

Chapter nine consists of the review of the Pathology and Laboratory Section of the CPT manual.

The focus is on the arrangement of this section and the content of each subsection. Specifically reviewed is the difference between quantitative and qualitative testing and the different levels of surgical pathology.

Chapter ten is the review of the last section of the CPT Manual, the Medicine Section.

Primary focus involves the special nature of the Medicine section and the medical specialties. Special emphasis is placed on the pertinent notes that accompany subsections and categories. The difference between noninvasive and minimally invasive procedures is reviewed along with the reporting guidelines for immunization administration.

Chapter eleven presents the overview and review of HCPCS level II codes.

Reviewed in this chapter are the history and usage of HCPCS Level II codes, how to locate and index the codes, the special modifiers that accompany the codes, and their application to CPT codes.

Chapter twelve is the comprehensive review of ICD-9 CM coding.

This chapter contains two parts. Part I consists of the review of the organization of the ICD-9 Tabular List of Diseases, Index to Diseases, Index to Procedures and Tabular List of Procedures. A primary focus for both Part I and Part II consist of the concentration of the ICD-9 coding guidelines and conventions. Reviewed in depth in Part I of this chapter are E-Codes, V-Codes, Infectious and Parasitic Diseases, Neoplasms, Endocrine System Diseases, Diseases of the Blood, Mental Disorders, Diseases of the Nervous System, Disease of the Circulatory System, and Diseases of the Respiratory System. The review of HIPAA, coding from abstracts and the Uniform Hospital Data Discharge Set are presented.

Chapter thirteen consists of the comprehensive review of all instructional notes as they appear in the Tabular List of Diseases.

Reviewed in depth of Part II is the review and application of all instructional notes as they appear in the Tabular List of Diseases. Special focus is centered on the Digestive System, Diseases of the Genitourinary System, Complications of Pregnancy, Diseases of the Skin, Diseases of the

Musculoskeletal System, Congenital Anomalies, Newborn, Signs, Symptoms, Injury and Poisoning. A review of Data Quality and Management are included along with many coding scenarios and problems.

Chapter fourteen, the final chapter, consists of the mock examination designed to include concepts from both the CPC (AAPC) and the CCS-P (AHIMA/CAHIIM) examinations.

The examination is timed and consists of 150 questions/problems, multiple choice, with four possible answers. Test items are written in consistent prose with incremental difficulty and mirror the parameters, attributes and properties of the CPC and CCS-P examinations.

Appendix A provides answers and rationale to all problems for "Think Like a Coder," "Applying Coding to Theory Practice," and the mock examination.

Rationale for coding problems is instrumental in increasing your awareness of coding theory, standards, guidelines, conventions, code descriptors and notes in the coding manuals. Appendix B provides a listing of commonly used abbreviations you will encounter as a medical coder while abstracting from health records, operative notes, progress notes, and pathology and radiology reports. Appendix C provides correlations to both the CPC and CCS-P examinations to specific chapters in this textbook.

Key Features of the Review Textbook

- **Objectives** are clearly stated at the beginning of each chapter to help set goals, set the stage for the review process, and incorporate into exercises the theory presented.

- **From the Author** provides you with insight into to how each chapter is relevant to your success in passing a national coding certification. It also explains and reviews how each chapter is arranged to aid you in the logical thinking process of a medical coder.

- **Indexing Tips** are used to provide you with expertise in finding medical codes quickly and accurately. Indexing Tips also help you with the process of logical thinking that begins with taxonomy (classification) of the diagnosis or procedure. When repeated in a consistent manner, you will begin consistently think in an organized and logical manner.

- **Coding Alert!** draws your attention to either a principle or coding note that can be easily overlooked or is unclear to you. Coding Alert! provides critical insight to the concept presented and aids your success in understanding more complex ideas.

- **Think Like A Coder** is the theme of this review textbook. It provides you with consistent reinforcement of organized and logical thinking. An organized and logical thinking process is the critical tool you need to be successful in passing a national certification; you must be consistent in the way you answer each question/problem.

- **Full color** is used to teach and reinforce visually each of the concepts presented in the review.

- **Figures, Tables, and Examples** are presented throughout the textbook. Each is titled and presents clear identification and location. Tables and examples assemble coding information in a logical, organized manner, showing relevance to the concept.

- **Applying Coding to Theory Practice** is specifically designed to enhance the application of reviewed theory in the chapters and to reinforce Coding Alerts!, "Indexing Tips", and scenarios in "Think Like a Coder." Applying Coding to Theory Practice is a "warm-up" for the mock examination.

- **Appendix A, Answers and Rationale** provides you with a learning tool that reinforces greater comprehension, and in-depth understanding of more complex coding situations and provides insight into the strengths and weaknesses of your medical coding.

- **Appendix B** presents common abbreviations used in the medical field that you can quickly access for clarity of a diagnosis or procedure.

- **Appendix C** presents tables that correlate the content of the CPC and CCS-P examinations with the relevant chapters of this text.

- **Challenge Questions** are provided for each chapter and test key concepts that have been presented in the review textbook. These Challenge Questions are located on the Online Learning Center at www.mhhe .com/HarmonCodingReview.

Supplements

Online Learning Center, www.mhhe.com/HarmonCoding Review provides access to practice exams, updates for ICD and CPT codes, and Challenge Questions.

Acknowledgments

I would like to thank Zachary Winston Tiller and Jacob Sean Tiller (my sons) for their work with some medical research for this textbook.

Reviewers

For insightful reviews and helpful suggestions, I would also like to acknowledge the following individuals.

Cathy M. Best, CMA, CPC
   Ivy Tech Community College Northeast

Gerry A. Brasin, CMA, AS, CPC
   Premier Education Group

Judy Hurt
   East Central Community College

Carol Hinricher
   University of Montana, College of Technology

Cheryl L. Javer, MS, MHA
   The Chubb Institute

Naomi Kupfer, CMA
   Heritage College

Janice Manning, MBA, CPC
   Baker College

Wilsetta McClain, NR-CMA, RMA, NCPT, NCICS, MBA
   Baker College

Michael Meyer, DO, CCS, CPC
   Everest University

Stacey Mosay, RHIA, CCS-P, CPC-H
   Trident Technical College

Kathleen Peterson, MS, RHIA, CCS
   Santa Barbara City College

Lori Rager Anderson, CMA (AAMA), CPC (AAPC)
   Salt Lake Community College

Susan Silberman Scalzi
   Delaware County Community College

Debra A. Slusarczyk, BS, RHIT
   Camden County College

Jim Wallace, MHSA
   Stars Behavioral Health Group

Walkthrough

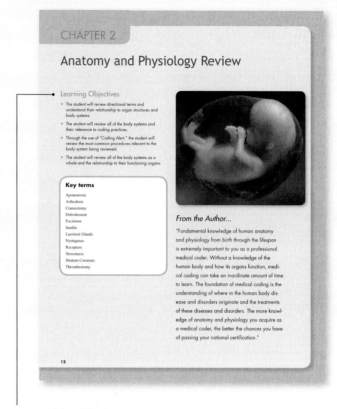

Learning Objectives

present the important points that you should focus on in the chapter.

Key Terms

assist in building the foundation of your medical coding vocabulary.

From the Author

provides you with insight into how this chapter is relevant to your success in passing a national coding certification exam.

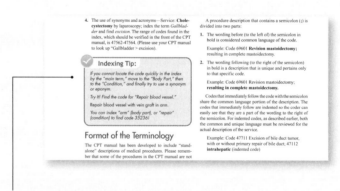

Indexing Tip

guides you in finding medical codes quickly and accurately.

Coding Alert!

emphasizes the importance of ideas or concepts that help you code in a logical manner

Think Like A Coder

reinforces the understanding of coding guidelines

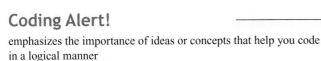

Medial: nearest the midline
Lateral: toward the side or away from the midline
Proximal: nearest point of attachment
Distal: farthest point of attachment
External: on the outside
Internal: on the inside
Superficial: toward or at the body surface

Coding Alert!
Knowing directional terms can provide a better understanding of where, in relation to the body, procedures are taking place in an operative note. Example: "A small incision was made in the midline proximal to the bladder. . . ."

Anatomy and Physiology Overview

Anatomy is defined as the study of the structures of the

- *Lungs* are located on either side of the heart and are enclosed by the rib cage. The left lung has two lobes and the right lung has three lobes.
- The *pleura* is the double-layered membrane that surrounds the lungs. It consists of the parietal and visceral pleura.

Think Like A Coder 2.1
A group of disorders that obstruct the bronchial airflow is known as:
- Bronchitis
- Asthmatic bronchitis
- COPD
- Lobar pneumonia

The Urinary System

The urinary system is made up of the kidneys, ureters, urinary bladder, and urethra. The function of the urinary system is to regulate the volume and composition of fluids in the body and remove waste products from the blood (see Figure 2.5).

Figure 2.1
Body Sections Broken Down into Planes
From D. Shier et al., *Hole's Human Anatomy & Physiology*, 11e. Copyright © 2007

the body as a whole. A professional medical coder must have a knowledge of anatomy and physiology so that coding assignment is quick and accurate. For example, if you were having trouble finding the procedure bilateral oophorectomy in the index, with your knowledge of medical terminology and anatomy and physiology you would know that *oophr/o* means "egg" and *-ectomy* means surgical removal. In medical terms this would be a partial hysterectomy. Therefore, you would look to look in the CPT manual under Surgery, Female Genital System.
Figure 2.2 is an illustration of all the body organ systems and the organs that make up these systems in relations to the body as a whole.

The Integumentary System

In the Surgery section of the CPT manual, the first body bladder. The function of the ureters is to transport urine from the kidneys into the urinary bladder for eventual elimination.

- The *urinary bladder* is a hollow, muscular organ that is located in the pelvic cavity posteriorly to the pubic symphysis and acts as a reservoir, storing urine until it is expelled.
- The *urethra* is the tube that extends from the bladder to the outside of the body and is the means by which urine is eliminated.

Coding Alert!
In the Surgery section of the CPT manual under Urinary System, the most common procedures include catheterization, laparoscopies, cystoscopies, and urethroscopies.

The Male Reproductive System

The male reproductive system can be divided into two parts consisting of primary and accessory organs. The primary organs are the testes, the male gonads. The accessory organs include a series of ducts that provide the transport of various cells to exocrine glands. The function of the male

Examples

provide coding information in a logical, organized manner showing relevance to the concept.

Research and Development, provides staff support for the process of adding, modifying, and deleting CPT codes. The 16-member CPT Editorial Panel meets four times a year and considers proposals for changes to CPT. The Editorial Panel is supported in its efforts by the CPT Advisory Committee, which is made up of representatives of more than 90 medical specialty societies and other health care professional organizations.

In addition to preparing an annual update of CPT, the American Medical Association provides several additional resources on CPT, including *CPT Assistant*, a monthly newsletter; *CPT Changes: An Insider's View*, an annual publication explaining the intent and use of new and revised procedures/services; *CPT Principles of Coding*, an educational primer covering the basic concepts of CPT coding; *CPT Information Services*, a telephone service that provides users with expert advice on code use; and an annual CPT coding symposium. Each year changes occur within the CPT system. The change can be the revision of the narrative description of the code of the addition or deletion of a code. It is crucial that the health care providers maintain up-to-date codes.

Section Numbers and Their Sequence

The eight sections of the CPT manual are as follows:

- Evaluation and Management
- Anesthesia
- Surgery
- Radiology
- Pathology and Laboratory
- Medicine
- Category II Codes
- Category III Codes

The first and last code numbers and the subsection name of the items appear at the top of most pages in the CPT manual.

Example
Cardiovascular System/Surgery **33010 – 37785**

Within the main body of the CPT manual, each section has a structure that is progressive. Each of the eight major sections of the CPT manual has codes grouped into subsections, with the exception of the Evaluation and Management section, which is divided into category levels.

Think Like A Coder 4.1
Section: *Radiology;* **subsection** to Radiology Section: *Radiation Oncology;* **heading** in subsection: *Consultation: Clinical Management*
Section: *Evaluation and Management: Office or Other Outpatient Services;* **Category Levels:** *New Patient, Established Patient, and Severity of Diagnostics*

Codes are further divided into smaller categories under subheadings, such as the type of procedure being performed. The final subdivision is the service of procedure code and its descriptor.

Applying Coding Theory to Practice

enhances the application of coding theory and reinforces Coding Alert!, Indexing Tips, and scenarios encountered in Think Like A Coder.

APPLYING CODING THEORY TO PRACTICE

Please answer the following questions on the basis of the information provided to you in this chapter. (Please see Appendix A for answers and rationale.)

1. Where will you find all the instructions necessary to properly code a procedure in the CPT code book?
   A. ▢ Appendix A
   B. ▢ Guidelines
   C. ▢ Index
   D. ▢ Unlisted Procedures

2. Why is it necessary for a medical coder to use a current editor of the AMA's CPT manual?
   A. ▢ It is the law
   B. ▢ For accurate coding
   C. ▢ Reimbursement will be less
   D. ▢ Reimbursement will be more

3. What is a two-digit modifier used for in CPT coding?
   A. ▢ Add-or code
   B. ▢ Conscious sedation
   C. ▢ Code changes
   D. ▢ Alteration of a procedure or service

4. Please list the three most important coding conventions, and identify them.

5. Please describe the difference between a "stand-alone" code, and an "unlisted procedure."

6. Please list the 8 sections of the CPT manual in order and their code ranges.

11. What modifier would be assigned to an office consultation when the physician's care exceeded the criteria listed under code 99275?
    A. ▢ Modifier 22
    B. ▢ Modifier 53
    C. ▢ Modifier 21
    D. ▢ Modifier 25

12. What modifier would be assigned to an anterior packing of both nares for a nose bleed?
    A. ▢ Modifier 51
    B. ▢ Modifier 50
    C. ▢ Modifier 21
    D. ▢ Modifier 59

13. In what appendix would you find Add-Or Codes?
    A. ▢ Appendix F
    B. ▢ Appendix B
    C. ▢ Appendix D
    D. ▢ Appendix I

14. The symbol "◄ ►" is used to indicate:
    A. ▢ New and revised text
    B. ▢ Conscious sedation
    C. ▢ Special report indicated
    D. ▢ Modifier indicated

15. What section of the CPT manual includes the range of codes 90281-99607?
    A. ▢ Anesthesia

Appendix A

provides answers and rationales that serve as a learning tool to increase comprehension and understanding of more complex coding situations.

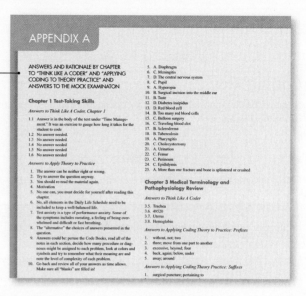

Appendix B

presents common abbreviations used in the medical field and provides quick access for clarity of a diagnosis or procedure.

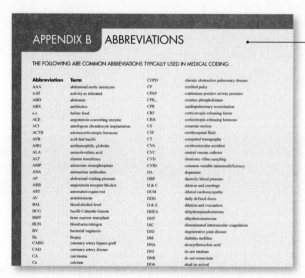

Appendix C

features correlations to the CPC and CCS-P examinations and their relevant chapters.

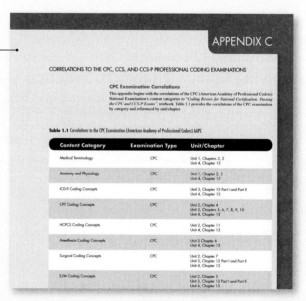

Foundation for Taking the Coding Examination

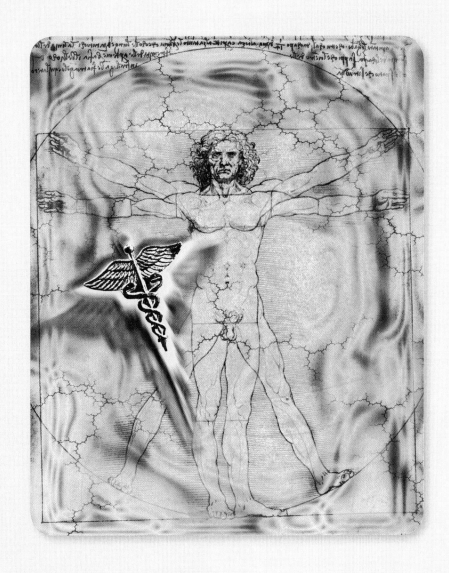

Chapter 1: Test-Taking Skills

Chapter 2: Anatomy and Physiology Review

Chapter 3: Medical Terminology and Pathophysiology Review

Test-Taking Skills

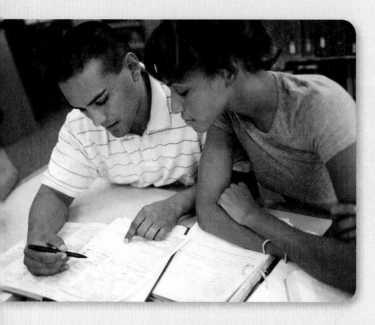

Learning Objectives

- The student will learn sound test-taking techniques that will enable him or her to complete a national examination with confidence, awareness, and skill.

- The student will learn how to manage study time through scheduling for weekly and daily planning.

- The student will become acquainted with examination content areas for better test-studying preparation.

- The student will learn study skill strategies that are focused on examination content.

Key Terms

Adrenaline	Peruse
Conjunctivitis	Protocol
Conventions	Pustulent
Furuncle	Superlatives
Lidocaine	Symbology
Ophthalmologist's	Synthesize

From the Author...

"Motivation is the key element of and is central to learning and passing professional coding examinations. You can increase your motivation level by regarding the examination as a stepping stone to greater responsibility at your place of employment and to opportunities for accomplishing more in your medical coding position, resulting in a more satisfying and higher paying career.

Time is of the essence when you have a full-time job, family, and all the other responsibilities of maintaining your life beyond the studying required for passing your professional coding examination. Time management is one of the major issues facing students who are studying for a national examination and do not have the luxury of studying when it is convenient. However, this does not mean that budgeting your time has to be difficult. You were disciplined enough to gain your experience as a medical coder through commitment in the workplace or completion of an educational coding program. Time management had to be part of your life, or you would not be ready to take this professional examination. It should not be difficult implementing effective study habits to complete and pass a professional coding examination. When you understand how you learn, you can formulate a plan for studying that will be the first step to your success in passing a national coding certification examination!"

Recommended Time for Study

For those pursuing professional coding status while working a full-time job and/or raising a family, developing successful study habits comes down to one word: balance. The necessity for maintaining a healthy balance between school, work, and family cannot be overstated. Unfortunately, it is not always easy to do this, and many people make the mistake of not setting a schedule for their busy lives to include everything that is necessary to accomplish goals. If you can plan ahead and manage to arrange the hours of your day before the day arrives, you will be able to better manage time and accomplish everything you had intended. When you actually plan out your daily schedule, don't budget too much time for one particular area. Make sure you leave enough time for all of the aspects of your life.

Time Management

The amount of time you study for your coding examination cannot be set by anyone other than yourself. Each individual's learning level is different. Some individuals need more time to study than others. It may take a colleague of yours twice the amount of time to assign codes to an operative note than it takes you. The question is, "How much time does it take you to study?" You can begin by understanding how quickly you retain information and assess coding problems. Does it take you 2 minutes to read the problem and 3 to 5 minutes to assign codes? Or does it take 3 minutes for reading and assigning? If you are not sure, adjust your "study schedule" accordingly so that all aspects of your life, including studying, are well thought out and planned in advance. How long does it take you to assign codes to a problem of moderate complexity? Let's try an exercise so that you can gauge the amount it takes you to assign codes. Please keep in mind that all professional coding examinations have time limits, so time is critical when you are testing. Below are two problems that are moderately complex to code. Position yourself in front of a clock with a second hand, use the second hand of your watch, or use your cell phone's "stop watch" feature to time yourself. Only time yourself for the first problem and then stop and check the amount of time that elapsed. In "Think Like A Coder," write your time down and go to the next problem and repeat the same procedure. Ready...Set...Go...

Finished! How long did it take you to code each of these problems correctly? The answers are (1) 10061 and (2) 99215. Did you code correctly? Next, add the times needed to code both these problems and divide by 2. If you needed 10 minutes total to code both problems, then your average coding time per problem is five minutes. You are now ready to begin creating a study schedule that will work for you. A rule of thumb when studying for a coding exam is to try to code at least 20 problems per study

session. If it takes you five minutes to code a problem, then you might want to set aside 1 hour and 45 minutes per study session.

Making the Most of Your Time

Begin to develop blocks of study time that work for you in your busy schedule. It is best to use a planner so that you can organize and prioritize all of the activities in your busy life. Blocks of study do not have to be gauged by the time it takes you to code a problem; it is just a place to start. You might want to consider the following when creating, scheduling, and managing your study time.

- How long does it take for you to become restless or bored?
- Are you taking too many "day trips" during the time you study?
- You may need more frequent short breaks instead of less frequent long breaks.
- Schedule weekly study sessions.

- Develop alternative plans in case your personal study place is not accessible.
- If you have free time, try to sneak in a few minutes of study.
- Review coding guidelines just before beginning your study session.

Finally, use effective aids when making the most of your time while you prepare for your coding examination. Use your planner (see Figure 1.1) to organize all activities that occur on a daily and weekly basis. Write down appointments and meetings that are both personal and professional. Keep a daily "to do list" in your planner and prioritize your "to do list" in order of importance. Not all items in your daily planner should be "high priority" or a "1" on your list. If you have too many "1s" in your daily planner, you are not managing your time efficiently. At the beginning of your day, check what must be accomplished, implement it, and always go to sleep knowing you are prepared for tomorrow!

Friday, April 7, 2008

1,2,3 Priority

✓ Completed

Write in time if appointment is on the 1/2 hour

✓	1,2,3	Daily To Do List	Daily Appointment Schedule	
✓	1	Kids to soccer practice	9:00	
		from 9—11	10:00	Soccer practice
✓	1	Send taxes	11:00	
	2	Grocery	12:00	
	2	Pay bills	1:00	
	3	Call sister	2:00	Dr. appointment
✓	3	Pick up dry cleaning	3:00	
			4:00	
			5:00	
			6:00	
			7:00	Study
			8:00	
			9:00	

Figure 1.1

Example of Daily Planner

Table 1.1 Daily Life Schedule

Daily life schedule (Weekly) Including study schedule							
Daily Activities:	**Mon**	**Tues**	**Wed**	**Thu**	**Fri**	**Sat**	**Sun**
Work, if Applicable							
Study Sessions for Coding							
Classes, if Applicable							
Exercise							
Sleeping							
Family Commitments							
Personal Care							
Meal Preparation/Eating							
Transportation (school, kids, work, etc.)							
Relaxation (TV, hobby, etc.)							
Socializing & Personal Commitments							
Other							
Total Amount of Hours in a Day							

Table 1.1 provides an example of a daily life schedule that includes all aspects of living. This will help you understand how to create time for study sessions. Here is how to begin:

- Make a copy of your work or school schedule.
- Develop a calendar of your study session.
- Develop a schedule to include exercise.
- Develop a schedule for sleeping and try to include at least 7 hours per night.
- Enter important dates for your family commitments.
- Enter time for personal issue and appointment.
- Enter time for meals.
- Enter time for transportation for yourself and children if applicable.
- Enter time for relaxation and your hobbies.
- Enter time for socializing.
- Each evening review your schedule.
- Review how you spend your time in order to help you prioritize your goals and objectives.

Examination Content

Before you can effectively study for your coding examination, you must understand the examination content. Once you are aware of the content areas included in the coding examination, you can begin to create a study plan. The American Academy of Professional Coders CPC examination content areas include Medical Terminology, Anatomy, ICD-9, HCPCS, Coding Guidelines, and coding cases for all sections of the CPT manual. The examination is broken down into three parts. Part I consists of Medical Terminology, Anatomy, ICD-9 CM Coding, HCPCS Coding, and Coding Guidelines. Part II consists of coding in the Surgery section and Modifiers. Part III consists of coding in the Evaluation and Management section, Anesthesia section, Radiology section, Laboratory and Pathology section, and Medicine section. The examination is 5 hours in length and contains 150 questions.

The American Health Information Management Association's CCS-P content areas include health information documentation, diagnostic coding guidelines, procedural coding guidelines, HCPCS coding guidelines, reimbursement methodologies, and data quality. The examination consists of two parts. Part I includes 60 four-option multiple choice questions. Part II consists of medical record coding and contains 16 cases of ICD-9 and CPT physician-based coding with a time limit of 4 hours.

Study Skills Strategies

Now that you have created a study schedule, have planned study sessions, have acknowledged your coding speed, and are aware of examination content, you are ready to study! Learning study skills and strategies will allow you to maximize the amount of time you must set aside for study.

Focusing

Focusing and concentrating is the ability to direct your thinking to the task at hand to eliminate distraction. Create a personal "space" for yourself, desk, and chair with proper lighting and environment. Keep the children busy or send them to the babysitter and avoid your cell phone or telephone. Play music or the television only if the background noise enhances your productivity instead of distracting you. Make sure you follow your study schedule and keep in mind your varied levels of energy.

Before you begin studying, take a few minutes to summarize a few objectives and gather what you will need, such as the CPT, ICD-9, and HCPCS manuals and a medical dictionary. Create a general strategy of accomplishment that might include coding two problems from each section of the CPT manual. Create an incentive for yourself when your study session is supposed to end. Plan to watch a favorite TV show, take a walk, soak in a hot bath tub, or engage in whatever activity you find enjoyable. Make sure you change topics while studying. Don't concentrate in one area too long and vary your study activities. Alternate your study habits by studying alone, having a family member quiz you, or even facilitating group studying if possible. Make sure you take regularly scheduled breaks and do something different like walking around or getting a quick snack in a different area.

Pre-reading Strategies

Pre-reading strategies aid in the overall comprehension of the subject currently being studied. Examine the title of the selection you are about to read. **Peruse** all of the sections and subsections of the CPT and ICD-9 manuals. Mentally list all of the information that comes to mind when you peruse all of these sections. If you come across a section that you are not very familiar with, begin a list that includes topics for further study. As you mentally list all of these categories, try to relate these sections to something you already know about them. Look at the key words, special notes, colors in the ICD-9 manual, and symbols in both manuals for mental recall of their use while coding.

Before reading a coding record, basic frameworks that are included should be mentally noted or written down. Use a mental framework such as (1) noting how many diagnoses are involved and in what section of the ICD-9 manual you would generally find each diagnosis; (2) noting how many procedures are involved and in what section of the CPT manual you would generally find each procedure; (3) noting the level of complexity and how the problem is constructed; and (4) mentally beginning to break down the coding problem one step at a time. Once you have "pre-read" your coding problem, you are ready to begin coding assignment.

Open Book Tests

Both the CPC and CCS-P examinations allow you to use the CPT, ICD-9 CM, and HCPCS coding manuals. These examinations are similar to the "open book" tests. An open book examination evaluates you on understanding rather than recall and memorization. You will be expected to apply material to new situations. All coding situations on examinations are vastly differentiated, and you are introduced to new coding scenarios all of the time. You will need to analyze all of the elements in a coding record. Try to create mental relationships among former coding scenarios that will help you quickly assess where you need to search for a code. You need to **synthesize** and structure your method of finding a code by quickly referring to the correct manual and searching in the correct sections.

 Think Like A Coder 1.2

In "Think Like A Coder 1.1," coding problem number one immediately indicates that the patient presented with *multiple boils*. You should immediately synthesize your thinking and turn to the Integumentary System section of the CPT manual (see Figure 1.2). This will allow you to narrow down your search. In the index you will immediately know if you reference "boil or **furuncle**" that the code you are searching for should begin with 10021–19499. Once you have located the range of codes in the index, you will need to verify the code you have chosen is accurate. You do this by reading the descriptor that accompanies the code you have chosen to make sure it is correct. This code will be found in section "Surgery" under the sub section, "Integumentary." Always try to "connect" your coding assignments mentally with the section of the CPT manual in which the code belongs.

In preparation for the open book examination, you need to keep current on all coding standards, guidelines, updates, deletions, revisions, and **symbology.** While you study, prepare brief notes for all CPT guidelines, add-on codes, modifiers, unlisted procedures, special reports, and code symbols. For ICD-9 CM prepare brief notes on all tabular lists, alphabetic index, coding **conventions,** Medicare requirements, special tables, classifications, supplementary classifications, instructional notations, abbreviations, punctuations, e-codes, and v-codes. Include your own commentary on the brief notes you created and annotate anything significant about them. Study and memorize your brief notes and become an expert with the format, layout, and structure of all your coding reference manuals. Organize your notes for speedy retrieval. Use sticky notes in your coding reference manuals as reminders. This will provide quick retrieval for coding assignment and will cut down on the amount of time spent on each problem. Once you are comfortable knowing where the coding information is located, remove the sticky notes.

Test-Taking Skills

Test-taking skills are those skills not related to medical coding knowledge. Test-taking skills include your attitude and the approach you use while taking an examination. When you acquire good test-taking skills, your chances of passing an examination are increased. There are six major areas for developing better test-taking skills. They include:

1. Knowing the different kinds of test items and how the test will be graded.
2. Following the proctor's directions.
3. Establishing a good attitude when taking a test.
4. Knowing your personal strengths and weaknesses.
5. Moving through the examination without wasting time.
6. Attacking difficult questions/guessing.

Knowing the Different Kinds of Test Items

Knowing the different kinds of test items on your coding examination will help you be more prepared. Become familiar with the most common kinds of items given on tests. Both coding examinations consist of multiple choice questions and the assignment of codes from medical records or case studies. The examinations have you choose the correct coding assignment, usually in four-option choice format. Later, we will learn test-taking tips for multiple choice questions.

Following the Proctor's Directions

Understanding and following directions are very important to your success on an examination. Read the directions carefully and listen to your proctor attentively. Ask questions about any **protocol** you do not understand before beginning the examination. Take time to understand the exact meaning of all examination directions. Sometimes the language used for directions in an examination can be confusing. If you are unsure of the directions, please ask your proctor. Understand exactly how to mark on your test booklet or how to indicate your answer in a computerized testing environment.

Establishing a Good Attitude

Learn to control your nervousness and take one step at a time. Remember, a little nervousness is natural, but nervousness may cause poor performance and memory lapses during the examination. Do not dwell on the things you think you don't know. Constantly remind yourself of all of the things about coding you do know. Use the "brief notes" you have created

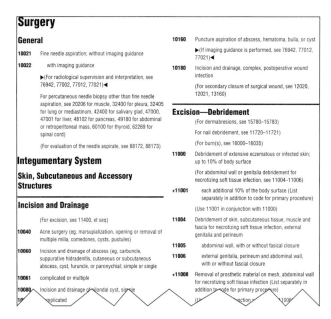

Figure 1.2

Sample of CPT Manual, Integumentary System

Source: *Current Procedural Terminology, CPT 2008, Standard Edition,* American Medical Association.

in your study session to enforce positive study habits. If you are a person who tends to be nervous, remember to stay away from caffeine a few days before your coding examination. Caffeine may stimulate you to stay awake and be alert; however, it also tends to make you more nervous. Keep a positive attitude about your upcoming coding examination!

Personal Strengths and Weaknesses

Everyone has a weakness they are aware of, so plan ahead by identifying those areas in coding that are more difficult for you. For example, after running through the practice questions in this textbook, you may identify an area of weakness such as Evaluation and Management (E&M) codes. Make sure you focus on this weakness and provide yourself with extra studying time for E&M codes. Before the coding examination, make mental lists of (memorize) all the sections, subsections, categories, subcategories, levels of service, and their elements. This will provide you with quicker access to the correct area of the E&M section. Quicker access to the correct area will provide you with more time to decide the levels of service. The more you familiarize yourself with material or concepts you find difficult, the better the chances you have of performing at a higher level on the examination.

Moving Through the Examination

Have you ever become upset or panicked when you think you have run out of time when taking a test? This is very common and usually occurs because you are spending too much time on difficult questions, coding scenarios, or operative notes during the test. Use this textbook to gauge the time it takes you to code a problem and use this information to help you manage your time when taking a test. Learn to briefly look over the section of the test you are about to take and identify the coding problems or questions that will be easy for you. After you answer the easy problems, go back through and work the more difficult problems, keeping time in mind. Do not make the mistake of spending a lot of time on one coding problem; you need to keep moving. Answer every question even though you do not know the answer. You should understand that, if your test is computerized, you cannot go back to a section once you have completed it and moved to a new section. If you are using an answer sheet and skip a problem on the test, be sure to mark the skipped item on the answer sheet. This will avoid marking the next problem in the wrong answer space.

Attacking Difficult Questions/Guessing

During the examination you may not know the answer to some problems or questions. Remember, it is always better to guess than to leave a question/problem unanswered. "Think Like A Coder 1.3" will help you make a more educated guess when answering an unknown question or problem.

 Think Like A Coder 1.3

- With multiple choice questions, the correct answer is often more carefully stated than the incorrect choices.
- On a multiple choice test, a positive statement is more likely to be correct than a negative statement.
- On a four or five-choice multiple choice test, there are usually more "c" answers than any other choice.
- On a multiple choice test, if the last word in the stem ends with "a," then you know the answer must begin with a consonant.

Studying/Comprehending Medical Records

At a Glance

The main purpose of glancing at or perusing the medical record is simply to read and get a good idea of the material presented in the medical record. Sometimes the medical record will present new and complex material that may be difficult to understand. Read carefully. Ascertain what you know and do not know about the scenario. Ask yourself the following questions: (1) Where is this procedure taking place? (2) What is the principle diagnoses? (3) What procedures are indicated? Use these three questions as a format for thinking logically. After practice, glancing or perusing becomes automatic as long as you are intentionally striving for meaning.

Deeper Meaning

Once you have ascertained the general idea of the medical record, you are ready to begin the coding assignment process by reading for deeper, more detailed meaning. Look back and forth between words, diagnoses, and procedures until you can understand the relationship between the words and the codes.

From time to time, ask yourself if you are "on track"—if you understand the information presented in the medical record. If you find yourself reading without understanding, stop and ask yourself why. Is it a question of complexity, distraction, or the terminology? If you are tired and meanings come very slowly into your mind and you are taking longer than you normally do to assign codes, take a break! If you return to reading after a break, scan the medical record again before reading to cue associations you have previously ascertained. Return to what you do not understand or what you want to enforce so that memorization (if necessary) will become easier later. Mark or highlight what you found to be important in the medical record, such as the diagnosis and the procedures taking place in the scenario. Write a "d" over the diagnoses and a "p" over the procedures in the reading so that you can get into the habit of quickly identifying coding assignments. Write down new medical terms that are unfamiliar to you. Using your medical dictionary, define these terms in order to relate them to the coding scenario.

Read the material again only if you do not understand it. If you are comfortable with what you comprehend, proceed to the task of coding assignment. Always begin with the diagnosis and move to the procedures. Make sure the procedure fits the diagnosis. Always review your notes for what you need to memorize, such as a coding note, symbol, modifier, etc. Create or find "like" coding problems that are difficult for you while you study; this reinforces your knowledge.

Multiple Choice Questions

Both the CCS-P and the CPC examination contain multiple choice questions. In order to be successful on these examinations, you need to become an expert when answering multiple choice questions. The first "rule of thumb" when answering multiple choice questions is *read the directions carefully.* The directions usually indicate that some alternatives may be partly correct or correct statement themselves but not when joined to the stem. The directions may say, "choose the *most* correct answer" or "mark the *best* answer." Sometimes you may be asked to "mark *all* correct answers." There are two parts to a multiple choice question: the *stem* and the *alternatives.* The stem and alternatives are shown in "Think Like A Coder 1.4" in the multiple choice question.

You should use several steps to increase your chances of correctly answering multiple choice questions.

1. Read *all* of the stem and *every* alternative.

2. Use the process of elimination procedure to eliminate the obviously incorrect alternatives.

3. Consider *"all of the above"* and *"none of the above."* Examine the *"above"* alternatives to see if all of them or none of them apply *totally.* If even one does not apply totally, do not consider *"all of the above"* or *"none of the above"* as the correct answer.

4. If a negative such as *"none," "not," "never,"* or *"neither"* occurs in the stem, know that the correct alternative must be a fact or absolute and that the other alternatives could be true statements or codes but not the correct answer.

Think Like A Coder 1.4

Stem and Alternatives

Stem

A 32-year-old male new patient presented in the **ophthalmologist's** office with a red, swollen, and draining right eye and blurred vision that had begun 3 days previously. The physician performed an intermediate examination and the patient was diagnosed with **conjunctivitis.**

Alternatives

Choose the best "alternative" for the coding assignment. Hint: Some of the alternatives (answers) may be partially correct, however, they must be entirely correct or the answer will be marked wrong.

- 99203, 99204
- 99203, 92002
- 99205, 92002
- 92002

Answer: 99202, intermediate opthalmological examination for a new patient.

5. Words such as *"every," "all," "none," "always,"* and *"only"* are **superlatives** that indicate the correct answer must be an undisputed fact.

6. Note that words such as *"usually," "often," "generally," "may,"* and *"seldom"* are qualifiers the *could* indicate a true statement.

7. Break the stem down into parts. Pull out the "where it took place," such as the hospital or a physician office; pull out the diagnoses and procedures. This process will ensure that you have examined every part of the stem and are ready for the alternatives.

8. Feel free to change your answer on a multiple choice question. If you have a good reason for changing your answer and you have the time, change it.

Think Like A Coder 1.5

Stem Parts

A 20-year-old female established patient presented in the hospital emergency room *(where it took place)* with symptoms of premature labor with vaginal bleeding and severe pain in the lower left quadrant *(diagnoses)*. The ER physician performed an intermediate exam of moderate complexity. The patient was monitored for 6 hours and released on bed rest *(procedures)*.

9. "Look alike options" are similar alternatives, one of which is most likely correct. Choose the best codes, but eliminate alternatives that basically indicate the same coding assignment.

10. If two answers are the direct opposite of each other, chances are one of them is the correct answer.

Think Like A Coder 1.6

Look Alike Options

Below are "look alike options" for alternatives to coding problems. Always be cautious when choosing an answer that is similar in numeric value to all other alternatives. Below is an example of a coding problem that has "look alike options." You do not want to make a "silly" error on your examination because you were not careful when choosing your answer.

Problem

Choose the correct code for an open treatment of fracture to the great toe on the left foot that includes internal fixation that requires anesthesia.

- 28545
- 28505
- 28454, 29450
- 28454, 29450, 73620

Answer: 2

How to Overcome Test Anxiety

Test anxiety is actually a type of performance anxiety, a feeling you might have in a situation in which performance really counts or when the pressure is on to do well. Test anxiety can bring on physical symptoms such as feeling shaky, a stomachache, or a tension headache. Some individuals might feel sweaty or feel their heart beating quickly as they wait for the test to be given out. A person with really strong test anxiety may even feel like passing out or vomiting.

Anxiety is a reaction to anticipating something unknown, frightening, or stressful. Like other anxiety reactions, test anxiety affects the body and the mind. When you are under stress, the physical symptoms you experience are from the **adrenaline** your body releases when it is in danger. These physical symptoms can be mild or very intense. Just like other types of anxiety, test anxiety can create a vicious cycle. The more you focus on the bad things that could happen, the stronger the feeling of anxiety becomes. Negative thoughts will make you feel worse. If your head is filled with distracting thoughts and fears, it can increase the possibility that you will perform poorly on the test and experience memory lapses.

Test anxiety for the coding examination can be a real problem if you cannot overcome nervousness. Feeling ready to meet the challenge can keep test anxiety at a manageable level. Make sure you are prepared! Earlier in this chapter we created a study schedule to manage time for all activities including study. If you kept to your schedule and studied, you *know* you are prepared. Studying consistently and over a period of time creates a deeper level of learning. This deeper level of learning provides you with confidence and therefore relieves stress.

Control your thinking. Be positive. If expecting to do well on a test can help you relax, think about it. Do not dwell on what could go wrong. Concentrate on the material you know and understand. Watch out for any negative messages you might be sending yourself about the test. They can contribute to your anxiety. If you find yourself thinking negative thoughts such as "I am not good at test taking" or "I always draw a blank on a test," replace them with positive messages to yourself. A positive message can be, "I have studied hard and I know this material" or "I know all of the coding conventions in the ICD-9 CM manual."

Take care of yourself physically by getting plenty of rest and exercise and following a sensible diet. Try not to eat too many foods with a high fat content and keep the caffeine down to a minimum. Keeping physically healthy can help you learn ways to calm yourself down and get centered when you are tense or anxious. Breathe slowly and take deep breaths; do not think about the fear. Stop and think about the next step at hand in your examination and use positive reinforcement messages to yourself to help you continue the examination.

Preparing for Your Examination

Approach the coding examination with confidence. Use whatever strategies or methods necessary to believe in your success. Visualize your testing environment, think with logic, maintain positive thoughts, review overall information, and keep your mind on your goal: passing the coding examination. Consider the coding examination an opportunity to show yourself and potential employers you are a professional. Be prepared and organize the materials you will need for your coding examination. Make sure you have your ICD-9 CM manual, CPT manual, HCPCS manual, medical dictionary if applicable, and your favorite pen or pencil.

On the morning of the examination, get up early enough so that you have plenty of time to prepare mentally and eat a good breakfast and so that you'll be alert during the examination. Never go to an examination on an empty stomach. Fresh fruits and vegetables are often recommended to reduce stress. Stay away from foods that can increase stress

such as processed foods, carbonated soft drinks, chocolate, eggs, fried foods, junk food, sugar, potato chips, and foods containing preservatives or heavy spices. Take a small snack with you in the event you receive a break during your examination; this will help you reduce stress.

The Day of the Examination

Arrive a few minutes early for your examination, but do not arrive too early or you will find yourself worrying and experiencing unnecessary stress. Approach the examination with confidence, knowing that you have prepared well in advance and are ready for the challenge! Choose a comfortable location in the testing room with good lighting and minimal distractions. Avoid thinking that you should have crammed the night before and strive for a relaxed state of mind. Avoid speaking with any fellow examinees who have not prepared, who express negative thoughts, and who will distract you from your preparation.

Listen to the proctor carefully and ask questions if you are unsure of any testing direction that has been presented. If you are taking a computerized test, make sure you understand how the computerized test works and how to navigate during the test. Read all directions carefully; this may help you avoid careless errors. If you have time and it is applicable, work through testing examples carefully and quickly look through the examination for an overview.

Remember your coding examination is timed. Answer questions in strategic order by answering the easiest questions first. This builds confidence and allows you to mentally orient yourself to the medical terminology and coding concepts that help you make associations with more difficult coding scenarios. Next, proceed to the questions, coding records, or coding scenarios that are more difficult. Remember when answering multiple choice questions to eliminate answers (alternatives) that you know are wrong or likely to be wrong, that don't seem to fit, or that seem to be too excessive.

If you complete the examination and there is time available, review your test answers! Some computerized tests will not allow you to return to a section once you have completed it. If this is the case, always review each computerized section when you still have time available before moving to the next section. If your test is not computerized and you have time available after you have completed it, review your test to make sure you have answered all questions. Also check for answers marked in the wrong order on the answer sheet. Quickly review the coding assignments you found to be more difficult to ensure accuracy. Change your answers to questions if you feel that you have made a mistake. Once you have completed the coding examination, follow your proctor's directions and feel confident you did your best!

Please answer the following questions.

1. What type of environment is best for you to study in? Is it in a quiet room alone with no TV or music, or do you prefer to have noise with people surrounding you?

2. Is it best to leave an answer blank when you do not know the answer or should you try to answer anyway?

3. When you do not understand something that you have just read, what should you do?

4. What is the "key element" to studying and passing a professional coding examination?

5. Who can tell you how much time it takes you to study?

6. When setting up a Daily Life Schedule, is it "ok" to not include time for socializing?

7. What is "test anxiety" and what are some of the symptoms?

8. What is an "alternative" in a multiple choice question?

9. Give an example of a "pre-reading" strategy?

10. If you complete the examination early, what should you do?

CHAPTER 2

Anatomy and Physiology Review

Learning Objectives

- The student will review directional terms and understand their relationship to organ structures and body systems.
- The student will review all of the body systems and their relevance to coding practices.
- Through the use of "Coding Alert," the student will review the most common procedures relevant to the body system being reviewed.
- The student will review all of the body systems as a whole and the relationship to their functioning organs.

Key terms

Aponeurosis

Arthodesis

Craniectomy

Debridement

Excisions

Insulin

Lacrimal Glands

Nystagmus

Receptors

Stereotaxis

Stratum Corneum

Thrombectomy

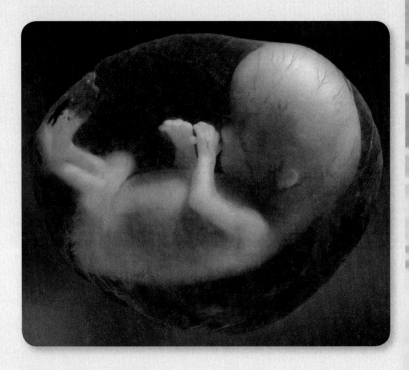

From the Author...

"Fundamental knowledge of human anatomy and physiology from birth through the lifespan is extremely important to you as a professional medical coder. Without a knowledge of the human body and how its organs function, medical coding can take an inordinate amount of time to learn. The foundation of medical coding is the understanding of where in the human body disease and disorders originate and the treatments of these diseases and disorders. The more knowledge of anatomy and physiology you acquire as a medical coder, the better the chances you have of passing your national certification."

Directional Terms

When reading operative notes, physician notes, and medical charts, you must be able to make reference to certain positions in regard to the body as a whole. The body can assume many positions and therefore have a variety of orientations. To establish a standard by which to study human anatomy, the anatomical position was developed. In the anatomical position, the individual is standing erect, with feet parallel, arms hanging to the side with palms out, and face forward. Sometimes it is necessary to divide the body by drawing imaginary lines through it to separate it into specific sections. Figure 2.1 shows the sagittal, midsagittal plane, transverse, and coronal planes.

The following directional terms are commonly used to facilitate types of references in accordance with the anatomical position.

Superior: uppermost or above

Inferior: lowermost or below

Anterior: toward or on the front

Ventral: another term to describe anterior

Posterior: toward or on the back

Dorsal: another term to describe posterior

Cranial: toward the head

Medial: nearest the midline

Lateral: toward the side or away from the midline

Proximal: nearest point of attachment

Distal: farthest point of attachment

External: on the outside

Internal: on the inside

Superficial: toward or at the body surface

Coding Alert!

Knowing directional terms can provide a better understanding of where, in relation to the body, procedures are taking place in an operative note. Example: "A small incision was made in the midline proximal to the bladder. . . ."

Anatomy and Physiology Overview

Anatomy is defined as the study of the structures of the body; closely related is physiology, which is the study of how these body structures function, what their role is in the body, and how they work together. All living material is organized into different levels from the simplest form of organism to the most complex. Specialized chemicals and complex substances form living cells. Cells are organized into tissues, and the tissues are further organized into organs. These organs make up the major systems of the body; called *organ systems,* they work together to maintain

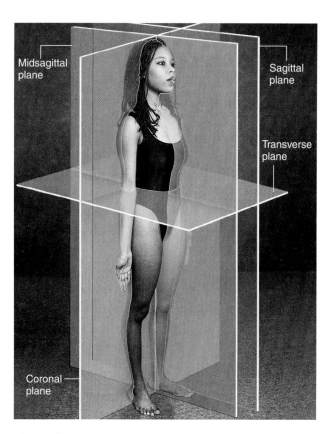

Figure 2.1

Body Sections Broken Down into Planes

From D. Shier et al., Hole's *Human Anatomy & Physiology,* 11e. Copyright © 2007 The McGraw-Hill Companies. Reprinted with permission.

the body as a whole. A professional medical coder must have a knowledge of anatomy and physiology so that coding assignment is quick and accurate. For example, if you were having trouble finding the procedure bilateral oophorectomy in the index, with your knowledge of medical terminology and anatomy and physiology you would know that *oophr/o* means "egg" and *-ectomy* means surgical removal. In medical terms this would be a partial hysterectomy. Therefore, you would know to look in the CPT manual under Surgery, Female Genital System.

Figure 2.2 is an illustration of all the body organ systems and the organs that make up these systems in relations to the body as a whole.

The Integumentary System

In the Surgery section of the CPT manual, the first body system for which medical procedures are described is the integumentary system. The integumentary system consists of two layers of skin, the epidermis and dermis, and its accessory structures such as hair, nails, and sweat and oil glands. The epidermis is the outermost layer of the skin in which cells are constantly lost through normal everyday movement. The epidermis contains hair shafts, sweat gland pores, and **stratum corneum,** which consists of dead layers of cells. The dermis, the second layer of the skin, is

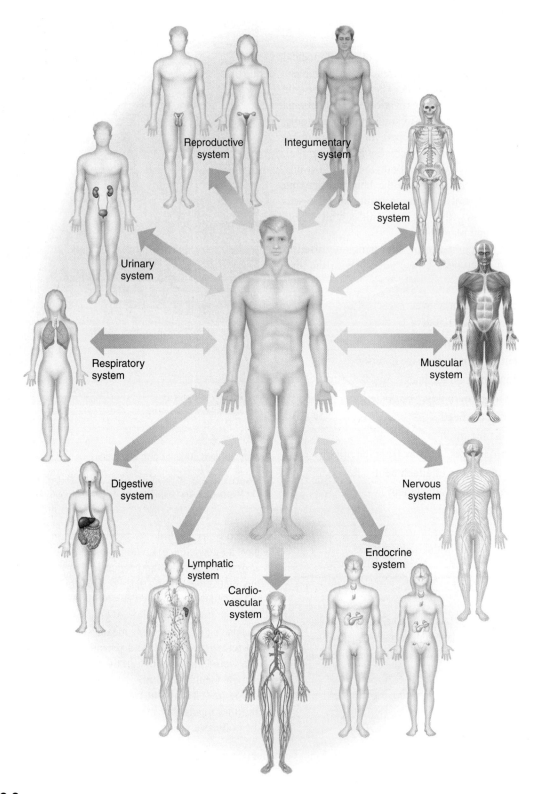

Figure 2.2

Body Organ Systems – The organ systems as depicted are broken down in the surgery section of the CPT Manual

From D. Shier et al., Hole's *Human Anatomy & Physiology,* 11e. Copyright © 2007 The McGraw-Hill Companies. Reprinted with permission.

made up of elastic connective tissue with blood vessels and nerves. These nerves and blood vessels play an important role in the regulation of body temperature. For example, when the body experiences heat, nerves send impulses to trigger the dilation of blood vessels that stimulate the sweat glands to produce sweat, which in turn cools the body. The dermis also consists of sebaceous glands, arrector pili muscle, and sweat glands. The subcutaneous layer of the skin

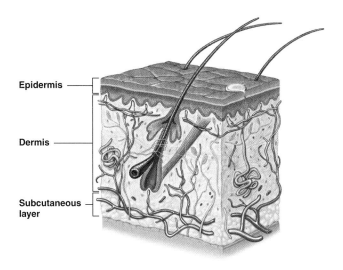

Figure 2.3

Layers of the Skin

From D. Shier et al., Hole's *Human Anatomy & Physiology,* 11e. Copyright © 2007 The McGraw-Hill Companies. Reprinted with permission.

is sometimes referred to as the superficial fascia, which connects the skin to the surface muscles. The subcutaneous layer consists of adipose tissue into which many fat-soluble drugs and medications are injected. A subcutaneous injection is often used as a route of administration for many drugs (see Figure 2.3).

> ## Coding Alert!
>
> The most common procedures, located in the Integumentary System portion of the Surgery section include **excisions, debridement,** and drainage of various skin lesions. Repair of wounds is a large part of this section, consisting of levels of repair that include simple, intermediate and complex. Excision of pressure ulcers and destruction of malignant or premalignant lesions are also very common.

The integumentary system has several functions. The first is to cover and protect tissue from infection and dehydration. The skin also regulates body temperature and acts as a site for nerve **receptors.** Finally, the skin screens out harmful sunlight and acts as a site for storage of glucose, water, fat, and salt.

The Respiratory System

The structures of the respiratory system facilitate the exchange of carbon dioxide and oxygen for use by the cells of the body. The respiratory system is divided into the upper and lower respiratory tracts. The upper respiratory tract consists of the nose, pharynx, larynx, and upper trachea. The lower respiratory tract consists of the lungs, bronchial tubes, pleura, and alveoli (see Figure 2.4).

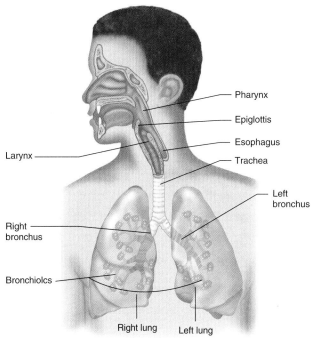

Figure 2.4

Organs of the Respiratory System

From D. Shier et al., Hole's *Human Anatomy & Physiology,* 11e. Copyright © 2007 The McGraw-Hill Companies. Reprinted with permission.

- The *pharynx,* or throat, is a tube that is a common passageway for air and food. It is located posteriorly to the nasal and oral cavities.
- The *esophagus* is the muscular tube that takes food from the lower end of the pharynx to the stomach.
- The *larynx* is the voice box located posteriorly to the nasal and oral cavity; it also functions as an air passage.
- The *trachea,* or windpipe, is a tube-like passageway that extends from the larynx to the bronchi and is found anterior to the esophagus.
- The lower end of the trachea separates into the right and left *bronchi,* the primary branches of the trachea. Bronchi and bronchioles are found at the lower end of the trachea, which divides into right and left bronchi, which further subdivide into bronchioles. These bronchioles further divide into the segments of each lobe of the lung. This continuous branching of bronchioles is commonly referred to as the bronchial tree.
- The *epiglottis* is the flap of cartilage lying behind the tongue and in front of the entrance to the larynx that allows air to pass through the larynx and to the lungs.
- *Alveolar ducts* are a further subdivision of terminal bronchioles; at the end of each alveolar ducts is an alveolar sac that resembles a cluster of grapes.
- *Alveoli* are pouches lined with epithelium that are clustered like grapes at the end of each alveolar duct. The exchange of respiratory gases between the blood and lungs take place across the alveoli.

- *Lungs* are located on either side of the heart and are enclosed by the rib cage. The left lung has two lobes and the right lung has three lobes.
- The *pleura* is the double-layered membrane that surrounds the lungs. It consists of the parietal and visceral pleura.

Think Like A Coder 2.1

A group of disorders that obstruct the bronchial airflow is known as:

- Bronchitis
- Asthmatic bronchitis
- COPD
- Lobar pneumonia

The Urinary System

The urinary system is made up of the kidneys, ureters, urinary bladder, and urethra. The function of the urinary system is to regulate the volume and composition of fluids in the body and remove waste products from the blood (see Figure 2.5).

- The *kidneys* extract wastes from the blood, balance body fluids, and form urine. They are located against the muscles of the back and are inferior to the diaphragm and protected by the lower ribs.
- The *ureters* are two narrow tubes running from the kidney down to and through the lower part of the urinary

bladder. The function of the ureters is to transport urine from the kidneys into the urinary bladder for eventual elimination.

- The *urinary bladder* is a hollow, muscular organ that is located in the pelvic cavity posteriorly to the pubic symphysis and acts as a reservoir, storing urine until it is expelled.
- The *urethra* is the tube that extends from the bladder to the outside of the body and is the means by which urine is eliminated.

Coding Alert!

In the Surgery section of the CPT manual under Urinary System, the most common procedures include catheterization, laparoscopies, cystoscopies, and urethroscopies.

The Male Reproductive System

The male reproductive system can be divided into two parts consisting of primary and accessory organs. The primary organs are the testes, the male gonads. The accessory organs include a series of ducts that provide the transport of various cells to exocrine glands. The function of the male reproductive system is to produce sperm for reproduction (see Figure 2.6).

- The *testes* are the primary reproductive organ. They lie outside the body in the scrotum, and they produce testosterone and sperm.
- The *scrotum* consists of loose skin that resembles a pouch. It holds and protects the testes.

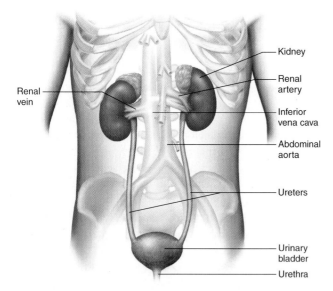

Figure 2.5

Urinary system includes the kidneys, ureters, urinary bladder, and uretha.

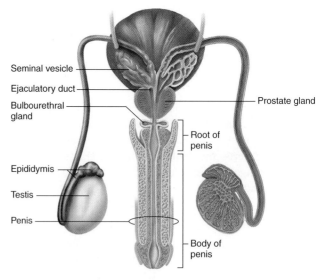

Figure 2.6

Male Reproductive Organs

- The *epididymis* is made up of a tightly coiled tube located inside the scrotum along the posterior border of the testes. It is the site where sperm cells mature.
- The *prostate* is located under the urinary bladder and is donut-shaped. It secretes alkaline fluid that makes up semen and plays a role in activating sperm cells to swim.
- The *bulbourethral glands,* or Cowper's Glands, are a pair of peanut-sized organs located beneath the prostate gland on either side of the urethra. They secrete mucus to lubricate the urethra and tip of the penis during sexual arousal.
- The *ejaculatory duct* is located posteriorly to the urinary bladder. It serves as a common passageway for both spermatozoa and urine.
- Seminal vesicles are attached to the connective tissue at the back of the urinary bladder. They are twisted, muscular tubes with outpouchings in which their linings produce secretions that act as nourishment for sperm.
- The *penis* is the external organ used to deliver spermatozoa into the female reproductive tract. The penis consists of a shaft and the glans penis.

Think Like A Coder 2.2

If you were coding a repair of the tunica vaginalis hydrocele, in what section of the CPT manual will you find the code?

- Surgery; Female Genital System
- Surgery; Male Genital System
- Surgery; Maternity Care and Delivery
- Surgery; Urinary System

The Female Reproductive System

The female reproductive system can be divided into two parts, the primary and accessory organs. The primary organs are the ovaries, the female gonads. The accessory organs include the fallopian tubes, uterus, vagina, and external genitalia. The function of the female reproductive system is to produce germ cells and the hormones estrogen and progesterone for reproduction and the birthing process. (see Figure 2.7).

- The *ovaries* are the primary sex organs of the female. They produce the hormones estrogen and progesterone and are located in the upper pelvic cavity on either side of the uterus.

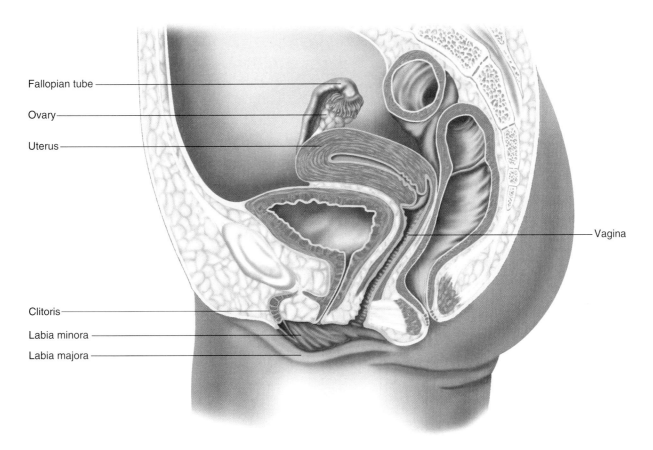

Figure 2.7

Female Reproductive Organs

From D. Shier et al., Hole's *Human Anatomy & Physiology,* 11e. Copyright © 2007 The McGraw-Hill Companies. Reprinted with permission.

- The *fallopian tubes* are two oviducts that are attached to one end of the uterus. The fringe of finger-like projections catch the ovum when ovulation occurs and propels the ovum down to the uterus.
- The *uterus,* or the womb, is located in the pelvic cavity between the rectum and the urinary bladder and can greatly expand to accommodate a fetus. The uterus is where the fertilized egg is implanted and where the fetus develops during pregnancy.
- The *vagina* is the short canal that extends from the cervix or the uterus to the vulva. It serves as a passageway for menstrual flow, is the receptacle for the penis during sexual intercourse, and serves as the lower portion of the birth canal.
- The *clitoris* is the small cylindrical structure at the urethral opening. It consists of erectile tissue containing many nerve endings.
- The *labia majora* are two folds of skin that contain sweat glands and adipose tissue that surround the vagina.
- The *labia minora* are two folds of skin containing few sweat glands and many sebaceous glands that surround the vagina.

> ## Coding Alert!
> In the Surgery section of the CPT manual under Female Genital System, the most common procedures include various endoscopies, laparoscopies, biopsies, hysteroscopies, and maternity care and delivery.

The Cardiovascular and Blood Systems

The cardiovascular system consists of the heart and numerous blood vessels. The heart pumps blood throughout the body via blood vessels. The heart has three layers: the endocardium, myocardium, and epicardium. The heart has two partitions, both of which act as a pump. The right side of the heart pumps blood low in oxygen to the lungs, and the left side pumps oxygenated blood to the remainder of the body. On either side of the heart are two chambers; the upper chambers are the right and left atrium, and lower chambers are the right and left ventricles (see Figure 2.8).

The blood vessels that lead to and from the heart are:

- The *superior* and *inferior venae cavae,* which bring deoxygenated blood to the right atrium.
- The *pulmonary vein,* which brings oxygenated blood from the lungs to the left atrium.
- The *pulmonary artery,* which takes deoxygenated blood from the right ventricle to the lungs for the exchange of carbon dioxide for oxygen.
- The *orta,* which takes blood from the left ventricle to the body.

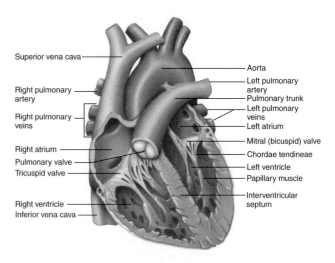

Figure 2.8

Sections of the Heart – Illustrates the connection between the right ventricle and the pulmonary trunk.

From D. Shier et al., Hole's *Human Anatomy & Physiology,* 11e. Copyright © 2007 The McGraw-Hill Companies. Reprinted with permission.

Valves of the Heart

1. The mitral, or bicuspid, valve is made up of two flaps and is the left *atrioventricular valve.*
2. Flaps of the valves project into the ventricles by the *chordae tendineae.*
3. Seminlunar valves are made up of three flaps.
4. The *pulmonary semilunar valve* lies at the entrance to the pulmonary artery.
5. The *aortic semilunar valve* lies at the entrance to the aorta.

Flow of Blood through the Heart

The blood flows into the left atrium of the heart from the pulmonary veins, through the bicuspid valve to the left ventricle, and through the aortic semilunar valve to the aorta. The blood flows into the right atrium of the heart from the superior and inferior venae cavae, through the tricuspid valve to the right ventricle, and through the pulmonary semilunar valve to the pulmonary artery, which takes the blood to the lungs for the exchange of carbon dioxide for oxygen.

The Conduction System of the Heart

The heart is a muscle with its own conduction system. The conduction system generates and distributes electrical impulses that cause the contraction of the heart (see Figure 2.9). The following describe the conduction system of the heart.

- The sinoatrial node (SA node), known as the natural pacemaker of the heart, is located in the upper wall of the right atrium. The SA node initiates each cardiac cycle and spreads electrical impulses over both atria, causing them to contract.

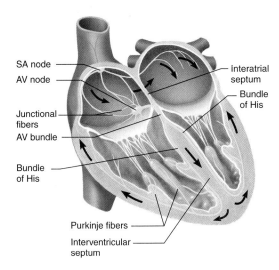

SA node
AV node
Junctional fibers
AV bundle
Bundle of His

Interatrial septum
Bundle of His

Purkinje fibers
Interventricular septum

Figure 2.9
The Conduction System of the Heart

From D. Shier et al., Hole's *Human Anatomy & Physiology,* 11e. Copyright © 2007 The McGraw-Hill Companies. Reprinted with permission.

- The atrioventricular node (AV node), located at the bottom of the right atrium, sends electrical impulses through the bundle of His to the top of the interventricular septum.
- The bundle of His, located at the top of the interventricular septum, has branches that extend to all parts of the ventricular walls that distribute electrical impulses over the surface of the ventricles.
- The Purkinje fibers, located off the bundle branches of the bundle of His, travel in a branching network and distribute the impulses to the cells of the myocardium of the ventricle, causing contraction.

> ## Coding Alert!
>
> In the Surgery section of the CPT manual under Cardiovascular System, the most common procedures will include pacemaker installation, cardiac valves, arterial and venous grafting and bypass, shunting procedures, endovascular repairs, intravascular procedures, and **thrombectomy.**

The Digestive System

The digestive system is composed of primary organs that include the mouth, pharynx, esophagus, stomach, small intestine, large intestine, and the anus (see Figure 2.10). The accessory organs of the digestive system are the salivary glands, liver, gallbladder, and pancreas. The function of the digestive system is the break down of food via hydrolysis into simpler substances that can be used as fuel for the body.

The primary organs of the digestive system are as follows:

1. The *mouth,* or the oral cavity, is where the food begins its passage through the digestive tract. It is composed of several parts. The hard palate or the roof of the mouth is formed from maxillary and palatine bones. The soft palate of the mouth is made from a movable mucous fold and separates the mouth from the nasopharynx. The uvula is the flap that hangs from the soft palate in back of the throat.

2. The *pharynx,* or throat, extends upward to the nasal cavity and downward to the larynx. When food is chewed and reaches the pharynx, swallowing occurs involuntarily.

3. The *esophagus* is a muscular tube that begins at the pharynx and ends at the stomach. In the esophagus, food is lubricated with mucus and moved by peristalsis into the stomach.

4. The *stomach* is j-shaped and is located in the upper quadrant of the abdominal cavity. It serves as a storage unit for food and is the digestive organ for the breakdown of food. Special cells in the lining of the stomach secrete substances that mix together to form gastric juices, which aid in the breakdown of food.

5. The *small intestine* is the longest intestine in the body. It is smaller in diameter than the large intestine. The small intestine is made up of the duodenum, jejumum, and ileum. The main function of the small intestine is to complete the absorption process of digested food.

6. The *large intestine,* also known as the colon, can be divided into descending, ascending, and transverse parts. The sigmoid portion of the colon and the rectum are at the end of the colon.

7. The *rectum* opens exteriorly to the anus, which contains voluntary and involuntary muscle sphincters used for defecation.

The accessory organs of the digestive system are as follows:

- The *salivary glands* aid in the process of digestion by creating a watery mixture call salivary amylase that converts starch to sugar. The three pairs of salivary glands are the parotid glands located below the ear, the submandibular glands located near the lower jaw, and the sublingual glands located under the tongue.

- The *liver* is located in the upper right portion of the abdominal cavity under the diaphragm. The main digestive function of the liver is the production of bile.

- The *gallbladder* is a small organ or muscular sac on the inferior surface of the liver that serves as a storage unit for bile until needed for digestion.

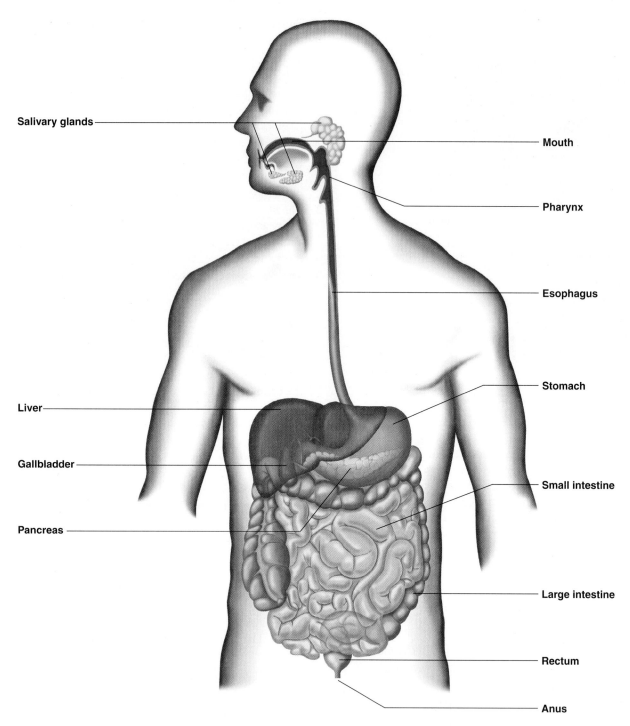

Salivary glands

Mouth

Pharynx

Esophagus

Stomach

Liver

Gallbladder

Small intestine

Pancreas

Large intestine

Rectum

Anus

Figure 2.10

Organs of the Digestive System

From D. Shier et al., Hole's *Human Anatomy & Physiology*, 11e. Copyright © 2007 The McGraw-Hill Companies. Reprinted with permission.

- The *pancreas* is a feather-shaped organ that extends from the duodenum to the spleen. The pancreas produces enzymes that digest proteins, fats, carbohydrates, and nucleic acid. The pancreas also secretes **insulin** and glucagon into the blood to control blood sugar levels.

Eyes, Ears, and Nose (Senses)

The five special senses that make up part of our nervous system are taste, smell, vision, balance, and hearing. Sensory receptors are found all over our body, such as in the tongue for our sense of taste. A receptor site is

Think Like A Coder 2.3

What is the procedure to describe the creation of an artificial opening between the stomach and jejunum?

- Gastrostomy
- Esophagogastroplasty
- Jejunotomy
- Gastrojejunostomy

stimulated; the impulse is sent to and interpreted by the brain; and some form of a reflex, sensation, or voluntary movement occurs.

The eye is the organ of vision. It consists of three layers: the sclera, retina, and choroid. The eye muscles are supplied by the oculomotor, trochlear, and abducens cranial nerves. The eyes are bathed in tears produced by the **lacrimal glands** (tear ducts). The parts of the eye include (see Figure 2.11):

The *iris* is the colored part of the eye consisting of smooth muscle that regulates the amount of light that enters through the pupil.

The *lens* is a biconvex, transparent structure that sits behind the pupil of the eye and flexes to accommodate vision of images that are near and distant.

The *pupil* is the central opening on the iris of the eye. Its function is to constrict when exposed to light and to dilate when exposed to the dark.

The cornea is the transparent, anterior portion of the sclera that is the first part of the eye that refracts light to facilitate vision.

The *optic nerves,* the second pair of cranial nerves, carry visual impulses from the rod and cones to the brain.

The *retina* is the innermost layer of the eye that receives images transmitted through the lens and contains the receptors for vision.

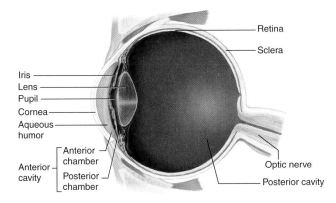

Figure 2.11

Major Structures of the Eye

From D. Shier et al., Hole's *Human Anatomy & Physiology,* 11e. Copyright © 2007 The McGraw-Hill Companies. Reprinted with permission.

The *sclera* is the outer layer of the eyeball made of fibrous tissue, usually considered the white part of the eye. The sclera is responsible for maintaining the shape of the eye.

The *aqueous humor* is the transparent liquid contained in the anterior and posterior of the eye.

Think Like A Coder 2.4

The inability of the eye muscles to coordinate their activity on one object is called:

- **Nytagmus**
- Astigmatism
- Strabismus
- Diplopia

The Musculoskeletal System

The Skeletal System

The skeletal system is the framework for the human body and is composed of 206 bones (see Figure 2.12). The major functions of the skeletal system are:

- Serving as an attachment point for muscles.
- Protecting internal organs.
- Storing minerals, phosphorous, and calcium for the body.
- Production of red blood cells.
- Providing aid in the process of movement.

The axial portion is shown in orange and the appendicular portions are shown in yellow.

The Long Bones

The long bones, the bones that make up the arms and legs, are comprised of the following components:

- The *diaphysis,* a long narrow shaft of the bone that has a central marrow cavity and two irregular ends.
- The *epiphysis,* the hollow cylindrical shaft of the bone.
- *Compact bone,* hard, thick bone that makes up the main shaft of the long bone and the outer layer of various other bones.
- *Spongy bone,* the bone that remains when hard bone dissolves.

Axial Skeleton

The axial skeleton consists of the skull, vertebral column, sternum, ribs, and hyoid bone. The skull is subdivided into 8 cranial bones and 14 facial bones. The vertebral column includes:

- Cervical vertebrae—7 bones
- Thoracic vertebrae—12 bones
- Lumbar vertebrae—5 bones

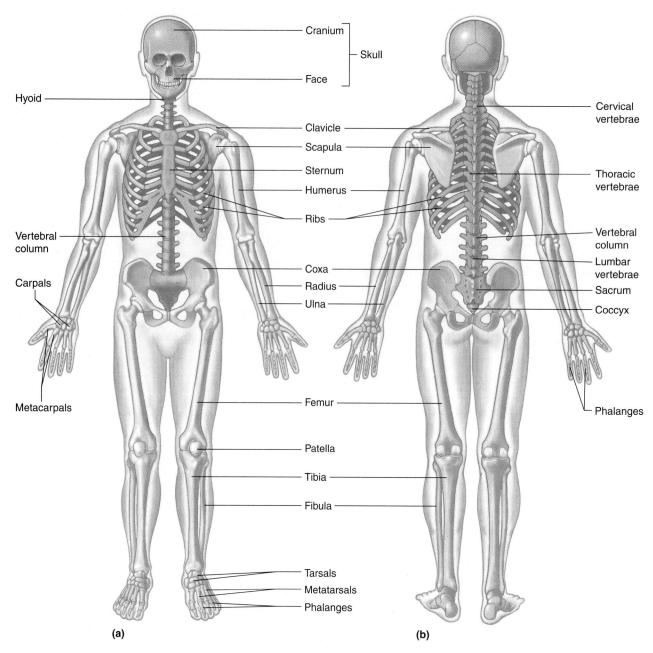

Figure 2.12

Major Bones of the Skeleton – (a) anterior view (b) posterior view.

From D. Shier et al., Hole's *Human Anatomy & Physiology*, 11e. Copyright © 2007 The McGraw-Hill Companies. Reprinted with permission.

- Sacrum—1 bone
- Coccyx—1 bone

The sternum includes the breastbone, and the ribs include seven true ribs, three false ribs, and two floating ribs. The hyoid bone is the U-shaped bone in the neck.

Appendicular Skeleton

The appendicular skeleton consists of the shoulder girdles, arms, wrists, hands, pelvic girdle, legs, ankles, and feet. The breakdown is as follows:

- The *shoulder girdle* consists of 2 scapulas and 2 clavicles.
- The *arm* consists of 2 humeruses, 2 radii, and 2 ulnae.
- The *hand* consists of 16 carpals, 10 metacarpals, and 28 phalanges.
- The *pelvic girdle* consists of the ilium, ischium, and pubic bone.
- The *upper leg* consists of the femur.
- The *lower leg* consists of 2 tibiae and 2 fibulae.

- The *ankle* consists of 14 tarsals and 2 calcaneous bones (heel).
- The *foot* consists of 10 metatarsals and 28 phalanges.

The Muscular System

The three kinds of muscles in the human body are smooth, skeletal, and cardiac. Smooth muscles are involuntary and striated and make up the walls of the hollow body organs as well as blood vessels. Cardiac muscle is striated and involuntary and makes up the wall of the heart. Skeletal muscle are voluntary and very heavily striated and are attached to the bones that aid in movement.

The functions of the muscular system are the movement of the skeleton, both appendicular and axial; the provision of body shape and posture; and the production of heat for the body. The attachments of the skeletal muscles are the tendons and **aponeurosis.** The tendons are connective tissue that attaches muscles to bone. The origin is the part of the muscle that is attached to a fixed structure with the least amount of movement. The insertion is attached to the movable part of the bone with the most amount of movement. Aponeurosis is the wide band of connective tissue that attaches muscles to bones and other muscles (see Figure 2.13).

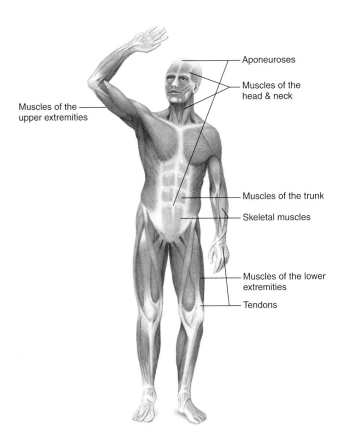

Figure 2.13

Muscle Groups

From D. Shier et al., Hole's *Human Anatomy & Physiology,* 11e. Copyright © 2007 The McGraw-Hill Companies. Reprinted with permission.

Muscle groups include:

- Muscles of the head and neck
- Muscles of the upper extremities
- Muscles of the trunk
- Muscles of the lower extremities

> ## Coding Alert!
>
> In the Surgery section of the CPT manual under Musculoskeletal System, the most common procedures include gunshot/stab wounds, replantation, grafts, fractures, dislocations, osteotomy, manipulation, **arthodesis,** spinal instrumentation, and amputation.

The Nervous System

The nervous system is made up of the brain, spinal cord, and nerves and serves as the control center of the body. The nervous system controls and directs all the functions of the body systems and interprets what is taking place in the external environment so that our muscles contract in relation to stimuli. The nervous system is broken down into two categories, the central nervous system (CNS) and the peripheral nervous system (PNS) (see Figure 2.14). The CNS controls the entire body and consists of the brain and spinal cord. The PNS consists of cranial and spinal nerves that connect the spinal cord and brain with muscles, glands, and receptors.

The nervous system's major function is to coordinate and facilitate body mechanics. The PNS accomplishes this through the somatic nervous system, which is responsible for the voluntary control of the skeletal muscle, and the autonomic nervous system, which controls cardiac and smooth muscle.

Nerve Cell Terms

- The *neuroglia* are connective tissue cells that help protect the nervous tissue and bind it to other structures as well as aiding in the repair of cells.
- The *neuron* is a functional cell of the nervous system that contains fibers called dendrites, which carry messages to the cell body and axons that carry messages away from the cell body.
- *Dendrites* are short and branched neuron fibers that conduct impulses to the cell body.
- *Axons* are long neuron fibers that conduct impulses away from the cell body.
- A *synapse* is the space between the junction of two neurons where the termination of the axon of one neuron comes into close proximity with the dendrites of another, thus ensuring that nerve impulses will travel in only one direction.
- A *neurotransmitter* is a substance that is released when the axon terminal of a neuron is excited and either inhibits or excites the target cell.

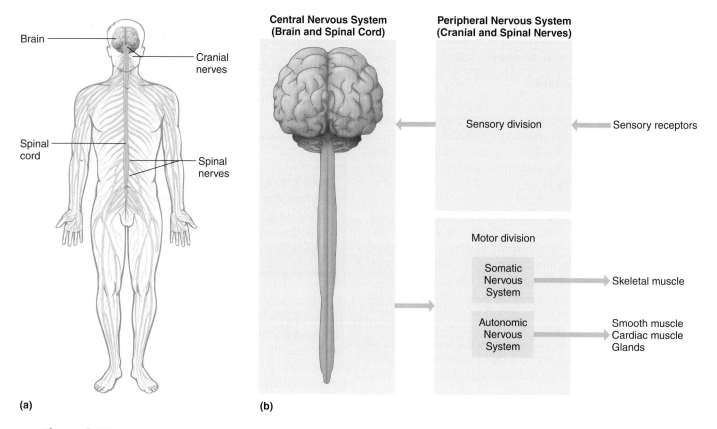

**Central Nervous System
(Brain and Spinal Cord)**

**Peripheral Nervous System
(Cranial and Spinal Nerves)**

Brain

Cranial
nerves

Spinal
cord

Spinal
nerves

Sensory division ← Sensory receptors

Motor division

Somatic
Nervous
System → Skeletal muscle

Autonomic
Nervous
System → Smooth muscle
Cardiac muscle
Glands

(a)   (b)

Figure 2.14

Nervous Systems — (a) The nervous system includes the central nervous system (brain and spinal cord) and the peripheral nervous system (cranial nerves and spinal nerves). (b) The nervous system receives information from sensory receptors and initiates responses through effector organs (muscles and glands).

From D. Shier et al., Hole's *Human Anatomy & Physiology,* 11e. Copyright © 2007 The McGraw-Hill Companies. Reprinted with permission.

- A *reflex arc* is the pathway through the nervous system that results in a reflex. The reflex arc has five basic parts: receptor, afferent (sensory) neuron, CNS, effector neuron (muscle), efferent (motor) neuron.

- *Adrenaline* (epinephrine) is the physiological response to stress, secreted by the adrenal gland when the sympathetic nervous system is stimulated.

- *Acetylocholine* is a neurotransmitter at somatic neuromuscular junctions.

Parts of the Brain

The brain is composed of neurons and neuroglia, which act as supporting cells. It is protected by the skull and meninges. The brain is made up of gray and white matter and consists of three major parts: the cerebrum, the cerebellum, and the brainstem. The brainstem consists of the medulla oblongata, pons, and midbrain.

The cerebrum is the largest part of the brain, consisting of two hemispheres that are separated by deep longitudinal fissures. The surface of each hemisphere is situated into numerous folds of convolutions called gyri, which are separated by furrows called fissures or sulci. Each hemisphere of the brain has four main lobes which are the frontal lobes, the parietal lobes, the temporal lobes, and the occipital lobes.

The frontal lobe is the anterior portion of the cerebral hemisphere and controls mood, smell, and motivation. The temporal lobe is located posteriorly to the occipital lobe and facilitates judgment, sense of hearing, and aid in memory. The parietal lobe is the division of each cerebral hemisphere lying beneath the parietal bones and controls and evaluates the senses of touch, taste, and pain. Finally, the occipital lobe is the posterior region of a cerebral hemisphere. It is pyramid-shaped and controls vision.

The cerebellum lies dorsal to the pons and medulla oblongata. It plays an important role in the skeletal muscles and helps coordinate voluntary movement. The cerebellum itself does not initiate voluntary movements; it interfaces with many brainstem structures that execute various movements, including posture, balance, and running.

The brainstem consists of three parts. The medulla oblongata is the lowest part of the brainstem and is continuous with the spinal cord above the level of the occipital bone. It regulates heart beat, swallowing, breathing, blood pressure, and other involuntary reflexes. The pons helps control the function of breathing and is located on the ventral surface of the brainstem between the medulla oblongata and cerebral peduncle. The midbrain connects

Table 2.1 Cranial Nerves

Cranial Nerve Number	Name of Cranial Nerve	Function
I.	Olfactory nerve	Sense of smell
II.	Optic nerve	Sense of sight
III.	Oculomotor nerve	Contraction of eye muscles
IV.	Trochlear nerve	Movement of eyeball
V.	Trigeminal nerve	Chewing, touch, pain
VI.	Abducens nerve	Movement of the eyeball
VII.	Facial nerve	Movements of the face
VIII.	Vestibulocochlear nerve	Sense of hearing
IX.	Glossopharyngeal nerve	Sense of taste and motor skill of swallowing
X.	Vagus nerve	Larynx and pharynx; also aids in the production of digestive juices
XI.	Accessory nerve	Swallowing and movement of the head
XII.	Hypoglossal nerve	Muscles of the tongue, swallowing, and speech

the pons and cerebellum with the hemispheres of the cerebrum. It is the reflex center for eye and head movements in response to stimuli.

There are 12 pairs of cranial nerves that are broken down into four categories: visceral motor impulses, somatic motor impulses, special sensory impulses, and general sensory impulses. The cranial nerves are denoted by the assignment of Roman numerals. See Table 2.1 (also see Figure 2.15).

Spinal Cord

The spinal cord is an integral part of the CNS. It begins at the end of the medulla oblongata and extends to usually the first or second lumbar vertebra. The spinal cord is the pathway for sensory impulses to the brain and motor impulses from the brain and is protected by the spinal meninges. There are 31 pairs of spinal nerves that emerge from the spinal cord. Figure 2.16 demonstrates the spinal nerves in relation to the body. The spinal nerves are as follows:

- 8 cervical nerves, C1-C8
- 12 pairs of thoracic nerves, T1-T12
- 5 pairs of lumbar nerves, L1-L5
- 5 pairs of sacral nerves, S1-S5
- 1 pair of coccygeal nerves, Co

Coding Alert!

In the Surgery section of the CPT manual under Nervous System, the most common procedures include skull base surgery, **craniectomy,** craniotomy, aneurysm, **stereotaxis,** laminectomy, neurorrhaphy, and nerve blocks.

 Think Like A Coder 2.5

The largest part of the brain is the:
- Cerebrum
- Cerebral cortex
- Brainstem
- Medulla oblongata

The Endocrine System

The endocrine system is made up of a group of glands, the endocrine and exocrine glands. The function of the endocrine system is to secrete hormones to coordinate and direct functions of the cells and organs. The exocrine glands secrete hormones through ducts before they reach cells or organs,

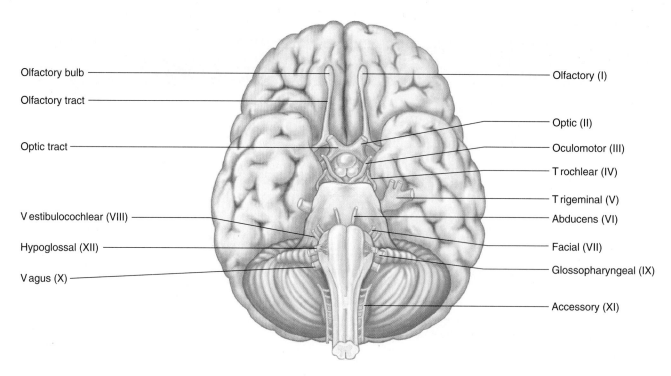

Olfactory bulb
Olfactory tract
Optic tract
Vestibulocochlear (VIII)
Hypoglossal (XII)
Vagus (X)

Olfactory (I)
Optic (II)
Oculomotor (III)
Trochlear (IV)
Trigeminal (V)
Abducens (VI)
Facial (VII)
Glossopharyngeal (IX)
Accessory (XI)

Figure 2.15

Cranial Nerves – The cranial nerves, except for the first two pairs, arise from the brainstem. They are identified by numbers indicating either their order, their function, or the general distribution of their fibers.

and the endocrine glands secrete hormones directly into the bloodstream. Ductless endocrine glands include the pituitary gland, thyroid gland, parathyroid gland, thymus gland, adrenal gland, pancreatic islets, ovaries, and testes.

- The *pituitary gland* is located in the sphenoid bone and controls the functions of other endocrine glands.
- The *thyroid gland* is located in the anterior portion of the neck and produces thyroxine.
- The *parathyroid gland* is located on the posterior side of the thyroid and produces parathormone.

    The *thymus gland* is located posteriorly to the sternum.

- The *adrenal gland* is located over the top of the kidneys.
- The *pancreatic islets* are located posteriorly to the stomach and produce glucagon and insulin.

- The *ovaries* are located in the upper pelvic cavity one on each side of the uterus and produce the hormones estrogen and progesterone.
- The *testes* are located on either side of the pelvic cavity inferior to the epididymis and produce the hormone testosterone.

 Think Like A Coder 2.6

When finding the code for excision of thyroglossal duct cyst, you would index first:

- Excision; duct, thyroglossal duct; cyst
- Excision; thyroglossal; duct; cyst
- Duct; excision; cyst; thyroglossal
- Thyroglossal duct; cyst

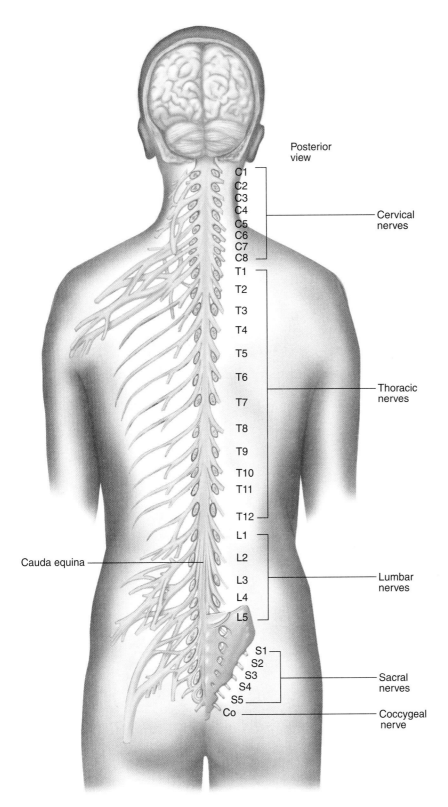

Posterior view

C1
C2
C3
C4
C5 — Cervical nerves
C6
C7
C8

T1
T2
T3
T4
T5
T6 — Thoracic nerves
T7
T8
T9
T10
T11
T12

L1
L2
L3 — Lumbar nerves
L4
L5

Cauda equina

S1
S2
S3 — Sacral nerves
S4
S5
Co — Coccygeal nerve

Figure 2.16

The Spinal Nerves – The 31 pairs of spinal nerves are grouped according to the level from which they arise and are numbered in sequence.

From D. Shier et al., Hole's *Human Anatomy & Physiology,* 11e. Copyright © 2007 The McGraw-Hill Companies. Reprinted with permission.

APPLYING CODING THEORY TO PRACTICE

Please answer the following questions on the basis of the information provided to you in this chapter. (Please see Appendix A for answers and rationale.)

1. The area of the body that is most commonly afflicted with decubitus ulcers is the:
   A. ❏ Elbow
   B. ❏ Buttocks
   C. ❏ Coccyx
   D. ❏ Sternum

2. The fibrous bands that connect muscles to bones are:
   A. ❏ Tendons
   B. ❏ Ligaments
   C. ❏ Joints
   D. ❏ Muscle fascia

3. The name of the disorder in which an accumulation of urate crystals affects the joints is:
   A. ❏ Ankylosis
   B. ❏ Gout
   C. ❏ Arthritis
   D. ❏ Bursitis

4. Skeletal muscle is referred to as:
   A. ❏ Smooth muscle
   B. ❏ Involuntary muscle
   C. ❏ Voluntary muscle
   D. ❏ Muscle tone

5. The muscle that is the most important for breathing is:
   A. ❏ Diaphragm
   B. ❏ Alveoli
   C. ❏ Pleural cavity
   D. ❏ Heart

6. Disease that causes the inflammation of the linings of the brain is:
   A. ❏ Encephalitis
   B. ❏ Parkinson's disease
   C. ❏ Meningitis
   D. ❏ Epilepsy

7. What system is inclusive of the brain and spinal cord?
   A. ❏ The peripheral nervous system
   B. ❏ The sympathetic nervous system
   C. ❏ The somatic nervous system
   D. ❏ The central nervous system

8. The central opening of the iris that contracts is called:
   A. ❏ Ciliary muscle
   B. ❏ Optic nerve
   C. ❏ Pupil
   D. ❏ Cornea

9. A person who cannot see objects up close is considered to have:
   A. ❏ Hyperopia
   B. ❏ Myopia
   C. ❏ Astigmatism
   D. ❏ Strabismus

10. A myringotomy is:
   A. ❏ Surgical incision into the meninges
   B. ❏ Surgical incision into the middle ear
   C. ❏ Surgical placement of a tube in the ear
   D. ❏ Surgical incision in the cochlear duct

11. The gustatory sense is:
   A. ❏ Smell
   B. ❏ Taste
   C. ❏ Vision
   D. ❏ Hearing

12. Excessive loss of water from the body occurs in:
   A. ❏ Hypertension
   B. ❏ Cretinism
   C. ❏ Seizures
   D. ❏ Diabetes insipidus

13. An erythrocyte is a(n):
   A. ❏ White blood cell
   B. ❏ Eosinophil
   C. ❏ Neutrophil
   D. ❏ Red blood cell

14. The condition of polycythemia is characterized by:
   A. ❏ Too many white blood cells
   B. ❏ Too many red blood cells
   C. ❏ Too few white blood cells
   D. ❏ Too few red blood cells

15. Another name for angioplasty is:
   A. ❏ Arteriovenous shunt
   B. ❏ Aortography
   C. ❏ Balloon surgery
   D. ❏ Septal defect repair

16. An embolism is a:
   A. ❏ Stationary blood clot
   B. ❏ Blood vessel that carries blood to the heart
   C. ❏ Traveling blood clot
   D. ❏ Blood vessel that carries blood away from the heart

17. A fatal allergic response is referred to as:
   A. ❏ Allergen
   B. ❏ Antihistamine response
   C. ❏ Hypersensitivity
   D. ❏ Anaphylactic shock

18. The condition in which the skin and blood vessels thicken is called:
    A. ❒ Hodgkin's disease
    B. ❒ Scleroderma
    C. ❒ Myasthenia gravis
    D. ❒ AIDS

19. The diagnostic test Mantoux is used to detect:
    A. ❒ AIDS
    B. ❒ Tuberculosis
    C. ❒ Mononucleosis
    D. ❒ Mucormycosis

20. An inflammation of the throat is called:
    A. ❒ Pharyngitis
    B. ❒ Laryngitis
    C. ❒ Bronchitis
    D. ❒ Rhinitis

21. The removal of the gallbladder is called:
    A. ❒ Colpectomy
    B. ❒ Ileostomy
    C. ❒ Cholecystotomy
    D. ❒ Cholecystectomy

22. Micturation is:
    A. ❒ Urination
    B. ❒ Breast feeding
    C. ❒ Tear drops
    D. ❒ Profuse sweating

23. The longest and strongest bone of the body is the:
    A. ❒ Tibia
    B. ❒ Fibula
    C. ❒ Femur
    D. ❒ Ulna

24. The area in the female between the vaginal opening and the rectum is referred to as the:
    A. ❒ Vagina
    B. ❒ Cervix
    C. ❒ Perineum
    D. ❒ Mons pubis

25. The vas deferens is a continuation of the:
    A. ❒ Ejaculatory duct
    B. ❒ Urethra
    C. ❒ Epididymis
    D. ❒ Prostate gland

26. A comminuted fracture is:
    A. ❒ More than one fracture, with splintered or crushed bone
    B. ❒ When the bone has been twisted apart
    C. ❒ A simple fracture with no open wound
    D. ❒ When broken ends of the bones are forced together by impact

CHAPTER 3

Medical Terminology and Pathophysiology Review

Learning Objectives

- The student will review and correlate the four word components—word roots, prefixes, suffixes, and combining forms—to medical terms.

- The student will review the most commonly used medical terms in each of the body systems.

- The student will review the most common diseases encountered in each of the body systems.

- The student will draw upon previous knowledge of medical terminology to put meaning to new medical terms encountered in the medical record.

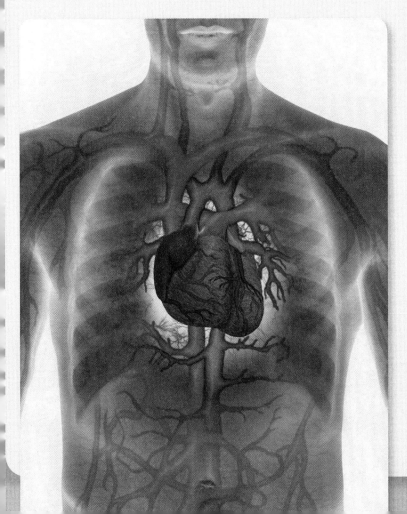

From the Author. . .

"Medical terminology is commonly known as the 'language of medicine.' This language is used in any profession that involves medicine or allied health. Being a professional medical coder is being part of the allied health care team. The foundation of medical terminology increases the comprehension of human anatomy, diseases, disorders, treatments, and the deciphering of medical records, operative notes, or laboratory reports. As you pursue your endeavor as a professional medical coder, increased knowledge of medical terminology will make abstracting and coding assignment much easier and quicker. Treat medical terminology as an ongoing skill that you will consistently learn and eventually your vocabulary will build which will aid in your comprehension of medical reports. Increased knowledge of medical terminology and coding will aid you in your process of passing your national certification!"

Key terms

Atrium	Inguinal Hernia
Embolus	Large Intestine
Gallbladder	Metabolism
Glomerulus	Microorganisms
Gonads	Nephron
Hysterectomy	Neuron

Medical Word Components

Word Roots Review

Medical words contain one or more word roots and are usually formed by combining with a suffix. A word root is the foundation of the medical term and is the source of meaning. Each body system has a core of word roots that are associated with it. Presented in this chapter are the cores of body system root words that will help you review for the medical terminology section of your coding examination (see Table 3.1).

 Think Like A Coder 3.1

Example of Word Roots

Gastrectomy   Arthritis
gastr/ectomy   arthr/itis
word root suffix   *word root suffix*

Combining Forms Review

A combining form is a word root with the combining vowel attached, separated by a "/".

> Example: hepat/o, lith/o, arthr/o.

The combining vowel is a word part, usually ending in an "o" used to make pronunciation easier. The combining vowel used to connect a word root and a suffix.

> Example: arthropathy – arthr/o/pathy – the combining vowel "o" is used between the word root "arthr" and the suffix "pathy."

A combining vowel is also used to connect two word roots.

> Example: schizophrenia – schizo/phrenia – the combining vowel, "o" is used between two root words, "schizo" and "phrenia."

Table 3.1 Most Commonly Used Word Roots

Word Root	Meaning	Word Root	Meaning
abdomin-	abdominal	mast-	breast
angi-	vessel	nat-	birth
append-	appendix	necr-	death
arthr-	joint	nephr-	kidney
bacteri-	bacteria	onco-	tumor
carcin-	cancerous	oste-	bone
cardi-	heart	path-	disease
cephal-	head/skull	pelv-	pelvis
cyt-	cell	radi-	x-ray
enter-	intestines	ren-	kidney
gastr-	stomach	sacr-	sacrum
gyne-	female	salping-	tube
hemat-	blood	sarc-	flesh, skin
hepat-	liver	therm-	heat
immun-	immunity	thorac-	thorax
irid-	iris	thromb-	clot
jejun-	jejunum	trache-	trachea
kerat-	cornea	urethr-	urethra
lip-	fat	uter-	uterus

Please note that a combining vowel is NOT used to connect a prefix and a word root.

Example: semicomatose – semi/comatose.

Prefixes Review

A prefix is a word part that comes before the root and begins the term. Prefixes modify the word root and often give an indication or direction, time, or orientation. (See Table 3.2).

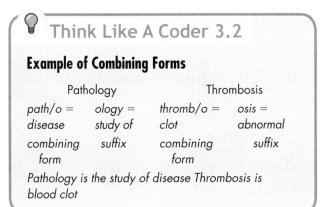

Think Like A Coder 3.2

Example of Combining Forms

Pathology		Thrombosis	
path/o = disease	ology = study of	thromb/o = clot	osis = abnormal
combining form	suffix	combining form	suffix

Pathology is the study of disease Thrombosis is blood clot

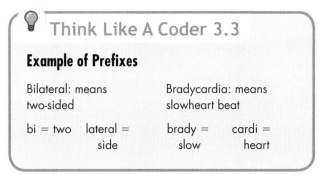

Think Like A Coder 3.3

Example of Prefixes

Bilateral: means two-sided		Bradycardia: means slowheart beat	
bi = two	lateral = side	brady = slow	cardi = heart

Table 3.2 Most Commonly Used Prefixes

Prefix	Meaning	Prefix	Meaning
a-	without, not	hemi-	half
ab-	away	hyper-	excessive; above
ad-	toward, near	hypo-	deficient; below
ante-	before	inter-	between
anti-	against	meta-	moving from one part to another
bi-	two	micro-	small
bio-	life	neo-	new
brady-	slow	pan-	all
circum-	around	poly-	many
con-	with or together	quadri-	four
dia-	across or through	re-	back; again
dys-	painful; bad	sub-	below; under
ecto-	outside	super-	above; excessive
en-	inside	tachy-	fast
epi-	upon	tri-	three
ex-	out, from	ultra-	excessive; beyond

Suffixes Review

Suffixes are word endings. Adding different suffixes to the word root changes the meaning of the medical term. A suffix can be a single letter or a group of letters and cannot be the foundation of a medical word. A suffix will always begin with a hyphen to show that it is a word part, not a complete word (see Table 3.3).

Think Like A Coder 3.4

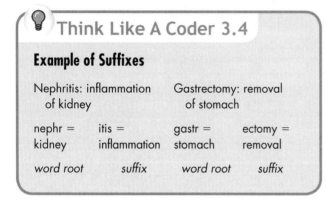

Example of Suffixes

Nephritis: inflammation of kidney

nephr = kidney	itis = inflammation
word root	suffix

Gastrectomy: removal of stomach

gastr = stomach	ectomy = removal
word root	suffix

Integumentary System Terminology Review

The skin and accessory organs such as the nails, hair, and skin make up the integumentary system (see Figure 3.1). The name comes from the Latin term "integumentum," which means to cover. The function of the integumentary system is to protect the body from infection and disease.

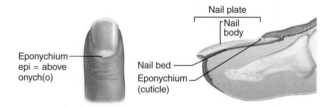

Figure 3.1
Structure of a Nail

From P. Besser & J. Fisher, Introduction to *Medical Terminology.* Copyright © 2006 The McGraw-Hill Companies, Inc. Reprinted with permission.

Table 3.3 Most Commonly Used Suffixes

Suffix	Meaning	Suffix	Meaning
-ac	pertaining to	-ia	condition, state, thing
-al	pertaining to	-ion	action; condition
-ar	pertaining to	-ism	process; disease from a specific cause
-ary	pertaining to	-itis	inflammation of
-ation	a process; being or having	-logy	study of
-centesis	surgical puncture	-megaly	enlargement
-cyte	cell	-meter	instrument to measure
-ectomy	surgical excision; removal	-metry	process of measuring
-graphy	process of recording	-oma	tumor, mass
-iatry	medical treatment	-osis	condition; abnormal condition
-itian	expert	-pathy	disease
-ous	pertaining to	-paralysis	loss of movement of feeling
-tic	pertaining to	-scopy	using an instrument to examine

Table 3.4 Review of Integumentary System Medical Terminology

Medical Term	Word Components	Definition of Word Component	Definition of Medical Term
adipose	adip/o -ose	fat full of	fatty tissue
arrector pili	rectus pil/o	to raise up hair	muscles that cause the hair to raise
cutaneous	cutane/o -ous	skin pertaining to	pertaining to skin
depilatory	de pil/o	away hair	agent used to remove hair
dermatology	dermat/o -ology	skin the study of	the study of the skin
elastin	elast/o -in	flexing substance	connective tissue protein
epithelium	epi- theil/o -um	upon; above cellular layer a structure	layer of cells forming the epidermis
follicle	follicle	small sac	a small sac or cavity
keratin	kerat/o -in	hard fibrous protein substance	protein polymers found only in epithelial cells
lipocyte	lip/o -cyte	fat cell	fat cell
melanin	melan/o	black	pigment in the skin
nevus	mole; birthmark		hyperpigmented area of the skin
sebaceous gland	seb/o -aceous	sebum pertaining to	gland that produces oily secretion
subcutaneous	sub- cutane/o -ous	below skin pertaining to	beneath the skin

Table 3.5 Review of Integumentary System Disease

Disease	Definition
basal cell carcinoma	tumor of epithelial tissue in the epidermis
cellulitis	inflammation of cellular or connective tissue caused by infection
dermatitis	inflammation of the skin
eczema	inflammatory condition of the skin marked by scaling and erythema
fissure	a deep furrow or slit in the skin
furuncle	a localized infection caused by *Staphylococcus aureus* that originates in the hair follicle
gangrene	death of tissue caused by lack of blood supply and infection
impetigo	a contagious skin infection caused by *Staphylococcus aureus* that is characterized by a thick yellow crust
onychomalacia	abnormal softening of the nails
pediculosis	infestation of lice in the hair or on the body
scleroderma	a hardening and thickening of the connective tissue of the skin
urticaria	an eruption of itchy wheals on the skin usually caused by allergies

Respiratory System Terminology Review

The respiratory system is divided into the upper and lower tracts. The upper respiratory tract consists of the nose, pharynx, and larynx, upper airways that are outside the thoracic cavity or the chest. The lower respiratory tract consists of the thorax, trachea, bronchial tree, and the lungs. The purpose of the respiratory system is to provide oxygen into the body and expel carbon dioxide.

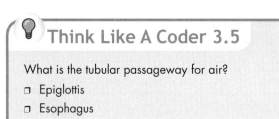

Think Like A Coder 3.5

What is the tubular passageway for air?
- ☐ Epiglottis
- ☐ Esophagus
- ☐ Larynx
- ☐ Trachea

Table 3.6 Review of Respiratory System Medical Terminology

Medical Term	Word Components	Definition of Word Component	Definition of Medical Term
alveolus	alveol/o	hollow sac	area where oxygen and carbon dioxide are exchanged
bronchial	bronch/o	bronchus	pertaining to the bronchus
	-al	pertaining to	
cavity	cav/o	hollow space	hollow space
	-ity	state; condition	

(Continued)

Table 3.6 Continued

Medical Term	Word Components	Definition of Word Component	Definition of Medical Term
epiglottis	epi- glottis	upon mouth of the windpipe	cartilage that acts as a valve of the glottis to prevent aspirated food
esophagus	esophagus	gullet	structure between the pharynx and the stomach
eupneic	eu- pne/o -ic	normal; good breathing pertaining to	pertaining to normal breathing
intercostal	inter- cost/o -al	between rib pertaining to	space between the ribs
larynx	laryng/o	larynx	voice box; structure that contains the vocal cords
lobe	lob/o	lobe	large division of the lung
mediastinum	mediastin/o	mediastinum	smaller cavity that contains the trachea and other respiratory structures
nasopharynx	nas/o pharyng/o	nose pharynx	part of the pharynx located above the soft palate
parietal pleura	pariet/o pleur/o	wall of a cavity lung membrane	membrane of the pleura that lines the thoracic cavity
sternum	stern/o	sternum; breast bone	bone that forms the anterior middle part of the bony thorax
thorax	thorac/o	thorax; chest	bony cage of ribs that surrounds and protects the lungs
trachea	trache/o	trachea	air passageway between the larynx and the bronchi

Table 3.7 Review of Respiratory System Disease

Disease	Definition
adenoiditis	inflammation of the adenoids
chronic obstructive pulmonary disease	a group of respiratory disorders that obstruct bronchial flow
emphysema	destruction of the alveoli, causing respiratory difficulty

(Continued)

Table 3.7 Continued

Disease	Definition
hemothorax	blood in the pleural cavity (chest)
lobar pneumonia	infection in one of the lobes of the lung
pansinusitis	the inflammation of all the sinuses
pleural effusion	excessive buildup of fluid in the pleural space between the parietal and visceral pleura
pneumothorax	air in the pleural space (chest) that causes the lung to collapse
pulmonary embolism	a blood clot that blocks circulation in the pulmonary artery
tracheostenosis	the narrowing of the trachea
upper respiratory infection	infection of the pharynx, larynx, and nasal cavity

Urinary System Terminology Review

The urinary system filters substances from the blood and eliminates waste. The urinary system begins with the kidneys. They are located in the retroperitoneal space, a small area behind the peritoneum of the abdominal cavity that is filled with fatty tissues that cushion the kidneys. The purpose of the urinary system is to remove waste products from the blood and maintain the body's internal environment by excreting urine. Figure 3.2 depicts a physician using a cystoscope to view the inside of the bladder. Cystoscopic viewing can lead to the diagnosis of many urinary disorders and diseases.

Think Like A Coder 3.6

What code(s) would you assign for the repair of a recurrent, reducible **inguinal hernia** in a 20-week-old infant?

☐ 49495

☐ 49520

☐ 49580

☐ 49505

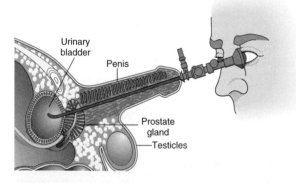

Figure 3.2

Cystoscope – A physician can view and diagnose diseases and disorders of the urinary bladder such as stone or calculi in the bladder.

From N. Thierer and L. Breitbard, *Medical Terminology, Language for Health Care,* 2e. Copyright © 2006 The McGraw-Hill Companies, Inc. Reprinted with permission.

Male Reproductive System Terminology Review

The male reproductive system is composed of external and internal genital organs. The external genitalia, located on the outside of the body, consist of the scrotum, testes, epididymis, penis, and urethra. The internal genitalia, located inside the body, consist of the vasa deferentia, ejaculatory duct, seminal vesicles, and prostate gland. The purpose of the male reproductive system is to produce sperm and fertilize the female ovum when appropriate.

Table 3.8 Review of Urinary System Medical Terminology

Medical Term	Word Components	Definition of Word Component	Definition of Medical Term
Bowman's capsule		eponym for a British anatomist	the first part of the **nephron** that surrounds the **glomerulus**
cortical	cortic/o -al	cortex; outer region pertaining to	pertaining to the thin layer of tissue beneath the renal capsule
excretory	excret/o -ory	removing having the function of	relating to the removal of waste the body
filtration	filtrate/o -ion	straining; filtering condition; action	passing a substance through a filter to separate particle matter
kidney	ren/o	kidney	organ of the urinary system that produces urine
micturition	micturio	desire to make	elimination of urine from the bladder
nephron	nephr/o	kidney; nephron	microscopic tubular structure that produces urine in the kidneys
pelvis	pelv/o	pelvis; hip bone; basin	large funnel-shaped cavity at the upper end of the ureter
proximal convoluted tubule	proxim/o tub/o	proximal; nearest pertaining to	tubule of the **nephron** that begins at the Bowman's capsule and ends at loop of Henle
retroperitoneal	retro- periteino -al	backward; behind stretch over pertaining to	indicating the area behind the peritoneum
secretion	cretus	separate	the release of substances by glands
ureter	ureter/o	ureter	tube that sends urine from the renal pelvis to the bladder
urethra	urethr/o	urethra	passageway for urine; tube that extends from the renal pelvis to the bladder
urinary meatus	urin/o meatus	urine passage	opening for the passage of urine out of the body
urination	urin/o -ation	urine a process; being	the process of eliminating urine from the body

Table 3.9 Review of Urinary System Disease

Disease	Definition
cystitis	inflammation of the bladder
cystocele	hernia (protrusion) of the bladder
glomerulonephritis	inflammation of the glomerulus and kidney
hypospadias	defect on the ventral surface of the penis
nephroblastoma	kidney containing a malignant tumor
nephrolithiasis	kidney stones
pyelonephritis	inflammation of the renal pelvis and kidney
renal hypertension	high blood pressure secondary to renal disease
uremia	blood in the urine
ureterolithiasis	stone or calculi in the bladder
urethrocystitis	inflammation of the urethra and the bladder

Table 3.10 Review of Male Reproductive System Medical Terminology

Medical Term	Word Components	Definition of Word Component	Definition of Medical Term
bulbourethral glands, also known as Cowper's glands	bulb/o urethra/o	bulb urethra	small bulb-like glands located below the prostate that secrete mucus into the urethra for lubrication
ejaculatory duct	ejaculat/o -ory ductus	to expel suddenly having the function of to lead	large collecting area for spermatozoa from each vas deferens
epididymis	epi- didym/o	upon; above testes; twin structures	structure attached to the testes that transports and stores sperm
gonad	gon/o	seed; ovum or spermatozoon	organ that produces sperm or ova
inguinal canal	inguin/o -al	groin pertaining to	passageway in the groin through which the testes travel as they descend into the scrotum
interstitial cells	interstiti/o -cyte	spaces within tissue cell	cells between the seminiferous tubules of the testes
perineum	perine/o -um	perineum structure	area of skin between the anus and the scrotum

(Continued)

Table 3.10 Continued

Medical Term	Word Components	Definition of Word Component	Definition of Medical Term
prostate	prostat/o	protector	small male gland located below the bladder that produces prostatic fluid
scrotum	scrot/o -um	scrotum; sac structure	sac of skin that holds the testes
semen	semen	seed	fluid that contains sperm
seminal vesicles	semen -al vesic/o	seed relating to small sac	glands along the posterior wall of the bladder that secrete seminal fluid
seminiferous tubules	semin/i fer/o tub/o	semen to bear tube	small tubes within each testis where spermatozoa develop
spermatocyte	spermat/o -cyte	sperm cell	immature spermatozoon in the wall of the seminiferous tubule
testis	testicul/o	testis	small, oval-shaped gland in the scrotum; male **gonad**
vas deferens	vas defero	vessel to carry down	tube that leads sperm from the epididymis and away from the scrotum

Table 3.11 Review of Male Reproductive System Disease

Disease	Definition
benign prostatic hyperplasia	an increased number of cells in the prostate gland causing nonmalignant enlargement of the prostate
cryptorchidism	failure of one or both of the testes to descend
epididymitis	inflammation of the epididymis
hydrocele	a collection of fluid that causes swelling of the scrotum
orchiepididymitis	inflammation of the testes and epididymis
phimosis	abnormal narrowing of the opening of the prepuce (fold of skin that covers the penis)
priapism	continuous erection of the penis causing pain
prostatitis	inflammation of the prostate gland
testicular carcinoma	cancer of the testicle
testicular torsion	a twisting or rotation of the spermatic cord cutting off blood flow to the testicles

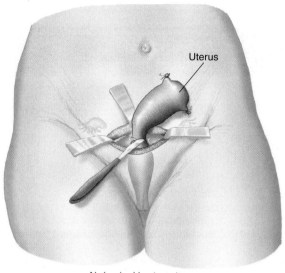
Uterus

Abdominal hysterectomy

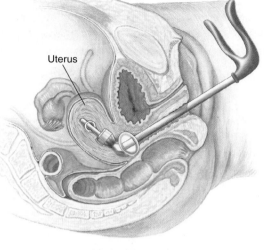
Uterus

Vaginal hysterectomy

Figure 3.3

Hysterectomy — A hysterectomy can be performed abdominally or vaginally. A surgical instrument is inserted through the cervix in a vaginal hysterectomy.

From N. Thierer and L. Breitbard, *Medial Terminology, Language for Health Care*, 2e. Copyright © 2006 The McGraw-Hill Companies, Inc. Reprinted with permission.

Female Reproductive System Terminology Review

The female reproductive system is a body system that is composed of the internal and external genital organs. The internal genitalia include the ovaries, uterus, fallopian tubes, and the vagina. The external genitalia include the area of the vulva, which is composed of several structures. The breasts also play a role in the female reproductive system. The purpose of the female reproductive system is to conceive and bear children. One of the more common medical procedures to be performed in relation to the female reproductive system is a **hysterectomy** (see Figure 3.3).

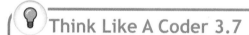

Think Like A Coder 3.7

What is the structure located in the pelvic cavity between the rectum and the urinary bladder, commonly referred to as the womb?

☐ Ovary

☐ Fallopian tube

☐ Cervix

☐ Uterus

Table 3.12 Review of Female Reproductive System Medical Terminology

Medical Term	Word Components	Definition of Word Component	Definition of Medical Term
amniotic	amni/o -tic	amnion; fetal membrane pertaining to	the fluid inside the amniotic cavity
areolar	areol/o -ar	small area around the nipple pertaining to	pertaining to the pigmented area around the nipple
clitoris	kleitoris	clitoris	a small erectile body located beneath the anterior labia
corpus luteum	corpus luteum	body yellow	a mass of tissue that forms in part of the ovary follicle after ovulation

(Continued)

Table 3.12 Continued

Medical Term	Word Components	Definition of Word Component	Definition of Medical Term
dilation	dilat/o -ion	widen; dilate action; condition	expansion of an orifice
effacement	efface/o -ment	do away with action; state	thinning of the cervix
embryonic	embryon/o -ic	immature form; embryo pertaining to	pertaining to the fetus
endometrium	endo- metr/o	within uterus	mucous membrane of the uterine wall
fallopian tube	fallopi/o -an tub/o	fallopian pertaining to tube	tube through which the ovum passes to the uterus
hymen	hymen	membrane	structure located at the inferior end of the vagina
menses	men/o	menstruation	process in which the lining of the uterus is sloughed, causing bleeding
neonate	neo- natus-	new born	newborn infant
obstetrics	obstetrix -ic	midwife pertaining to	the treatment of pregnancy
oocyte	oo/o cyt/o	egg, ovary cell	immature egg cell
perineum	perine/o -um	perineum structure	area between the vagina and the anus
salpinx	salping/o	tube	fallopian tube
uterus	uter/o	uterus	muscular organ that contains the growing fetus

Table 3.13 Review of Female Reproductive System Disease

Disease	Definition
adenomyosis	abnormal growth of adenomatous tissue in the muscle of the uterus
amenorrhea	absence of menstrual flow
cervicitis	inflammation of the cervix
endometriosis	abnormal endometrial tissue growth found in the female reproductive organs
fibroid tumor	benign fibroid tumor
mastitis	inflammation of the breast

(Continued)

Table 3.13 Continued

Disease	Definition
oophoritis	inflammation of the ovary
pelvic inflammatory disease	extension of infections from the reproductive organs into the pelvic cavity
prolapsed uterus	downward displacement of the uterus, with the cervix sometimes protruding from the vagina
vesicovaginal fistula	abnormal, tube-like passage from the opening of the bladder into the vagina

Cardiovascular System Terminology Review

The major components of the cardiovascular system include the heart, the organ that pumps the blood; the blood vessels, the passageways to transport the blood; and the blood itself. The purpose of the cardiovascular system is to direct blood throughout the body and transport nutrients, oxygen, and waste products in the blood.

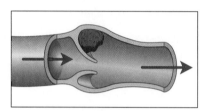

A thrombus.

Figure 3.4

Thrombus vs. Embolus — A thrombus is a stationary blood clot while an embolus is a traveling mass of material that blocks a blood vessel (at right).

From N. Thierer and L. Breitbard, *Medial Terminology, Language for Health Care*, 2e. Copyright © 2006 The McGraw-Hill Companies, Inc. Reprinted with permission.

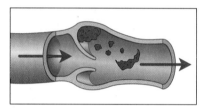

An embolus.

Table 3.14 Review of Cardiovascular System Medical Terminology

Medical Term	Word Components	Definition of Word Component	Definition of Medical Term
atrioventricular node	atri/o ventricul/o	artery ventricle	portion of the heart responsible for conduction of electrical impulses
bicuspid valve	bi- cusp/o -id valvul/o	two projection; point resembling; origin valve	heart valve with two cusps located between the ventricle and left **atrium**
Bundle of His	His	eponym for German physician	nerve fibers from the heart that conduct electrical impulses through the heart muscle
coronary artery	coron/o -ary arteri/o	encircling structure pertaining to artery	one of the blood vessels that sit on top of the heart and encircle it
depolarization	de- polar/o -ization	reversal of two opposites making; creating	a reversal of charges at a cell membrane

(Continued)

Table 3.14 Continued

Medical Term	Word Components	Definition of Word Component	Definition of Medical Term
diastole	diastole	dilation; expansion	resting period between contractions when the heart fills with blood
epicardium	epi- cardi/o -ium	upon; above heart structure or tissue	serous membrane that lines the chambers of the heart and heart valves
mitral valve	mitr/o -al valvul/o	structure like a miter; tall hat with two points pertaining to valve	valve located between the left atrium and ventricle
myocardium	my/o cardi/o -um	muscle heart structure	muscle layer of the heart
popliteal artery	poplite/o -al arteri/o	back of knee pertaining to artery	artery that runs behind the knee
Purkinje fibers	Purkinge	eponym of Bohemian anatomist	cells located in the walls of the ventricles that play a role in the heart's conduction
repolarization	re- polar/o -ization	again two opposite poles making; creating	restoration of the polarized state at a cell membrane
sinoatrial node	sin/o atri/o -al node	hollow cavity atrium pertaining to knob; mass of tissue	pacemaker of the heart that initiates electrical impulses
systolic	systol/o -ic	contracting pertaining to	pertaining to the contraction of the heart
tricuspid valve	tri- cusp/o -id valvul/o	three projection; point resembling valve	valve located between the right atrium and the right ventricle
vena cava	ven/o cava	vein plural for cavity	largest vein in the body
ventricle	ventricul/o	ventricle; lower heart chamber	one of the two larger lower chambers of the heart atrium

Table 3.15 Review of Cardiovascular System Disease

Disease	Definition
angioma	tumor, usually benign, consisting of blood vessels
arteriosclerosis	hardening, thickening, and loss of elasticity of the walls of the arteries
congestive heart failure	inability of the heart to pump enough blood to the organs
embolus	mass of undissolved matter (clot) that moves through the bloodstream until it is caught or lodged (see Figure 3.4)
fibrillation	quivering or spontaneous contraction of the atria or ventricles
hemophilia	hereditary disease in which the blood fails to clot and abnormal bleeding occurs
hypertensive heart disease	disease of the heart brought on by ongoing high blood pressure
ischemia	deficiency of blood supply caused by an obstruction
pericarditis	inflammation of the outer layer and around the sac of the heart
thrombus	stationary blood clot in the vascular system (see Figure 3.4)

Blood and Lymphatic System Terminology Review

Blood is the transporting fluid of the body. It contains cells, proteins, and clotting factors carrying nutrients from the digestive tract to the cells. The purpose of the blood is to transport oxygen, carbon dioxide, nutrients, and the waste products of **metabolism.** The lymphatic system is considered a supplement to the circulatory system. It is composed of lymph, lymph nodes, lymph vessels, spleen, thymus gland, tonsils, and lymphoid tissue in the intestinal tract. The purpose of the lymphatic system is to defend the body against **microorganisms** and cancerous cells via the immune system.

 Think Like A Coder 3.8

What is the iron-containing protein in red blood cells that transport oxygen?

- ☐ Hemoglobin
- ☐ Platelet
- ☐ Erythrocyte
- ☐ Leukocyte

Table 3.16 Review of Blood and Lymphatic Systems Medical Terminology

Medical Term	Word Components	Definition of Word Component	Definition of Medical Term
agglutinate	a- gluten	to glue	to form clumps
anemia	an- hem/o -ia	without blood condition of	decreased levels of hemoglobin in the blood
cytotoxic	cyt/o tox/o -ic	cell poison pertaining to	cells that engulf and destroy pathogens

(Continued)

Table 3.16 Continued

Medical Term	Word Components	Definition of Word Component	Definition of Medical Term
erythrocyte	erythr/o -cyte	red cell	blood cell that carries oxygen and carbon dioxide
glycoprotein	glyc/o protos	sugar first	substance consisting of protein and carbohydrates
granulocyte	granul/o -cyte	granule cell	WBC* that has a granular appearance
hemoglobin	hem/o glob/o	blood shaped like a globe	red, iron-containing molecule
hypoxia	hyp/o -oxy -ia	under; below oxygen condition of	decreased amount of oxygen
immunity	immun/o -ity	immune response state; condition	the quality of being unsusceptible to disease
leukocyte	leuk/o -cyte	white cell	any of five different types of WBC*
lymphocyte	lymph/o -cyte	lymph cell	type of agranular WBC* (basophile, eosinophil, neutrophil, and monocyte)
pathogen	path/o -gen	disease; suffering to make	disease-causing microorganism
phagocyte	phag/o -cyte	eating; swallowing cell	WBC* that engulfs and destroys cells
prothrombin	pro- thromb/o	before blood clot	protein essential for the clotting of blood
thrombocyte	thromb/o -cyte	blood clot cell	cell fragment that does not contain a nucleus

*Note: The acronym WBC stands for **White Blood Cell.**

Table 3.17 Review of Blood and Lympathic Systems Disease

Disease	Definition
aplastic anemia	insufficient amount of red blood cell production of the blood-forming tissue of the bone marrow
hematocytopenia	abnormal decrease of the red blood cells of the body

(Continued)

Table 3.17 Continued

Disease	Definition
Hodgkin's disease	neoplastic malignancy of the lymphatic system
leukemia	blood disease characterized by abnormal increase in the amount of WBC* in the body
lymphadenitis	inflammation of the lymph glands
lymphadenopathy	disease of the lymph nodes
lymphoma	group of malignant, solid tumors of the lymph tissues
splenomegaly	abnormal enlargement of the spleen
thrombophlebitis	inflammation of a vein associated with a thrombus usually occurring in an extremity
varicose vein	twisted, enlarged, superficial veins usually occurring in the lower legs

Digestive System Terminology Review

Digestion is performed by the digestive system, which includes the alimentary canal and accessory digestive organs. The alimentary canal consists of the mouth, pharynx, esophagus, stomach, small intestine, **large intestine,** and anus. Accessory organs include the tongue, teeth, salivary glands, pancreas, liver, and **gallbladder.** The function of the digestive system is to digest food and remove undigested matter from the body.

Table 3.18 Review of Digestive System Medical Terminology

Medical Term	Word Components	Definition of Word Component	Definition of Medical Term
bile	chol/e	bile; gall	yellow-green bitter fluid produced by the liver
cecum	cec/o	blind	first part of the **large intestine**
colon	colon/o	colon	longest part of the large intestine
duodenum	duodenum	twelve	first part of the small intestine
esophagus	esophag/o	esophagus	flexible, muscular tube that moves food from the pharynx to the stomach
gallbladder	gall- cholecyst/o bladder	bile; gallbladder receptacle	small, dark green sac posterior to the liver
hepatic	hepat/o -ic	liver pertaining to	pertaining to the liver
ileum	ileum	twist	third and last part of the small intestine

(Continued)

Table 3.18 Continued

Medical Term	Word Components	Definition of Word Component	Definition of Medical Term
jejunum	jejunum	empty	second part of the small intestine
large intestine	intestin/o	intestine	organ of absorption between the small intestine and the anal opening
mastication	mastic/o -ion	chewing action; condition	act of chewing
peristalsis	peri- stalsis	around contraction	contractions of the smooth muscle of the digestive tract that propel food
pyloric sphincter	pylorus -ic sphincter	gatekeeper pertaining to band	muscular band that holds food in the stomach during digestion
rugae	ruga	wrinkle	deep folds in the gastric mucosa
small intestine	intestin/o	intestine	organ of the digestive system between the stomach and the large intestine
visceral	viscer/o -al	internal organs pertaining to	pertaining to internal organs

Table 3.19 Review of Digestive System Disease

Disease	Definition
appendicitis	inflammation of the appendix
abdominal hernia	protrusion of an internal organ through an abnormal opening in the abdominal wall
cholecystitis	inflammation of the **gallbladder**
cholelithiasis	presence of gallstones within the gallbladder or bile ducts
Crohn's disease	chronic inflammation of the ileum causing bowel disorders
diverticulitis	inflammation of the pouch-like herniations in the intestinal wall
duodenal ulcer	lesion in the wide segment of the small intestine
gastroenteritis	inflammation of the stomach and the intestines
pancreatitis	inflammation of the pancreas that causes slow, progressive destruction of the pancreatic tissue
peritonitis	inflammation of the peritoneum

Terminology Review of the Senses

The senses are those organs and receptors that are associated with touch, taste, sight, hearing, and smell. Functions of the senses are to receive stimuli from the sensory receptors, eyes, ears, nose, and the tongue and to transmit these impulses to the brain for interpretation.

Table 3.20 Senses: Review of Eye Medical Terminology

Medical Term	Word Components	Definition of Word Component	Definition of Medical Term
aphakia	a- phak/o -ia	away from; without lens of eye condition, state	condition in which a lens of the eye has been surgically removed
canthus	kanthos	corner	part of the eye where the upper and lower eyelids meet
conjunctiva	conjunctus	joining of	transparent mucous membrane that covers the inside of the eyelids
cornea	corneus	horny membrane	transparent layer over the anterior part of the eye
intraocular	intra- ocul/o -ar	inside; within eye pertaining to	pertaining to the inside of the eye
iris	irid/o	iris; colored part of the eye	colored ring of tissue on the eye
lacrimal	lacrim/o -al	tears pertaining to	pertaining to tears
macula	macul/o	small spot	yellow-orange area with indistinct edges in the retina
nasolacrimal	nas/o lacrim/o -al	nose tears pertaining to	pertaining to the nasal or lacrimal ducts
optic nerve	opt/o -ic nerve	eye pertaining to nerve	sensory nerve that carries nerve impulses from the eye to the brain to enable vision
optometrist	opt/o -metrist	eye one who measures	one who tests visual acuity and prescribes lenses
pupil	pupa	doll	small opening in the iris
retina	retin/o	retina	membrane lining the posterior cavity of the eye that contains rods and cones

(Continued)

Table 3.20 Continued

Medical Term	Word Components	Definition of Word Component	Definition of Medical Term
sclera	scler/o	hard	white, tough, fibrous connective tissue that forms the outer layer of the eye
vitreous humor	vitre/o humor	glassy clear liquid	clear, gel-like substance behind the lens of the eye

Table 3.21 The Senses: Review of Ear and Nose Medical Terminology

Medical Term	Word Components	Definition of Word Component	Definition of Medical Term
auditory nerve	audi/o -ory nerve	hearing; sound having the function of nerve	nerve that conducts impulses to the brain for balance and hearing
cerumen	cera	wax	wax that traps dirt in the external auditory canal
cochlea	cochlea	snail	structure of the inner ear associated with the sense of hearing
ethmoid sinuses	ethm/o -oid	sieve resemblance to	groups of small air cells in the ethmoid bone
frontal sinuses	front/o	front	pair of sinuses above each eyebrow
incus	incus	anvil	second bone of the middle ear
malleus	malle/o	hammer-shaped bone	first bone of the middle ear
mastoid process	mast/o -oid	breast resemblance to	bony projection of the temporal bone behind the ear
maxillary sinuses	maxill/o	upper jaw	largest of the sinuses on either side of the nose
mucosa	mucos/o	mucous membrane	mucous membrane lining the nasal cavity
ossicles	ossicul/o	little bone	the three small bones in the middle ear
pinna	pinna	wing	external ear
stapes	stapes	stirrup	small bone of the middle ear
tympanic membrane	tympan/o -ic	drum pertaining to	eardrum

Table 3.22 Review of Diseases of the Senses

Disease	Definition
conjunctivitis	inflammation of the conjunctiva, also known as "pink eye"
glaucoma	abnormal increase of intraocular pressure causing damage to the optic nerve
hordeolum	stye; inflammatory infection of a sebaceous gland on the eyelid
oculomycosis	disease of the eye or part of the eye caused by fungus
nystagmus	the repetitive involuntary movement of the eye
strabismus	disorder in which one or both eyes cannot focus on the same object
impacted cerumen	abnormal accumulation of wax-like secretion found in the external ear canal that can lead to temporary hearing loss
Meniere's disease	chronic inner ear disease that causes tinnitus, vertigo, and progressive deafness
otitis media	infection caused by an accumulation of fluid found within the middle ear
otosclerosis	abnormal hardening of the stapes of the ear caused by unusual bone development

Terminology Review of the Musculoskeletal System

The musculoskeletal system gives the body strength, structure, and the capability of movement. The skeletal system is composed of 206 bones and is the framework on which the body is built. The muscle system is composed of 700 skeletal muscles and is the engine that moves the bony framework of the body.

> **Coding Alert!**
>
> ## Musculoskeletal System
> *When coding for fractures please be aware of the following terms:*
> - Closed treatment: fracture site is not surgically open
> - Open treatment: fracture site is surgically open or open remote from the fracture site
> - Percutaneous skeletal fixation: neither open nor closed treatment; fracture not visualized and fixation/pins are placed across the fracture

Table 3.23 Review of Skeletal System Medical Terminology

Medical Term	Word Components	Definition of Word Component	Definition of Medical Term
articulation	articul/o -ion	joint action or condition	joint where two bones come together and join
carpal bones	carp/o	wrist	eight small bones of the wrist
coccyx	coccyg/o	tail bone	small, fused vertebrae below the sacrum

(Continued)

Table 3.23 Continued

Medical Term	Word Components	Definition of Word Component	Definition of Medical Term
diaphysis	diaphysis	growing between	shaft of a bone
endosteum	end/ oste/o	within the bone	cells lining the inner structure of the bone
epiphysis	epi- -physis	upon growth	area of the long bone where growth takes place
ilium	ili/o	hip bone	most superior part of hip bone
metatarsal bones	tars/o	ankle	five long bones of the midfoot
occipital bone	occipit/o	back of head	bone that forms the back of the cranium
osteocyte	osse/o -cyte	bone cell	bone cell
parietal bones	pariet/o	wall of a cavity	bones that form the sides and roof of the cranium
synovial joint	synovi/o	membrane	fully movable joints
turbinates	turbin/o	scroll-like structure	facial bones in the nasal cavity
ulna	uln/o	forearm bone	forearm bone located on little finger side
zygomatic bones	zygoma	cheek bone	facial bones that form the sides of the eye sockets and cheek bones

Table 3.24 Review of Muscle System Medical Terminology

Medical Term	Word Components	Definition of Word Component	Definition of Medical Term
abduction	ab- duct/o	away from duct; move	away from the midline of the body
deltoid muscle	delt/o muscul/o	triangle muscle	muscle in the shoulder that raises and lowers the arm
extension	extens/o -ion	straightening action or condition	movement by which both ends of any part are pulled apart
flexion	flex/o -ion	bending action or condition	the act of bending (in contrast to extension)

(Continued)

Table 3.24 Continued

Medical Term	Word Components	Definition of Word Component	Definition of Medical Term
insertion	insert/o -ion	introduce; put in action or condition	moveable attachment of the distal end of a muscle
involuntary muscle	in- voluntas -ary muscul/o	not will relating to muscle	smooth muscle; muscle that cannot be voluntarily controlled
myofilaments	my/o filament	muscle thread	microscopic threads that make up striated muscle
neurotransmitter	neur/o trans- mitt/o	nerve across to send	chemical messenger between the nerves and muscles
pectoralis major muscle	pector/o muscul/o	chest muscle	muscle of the chest that moves the arm
sternocleidomastoid muscle	stern/o cleid/o mast/o -oid muscul/o	breast bone collar bone breast resemblance muscle	muscle in the neck that bends the head and allows it to rotate from side to side
tendon	tendin/o	tendon	connective tissue that serves for the attachment for muscles to bones
voluntary muscle	volunt/o muscul/o	done by free will muscle	skeletal muscle; muscle controlled by conscious thought

Terminology Review of the Nervous System

The nervous system is composed of the brain, nerves, and spinal cord and controls all bodily functions. The nervous system is divided into two parts: the central nervous system, which includes the brain and spinal cord, and the peripheral nervous system, which includes the 12 pairs of cranial nerves extending from the brain and the 31 pairs of spinal nerves extending from the spinal cord. The function of the nervous system is to receive nerve impulses from the body and the senses.

Table 3.25 Review of Musculoskeletal System Disease

Disease	Definition
ankylosis	stiffness of a joint resulting from chronic rheumatoid arthritis
kyphosis	abnormal outward curvature of the spine; humpback (see Figure 3.5)

(Continued)

Table 3.25 Continued

Disease	Definition
gout	chronic disease that causes excessive amount of uric acid in the body leading to sodium urate crystal buildup in the joints
lordosis	an exaggerated lumbar curvature; swayback (see Figure 3.5)
muscular dystrophy	muscle disease marked by muscle weakness and degeneration of the muscles and muscle tissue
myasthenia gravis	chronic, progressive neuromuscular disease
Paget's disease	chronic metabolic skeletal disease characterized by regrowth of bone with a coarse, irregular consistency that makes the bones softer
osteoarthritis	disease caused by inflammation of the bone and joint
osteocarcinoma	cancer of the bone; bone tumor
osteomalacia	abnormal softening of the bones
scoliosis	abnormal lateral curve of the spine (see Figure 3.5)
systemic lupus erythematosus	chronic, inflammatory connective tissue disease in which cells and tissues in the body are damaged

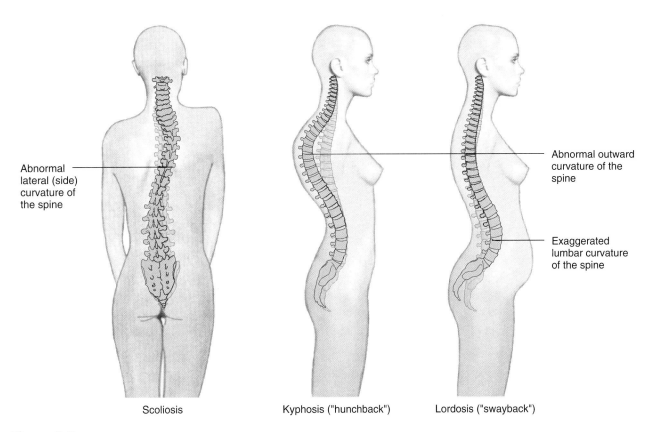

Abnormal lateral (side) curvature of the spine

Abnormal outward curvature of the spine

Exaggerated lumbar curvature of the spine

Scoliosis   Kyphosis ("hunchback")   Lordosis ("swayback")

Figure 3.5
Disorders of the Spine

Table 3.26 Review of Nervous System Medical Terminology

Medical Term	Word Components	Definition of Word Component	Definition of Medical Term
arachnoid membrane	arachn/o -oid	spider resemblance	spider-like middle layer of the meninges
cerebellum	cerebell/o -um	posterior part of the brain; little brain pertaining to	small back part of the brain that coordinates voluntary movements
cerebral cortex	cerebr/o cortic/o	brain outer layer	gray matter located on the outermost surface of the cerebrum and cerebellum
cerebrum	cerebr/o	largest part of the brain	largest part of the brain
frontal lobes	front/o lobe	front part of	areas in the front part of the brain
medulla oblongata	medulla oblongata	marrow long	lowest part of the brainstem, controlling breathing
meninges	mening/o	membrane	three membranes that cover the brain and spinal cord
myelin	myel/o	sheath of nerve fibers	cell membranes that forms the myelin sheath of neurons
neuron	neuron	nerve	nerve cell that passes electrical messages throughout the body
neurotransmitter	neur/o trans/o mitt/o	nerve across to send	chemical messenger that passes the electrical impulses from one **neuron** to another
occipital lobes	occipit/o -al lobe	back of head pertaining to part of	areas of the brain located posteriorly that receives sensory information from the eyes
parietal lobes	pariet/o lobe	wall of cavity part of	part of the cerebrum that receives information about the sense of touch
sympathetic nervous system	sym- pathet/o -ic	together suffering pertaining to	part of nervous system that prepares the body for "flight" or "fight"
temporal lobes	tempor/o -al lobe	side of head pertaining to part of	part of the cerebrum located laterally that contains the auditory receptive areas
visual cortex	vis/o cortic/o	sight outer layer	area in the cerebrum that receives nerve impulses from the eye

Table 3.27 Review of Nervous System Disease

Disease	Definition
Alzheimer's disease	chronic brain disease characterized the death of neurons in the cerebral cortex, which causes loss of memory and other bodily functions
Bell's palsy	disease of the facial nerves, thought to be viral, in which paralysis of the muscles on the face occur
cerebrovascular accident	disorder that occurs when the blood supply to the brain is shut off as a result of a cerebral thrombosis or **embolus**
encephalitis	disease characterized by the inflammation of the brain
hydrocephalus	abnormal enlargement of the cranium caused by an excessive amount of cerebrospinal fluid in the ventricles of the brain
meningitis	disease characterized by the inflammation of the meninges that surround the brain and spinal cord
Parkinson's disease	chronic, degenerative disease characterized by progressive muscle rigidity and involuntary tremors
poliomyelitis	disease marked by the inflammation of the gray matter of the spinal cord
subdural hematoma	collection of blood below the dura mater of the brain; blood tumor
transient ischemic attack	"little strokes," episodes in which the blood flow to the brain is obstructed; precursor to cerebrovascular accident

Endocrine System Terminology Review

The endocrine system is made up of one pituitary gland, one thyroid gland, four parathyroid glands, two adrenal glands, the pancreas, the thymus, and two gonads. The function of the endocrine system is to produce hormones and to keep the body in homeostasis.

Table 3.28 Review of Endocrine System Medical Terminology

Medical Term	Word Components	Definition of Word Component	Definition of Medical Term
adrenal glands	adren/o -al	adrenal gland pertaining to	endocrine glands on top of the kidneys
endocrine glands	end/o -crine	within secrete	glands that secretes directly into ductless glands
estradiol	estr/a	female	female hormone that is the most abundant of the estrogens
exocrine glands	exo- -crine	outside secrete	glands that secretes externally through ducts
follicle-stimulating hormone	follicle stimul/o hormon/o	little bad exciting hormone	hormone secreted by the anterior pituitary gland

(Continued)

Table 3.28 Continued

Medical Term	Word Components	Definition of Word Component	Definition of Medical Term
glycogen	glyc/o -gen	sugar to produce	the form glucose takes while in the liver
hypothalamus	hypo- thalam/o	decreased; below thalamus	endocrine gland in the brain located below the thalamus
insulin	insul/o	island	hormone secreted by beta cells in the pancreas
parathyroid glands	para- thyr/o	before shaped structure; thyroid	four small endocrine glands located on the back and lower edge of the thyroid gland
pineal gland	pine/o -al	shaped like a pine cone pertaining to	gland located in the center of the brain that secretes melatonin
pituitary gland	pituit/o	pituitary gland	small, rounded, gray gland attached to the lower surface of the hypothalmus
progesterone	pro- gest/o	before time from conception to birth	a female hormone obtained from the corpus luteum and placenta
testosterone	test/o	testis	a male hormone responsible for masculine characteristics
thymus	thym/o	thymus	endocrine gland located in the mediastinal cavity anterior to and above the heart
thyroid gland	thyr/o	shield-shaped	endocrine gland located on the base of the neck on both sides of the lower part of the larynx

Table 3.29 Review of Endocrine System Disease

Disease	Definition
acromegaly	disease in which hypersecretion of growth hormone is released by the pituitary gland, causing overgrowth of bones and disfigurement
Addison disease	disease in which deficiency of hormonal secretion causes depression, loss of appetite, and darkening of the skin
Cushing syndrome	disease characterized by hypersecretion of the adrenal cortex resulting in high levels of cortisol in the body
diabetes mellitus	disease characterized by insufficient production of insulin in the body
goiter	enlargement of the thyroid gland
Graves disease	condition caused by the oversecretion of hormones produced by the thyroid gland
hypercalcemia	disorder characterized by excessive calcium in the blood
hypoglycemia	disease characterized by an insufficient level of sugar in the blood
hypothyroidism	disorder characterized by an insufficient secretion of thyroid hormones
tetany	condition of low levels of calcium in the blood causing muscle spasms

APPLYING CODING THEORY TO PRACTICE

Please see Appendix A for answers and rationales.
Please fill in the correct meaning for each prefix.

1. a- _____   bi- _____

2. tri- _____   meta- _____

3. pi- _____   quadri- _____

4. re- _____   sub- _____

5. ab- _____   circum- _____

Please fill-in the correct meaning for each suffix.

1. -centesis _____   -ar _____

2. -scopy _____   -megaly _____

3. -oma _____   -ism _____

4. -iatry _____   -pathy _____

5. -ectomy _____   -graphy _____

Please choose the meaning for each medical term.

1. derm/o refers to:
   A. ❑ Skin
   B. ❑ Hair
   C. ❑ Nail
   D. ❑ Sweat

2. Thoracentesis refers to:
   A. ❑ Surgical incision into the chest wall
   B. ❑ Surgical puncture of the chest wall with a needle
   C. ❑ Surgical removal of the pleura of the lungs
   D. ❑ Surgical creation of an opening into the chest cavity

3. The term that means surgical incision for the removal of a stone from the bladder is:
   A. ❑ Cystectomy
   B. ❑ Nephrostomy
   C. ❑ Pyelotomy
   D. ❑ Lithotomy

4. The term dialysis refers to:
   A. ❑ Freeing a kidney from adhesions
   B. ❑ Surgical fixation of a floating kidney
   C. ❑ Removal of waste products from the blood
   D. ❑ Filtering waste products directly from a patient's blood

5. The term that describes what encloses and protects the testicles is:
   A. ❑ Genitalia
   B. ❑ Epididymis
   C. ❑ Scrotum
   D. ❑ Seminiferous tubules

6. The word root salping/o refers to the:
   A. ❑ Vagina
   B. ❑ Uterus
   C. ❑ Eggs
   D. ❑ Fallopian tube

7. The term meaning the external layer of the heart is:
   A. ❑ Myocardium
   B. ❑ Endocardium
   C. ❑ Pericardium
   D. ❑ Epicardium

8. The term phagocytosis refers to:
   A. ❑ Abnormal chest pain
   B. ❑ Process of engulfing and swallowing
   C. ❑ Clotting of blood
   D. ❑ Narrowing of arteries

9. The word root chol/e refers to:
   A. ❑ Green
   B. ❑ Bile; gall
   C. ❑ Carbon
   D. ❑ Enzyme

10. Lacrimal fluid is also known as:
   A. ❑ Choroid coat
   B. ❑ Tears
   C. ❑ Breast milk
   D. ❑ Ciliary body

11. The term tympanoplasty refers to:
   A. ❑ Disease of the eardrum
   B. ❑ Placement of tubes in ear canal
   C. ❑ Surgical correction of middle ear
   D. ❑ Surgical incision in the eardrum

12. The term used to describe the five long bones of the midfoot is:
   A. ❑ Maxillary bones
   B. ❑ Metacarpal bones
   C. ❑ Lacrimal bones
   D. ❑ Metatarsal bones

13. The term that refers to skeletal muscle, which is controlled by conscious thought, is:
   A. ❑ Involuntary muscle
   B. ❑ Muscle fascia
   C. ❑ Voluntary muscle
   D. ❑ Smooth muscle

14. The term that refers to the brain and spinal cord is:
   A. ❑ Peripheral nervous system
   B. ❑ Autonomic nervous system
   C. ❑ Central nervous system
   D. ❑ Parasympathetic nervous system

15. The word root glyc/o refers to:
   A. ❑ Stomach
   B. ❑ Hernia
   C. ❑ Insulin
   D. ❑ Sugar

UNIT 2

Procedures Review

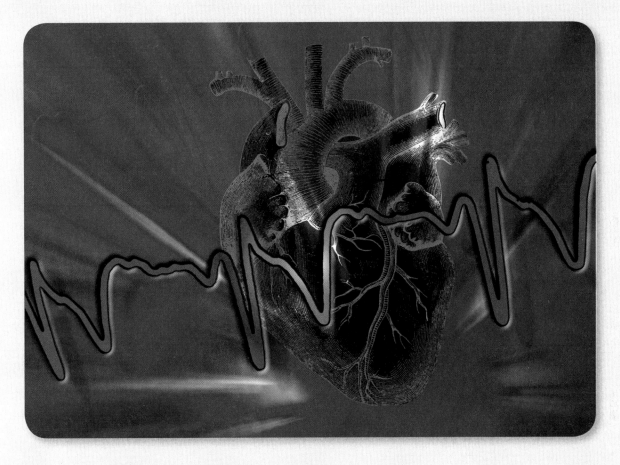

Chapter 4: CPT Guidelines Review

Chapter 5: Evaluation and Management Review

Chapter 6: Anesthesia Review

Chapter 7: Surgery Review

Chapter 8: Radiology Review

Chapter 9: Pathology and Laboratory Review

Chapter 10: Medicine Section Review

Chapter 11: HCPCS Level II Coding Review

CPT Guidelines Review

Learning Objectives

- The student will review *Current Procedural Terminology* as a set of codes, their descriptions, and guidelines so that he or she will be able to practice finding the correct codes(s) in an expeditious and accurate manner.

- The student will review the instructions for the use of the CPT Manual.

- The student will review and apply section numbers and their sequences.

- The student will review and apply the code symbols used in the CPT Manual.

Key terms

Aneurysm

Bilateral

Cholecystectomy

Concurrent

Lymphadenectomy

Mastectomy

Postoperative

Prognosis

Vascular

From the Author...

"Understanding the *Current Procedural Terminology* standards and guidelines is critical in your success for achieving a national coding credential. It is impossible to memorize all of the CPT codes; however, memorizing or gaining a complete understanding of the CPT guidelines can offer you a better chance at passing your national coding certification. *Current Procedural Terminology,* when broken down into 'bits and pieces,' can offer much more clarity to the understanding of all guidelines. You must try to achieve thinking that is organized and logical, the same way in which the CPT manual is arranged. If you can achieve in-depth understanding of these guidelines and all modifiers, then mastering your coding examination will become much easier."

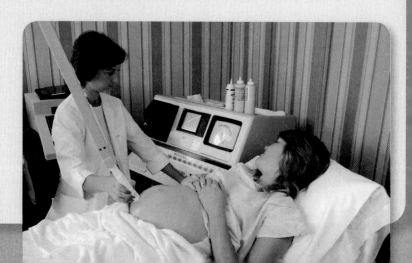

Introduction

CPT is an acronym for *Current Procedural Terminology,* which was developed by the American Medical Association in 1966. Each year, an annual publication is prepared that makes changes corresponding with significant updates in medical technology and practice. As you prepare to take a national examination, the most recent version of CPT, CPT 2009, which contains more than 8,000 codes and descriptors, is one of the tools you will need to be successful. Using an updated CPT manual is critical to ensure accurate coding assignment.

Current Procedural Terminology, fourth edition, is a set of codes, descriptions, and guidelines intended to describe procedures and services performed by physicians and other health care providers. Inclusion of a descriptor and its associated five-digit code number in the CPT book is based on whether the procedure is consistent with contemporary medical practice and is performed by many practitioners in clinical practice in several locations. The American Medical Association, through its Department of CPT Editorial Research and Development, provides staff support for the process of adding, modifying, and deleting CPT codes. The 16-member CPT Editorial Panel meets four times a year and considers proposals for changes to CPT. The Editorial Panel is supported in its efforts by the CPT Advisory Committee, which is made up of representatives of more than 90 medical specialty societies and other health care professional organizations.

In addition to preparing an annual update of CPT, the American Medical Association provides several additional resources on CPT, including *CPT Assistant,* a monthly newsletter; *CPT Changes: An Insider's View,* an annual publication explaining the intent and use of new and revised procedures/services; *CPT Principles of Coding,* an educational primer covering the basic concepts of CPT coding; *CPT Information Services,* a telephone service that provides users with expert advice on code use; and an annual CPT coding symposium. Each year changes occur within the CPT system. The change can be the revision of the narrative description of the code of the addition or deletion of a code. It is crucial that the health care providers maintain up-to-date codes.

Section Numbers and Their Sequence

The eight sections of the CPT manual are as follows:

- Evaluation and Management
- Anesthesia
- Surgery
- Radiology
- Pathology and Laboratory
- Medicine
- Category II Codes
- Category III Codes

Table 4.1 Range of Codes for Each CPT Section

Evaluation and Management	99201 – 99499
Anesthesiology	00100 – 01999,
Qualifying Circumstances for Anesthesia	99100 – 99140,
Moderate or Conscious Sedation	99143 – 99150
Surgery	10021 – 69990
Radiology	70010 – 79999
Pathology and Laboratory	80047 – 89356
Medicine	90281 – 99607
Category II Codes	0001F – 6020F
Category III Codes	0016T – 0183T

The first and last code numbers and the subsection name of the items appear at the top of most pages in the CPT manual.

> **Example**
>
> *Cardiovascular System/Surgery* **33010 – 37785**

Within the main body of the CPT manual, each section has a structure that is progressive. Each of the eight major sections of the CPT manual has codes grouped into subsections, with the exception of the Evaluation and Management section, which is divided into category levels.

> **Think Like A Coder 4.1**
>
> **Section:** *Radiology;* **subsection** to Radiology Section: *Radiation Oncology;* **heading** in subsection: *Consultation: Clinical Management*
>
> **Section:** *Evaluation and Management;* **subsection** to Evaluation and Management: *Office or Other Outpatient Services;* Category Levels: *New Patient, Established Patient,* and *Severity of Diagnostics*

Codes are further divided into smaller categories under subheadings, such as the type of procedure being performed. The final subdivision is the service of procedure code and its descriptor.

Think Like A Coder 4.2

Section Surgery
Subsection Mediastinum and Diaphragm
Heading Diaphragm
Subheading Repair

Code: 39502; Repair, paraesophageal hiatus hernia, transabdominal, with or without fundoplasty, vagotomy, and/or pyloroplasty, except neonatal.

Coding Alert!

The procedures and services with their identifying codes are presented in numerical order, (e.g., Anesthesia 00100-01999) with the exception of the first section of the CPT manual, Evaluation and Management Codes, which begins with the number assignment 99201-99499.

Review Instructions for Using the CPT Manual

When you are coding, choose the name of the procedure or service that accurately describes the service performed. Select a code that exactly identifies the service that was performed. If no code matches accurately matches the description of the service being performed, then assign an appropriate Unlisted Service or Procedure code. The alphabet index is the key to finding codes in the CPT Manual. Never assign a code directly from the index—it is only a reference to find the correct code and its descriptor in the front of the CPT manual. Always verify the code before assigning it to a service of a procedure. It is vital for accurate code assignment that the index is used properly. The index in the CPT manual (see Figure 4.1, #1) provides a specific code or a range of codes (Leg > Repair > Tendon; 27393-27400) for procedures and services listed by main term alone. Main terms are printed in bold font for quick access and identification.

The index is set up in such a way that it allows the user to locate CPT codes in various ways. Following are some ways in which the coder can use the index to find medical codes in a quick and accurate manner:

1. Body Part—Service: Lower leg biopsy; index the term *Leg* and find *Lower > Biopsy*. The range of codes found in the index, which should be verified in the front of CPT manual, is 27613-27614 (see Figure 4.1, #2).

2. The Condition—Service: Legionella antigen; index the term *Legionella* and find *antigen*. The range of codes found in the index, which should be verified in the front of the CPT manual, is 87277-87278, 87540-87542 (see Figure 4.1, #3).

3. Main Term—Service: Laser Surgery of a mouth lesion; index the term *Laser Surgery* and find *Lesion > mouth*. The code found in the index, which should be verified in the front of the CPT manual, is 40820 (See Figure 4.1, #4).

Anus 46614, 46917
Cautery
  Esophagus................. 43227
Lacrimal Punctum 68760
Lens Posterior 66821
Lesion
④ Mouth...................... 40820
  Nose 30117–30118
  Penis 54057
  Skin............... 17000–17111,
                    17260–17286
Myocardium.......... 33140–33141
Prostate 52647–52648
Spine
  Diskectomy 62287
Tumors
  Urethra and Bladder.... 52234
Urethra and Bladder........ 52214

Laser Treatment 17000-17286,
                    96920–96922
See Destruction

Lateral Epicondylitis
See Tennis Elbow

Latex Fixation. 86403–86406

LATS
See Thyrotrophin Releasing Hormone (TRH)

Latzko Operation
See Repair, Vagina, Fistula; Revision

LAV
See HIV

LAV Antibodies
See Antibody, HIV

LAV-2
See HIV-2

Lavage
Colon 44701
Lung
  Bronchial 31624
  Total 32997
Mammary Duct.... 0046T, 0047T
Penitoneal..................... 49080

LCM
See Lymphocytic Choriomeningitis

LD
See Lactate Dehydrogenase

LDH 83615–83625

LEEP Procedure 57460

LeFort Procedure
Vagina 57120

LeFort I Procedure
Midface Reconstruction............
  21141– 21147, 21155, 21160
Palatal or Maxillary Fracture
 21421-21423

Lefort II Procedure
Midface Reconstruction
  21150–21151
Nasomaxillary Complex Fracture
  21345–21348

Lefort III Procedure
Craniofacial Separation
  21431–21436
Midface Reconstruction
  21154–21159

Left Atrioventricular Valve
See Mitral Valve

Left Heart Cardiac Catheterization
See Cardiac Catheterization, Left Heart

Leg
Cast
  Rigid Total Contact 29445
Lower
  See Ankle; Fibula; Knee; Tibia
  Abscess
    Incision and Drainage
      27603
  Amputation............. 27598,
                    27880–27882
  Revision 27884–27886
  Angiography.......... 73706
  Artery
    Ligation 37618
② Biopsy 27613–27614
  Bursa
    Incision and Drainage
      27604
  Bypass Grafts 35903
  Cast .. 29405–29435, 29450
  CT Scan 73700-73706
  Decompression
    27600–27602
  Exploration
    Blood Vessel.......... 35860
    Fasciotomy.. 27600–27602,
                    27892–27894
  Hematoms
    Incision and Drainage
      27503
  Lesion
    Excision................... 27630
  Magnetic Resonance
  Imaging (MRI)
    73718–73720
  Neurectomy...27325-27326
  Repair
    Blood Vessel.......... 35226
    Blood Vessel with Other
    Graft 35286
    Blood Vessel with
    Vei...

X-Ray 73592
Upper
  See Femur
    Abscess............... 27301
    Amputation... 27580–27592
      at Hip........ 27290–27285
    Revision ... 27594–27586
  Angiography. 73706, 75835
  Artery
    Ligation 37618
  Biopsy 27323-27324
  Bursa 27301
  Bypass Graft 35903
  Cast 29345–29355,
                    29365, 29450
  Cast Brace 29358
  CT Scan .. 73700–73706,
                    75635
  Exploration
    Blood Vessel.......... 35860
    Fasciotomy............. 27305,
  27496–27499, 27892–27894
  Halo Application 20663
  Hematoma 27301
  Magnetic Resonance
  Imaging (MRI)
    73718–73720
  Neurectomy...27325-27326
  Removal
    Cast 29705
    Foreign Body......... 27372
  Repair
    Blood Vessel with
    Other Graft 35286
    Blood Vessel with
    Vein Graft 35256
    Muscle...... 27385–27386,
                    27400, 27430
① Tendon ...27393–27400
    Splint...................... 29505
    Strapping 29580
  Suture
    Muscle...27385–27386
  Tenotomy ... 27306–20307,
                    27390–27392
  Tumor
    Excision ... 27327–27329
  Ultrasound............... 76880
  Unlisted Services and
  Procedures 27599
  Urina Boot 29580
  X-Ray 73592
Wound-Exploration
  Penetrating............... 20103

Leg Length Measurement X-Ray
See Scanogram

Legionella
  Antibody..................... 86713
③ Antigen 87277–87278,
                    87540–87542

Legionella Micdadei
  Antigen Detection
  ...ity resp...

Figure 4.1

CPT Manual Index – 1. Range of codes. 2. Index "body parts."
3. Index "condition." 4. Index "main term."

Source: *Current Procedural Terminology,* American Medical Association, 2008.

4. The use of synonyms and acronyms—Service: **Cholecystectomy** by laparoscopy; index the term *Gallbladder* and find *excision.* The range of codes found in the index, which should be verified in the front of the CPT manual, is 47562-47564. (Please use your CPT manual to look up "Gallbladder > excision).

Indexing Tip:

If you cannot locate the code quickly in the index by the "main term," move to the "Body Part," then to the "Condition," and finally try to use a synonym or eponym.

Try It! Find the code for "Repair blood vessel."

Repair blood vessel with vein graft in arm.

You can index "arm" (body part), or "repair" (condition) to find code 35236!

Format of the Terminology

The CPT manual has been developed to include "stand-alone" descriptions of medical procedures. Please remember that some of the procedures in the CPT manual are not printed in their entirety but refer back to a common portion of a procedure that is listed before it (indented codes).

Think Like A Coder 4.3

| 58950: | Resection of ovarian, tubal, or primary peritoneal malignancy with bilateral salpingo-oopherectomy and omentectomy; |
| 58951: | with total abdominal hysterectomy, pelvic and limited para-aortic **lymphadenectomy** |

Code 58950 is the common portion of code 58951; therefore, the full procedure represented by code 58951 should read:
"Resection of ovarian, tubal or primary peritoneal malignancy with bilateral salpingo-oopherectomy and omentectomy with total abdominal hysterectomy, pelvic and limited paraortic lymphadenectomy"

Indexing Tip:

After indexing a procedure or service, verify the code in the front of the manual by reading the description. After reading the description, read the description of the two codes before the one you just verified. Next, read the description of two codes after the one you just verified to make sure you have chosen the correct coding assignment. This will aid in complete accuracy when taking a professional examination.

A procedure description that contains a semicolon (**;**) is divided into two parts:

1. The wording before (to the left of) the semicolon in bold is considered common language of the code.

   Example: Code 69601 **Revision mastoidectomy;** resulting in complete mastoidectomy.

2. The wording following (to the right of the semicolon) in bold is a description that is unique and pertains only to that specific code.

   Example: Code 69601 Revision mastoidectomy; **resulting in complete mastoidectomy.**

   Codes that immediately follow the code with the semicolon share the common language portion of the description. The codes that immediately follow are indented so the coder can easily see that they are a part of the wording to the right of the semicolon. For indented codes, as described earlier, both the common and unique language must be reviewed for the actual description of the service.

   Example: Code 47711 Excision of bile duct tumor, with or without primary repair of bile duct; 47112 **intrahepatic** (indented code)

Think Like A Coder 4.4

Code 17260	Destruction, malignant lesion trunk, arms, or legs; lesion diameter 0.5 cm or less
Code 17261	lesion diameter 0.6 to 1.0 cm
Code 17626	lesion diameter 1.1 to 2.0 cm

Coding Alert!

Be aware and pay special attention to the placement of the semicolon (**;**) in the code description. It is easy to make a mistake when trying to hurry and assign a code!

Guidelines

Specific guidelines are found at the beginning of each of the eight sections of the CPT manual. These guidelines, which are of utmost importance to you when taking an examination, aid in defining the specifics that are necessary to appropriately assign services and procedures that are contained in that section. An example would be the information in the "Supervision and Interpretation" subsection of the Radiology section of the CPT manual which states that, when a procedure is performed by two physicians, the radiological portion of

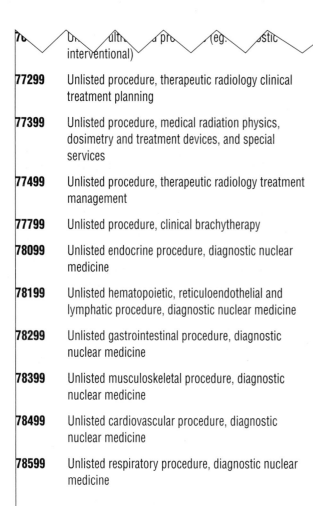

70... U... ult... pro... (eg... stic ...urrent ...s interventional)

77299 Unlisted procedure, therapeutic radiology clinical treatment planning

77399 Unlisted procedure, medical radiation physics, dosimetry and treatment devices, and special services

77499 Unlisted procedure, therapeutic radiology treatment management

77799 Unlisted procedure, clinical brachytherapy

78099 Unlisted endocrine procedure, diagnostic nuclear medicine

78199 Unlisted hematopoietic, reticuloendothelial and lymphatic procedure, diagnostic nuclear medicine

78299 Unlisted gastrointestinal procedure, diagnostic nuclear medicine

78399 Unlisted musculoskeletal procedure, diagnostic nuclear medicine

78499 Unlisted cardiovascular procedure, diagnostic nuclear medicine

78599 Unlisted respiratory procedure, diagnostic nuclear medicine

CPT Surgical Package Definition

The services provided by the physician to any patient by their very nature are variable. The CPT codes that represent a readily identifiable surgical procedure thereby include, on a procedure-by-procedure basis, a variety of services. In defining the specific services "included" in a given CPT surgical code, the following services are always included in addition to the operation per se:

- Local infiltration, metacarpal/metararsal/ digital block or topical anesthesia

- Subsequent to the decision for surgery, one related E/M encounter on the date immediately prior to or on the date of procedure (including history and physical)

- Immediate postoperative care including dictating operative ...lking ...e fam... oth... ...cian

- Follow-up care

Supervision and Interpretation

When a procedure is performed by two physicians, the radiologic portion of the procedure is designated as "radiological supervision and interpretation." When a physician performs both the procedure and provides imaging supervision and interpretation, a combination of procedure codes outside the 70000 series and imaging supervision and interpretation codes are to be used.

(The Radiological Supervision and Interpretation codes are not applicable to the Radiation Oncology subsection.)

Administration of Contrast Material(s)

The phrase "with contrast" used in the codes for procedures performed using contrast for imaging enhancement represents contrast material administered intravascularly, intra-articularly or intrathecally.

Materials Supplied by the Physician

Supplies and materials provided by the physician (eg, sterile trays/drugs), over and above those usually included with the procedure(s) rendered are reported separately. List drugs, trays, supplies, and materials provided. Identify as 99070 or specific supply code.

Reporting More than One Procedure/Service

When a physician performs more than one procedure/service on the same date, same session or during a post-operative period (subject to the "surgical package" concept), several CPT modifiers may apply (see Appendix A for definition).

Figure 4.2

CPT Guidelines — a. Radiology Guidelines excerpt. b. Surgery Guidelines excerpt.

Source: *Current Procedural Terminology,* American Medical Association, 2008.

the procedure is designated as "radiological" supervision and interpretation" (see Figure 4.2a). When a physician performs both the procedure and provides imaging supervision and interpretation, a combination of procedure codes outside the 70000 series and imaging supervision and interpretation codes should be used. Another example would be the information in the subsection "Reporting More Than One Procedure/Service" the Surgery section, which states that, when a physician performs more than one procedure or service on the same date, same session, or during a postoperative period, several CPT modifiers may apply (see Figures 4.2b). This information may be common to all guidelines; however, it is important for test-taking purposes to read and become familiar with all guidelines in all of the sections for accurate code assignment.

Add-on Codes

Add-on codes are for procedures that are always performed during the same operative session as another surgery in addition to the primary service/procedure and are never performed separately. Stand-alone codes must never be used to report such procedures. Add-on codes are usually secondary codes and can be found in Appendix D of the CPT manual. The CPT manual identifies these codes by placing a "+" sign before the code and adding specific descriptor nomenclature such as "each additional" or "list

separately in addition to primary procedure." All add-on codes found in the CPT manual are exempt from the multiple procedure concept.

Think Like A Coder 4.5

34825 Placement of proximal or distal extension prosthesis for endovascular repair of infrarenal abdominal aortic or iliac **aneurysm,** false aneurysm, or dissection; initial vessel
+34826 each additional vessel (List separately in addition to code for primary procedure)

Modifiers

A modifier (see Table 4.2) provides the means by which the reporting physician can indicate that a service or procedure that has been performed has been altered by some specific circumstance but not changed in its definition or code. It is easy to overlook assigning modifiers if you are in a rush, but do not make this mistake when taking your coding examination; read carefully and consider all indications. Modifiers are designed to give Medicaid and commercial payers the additional information needed to process a claim.

Table 4.2 Listing of Modifiers

Modifier	Description
-21	Prolonged Evaluation and Management Services
-22	Unusual Procedural Services
-23	Unusual Anesthesia
-24	Unrelated E&M Service by the Same Physician during a **Postoperative** Period
-25	Significant, Separately Identifiable E&M Service by the Same Physician on the Same Day for the Procedure or Other Service
-26	Professional Component
-32	Mandated Services
-47	Anesthesia by Surgeon
-50	Bilateral Procedure
-51	Multiple Procedures

(Continued)

Table 4.2 Continued

Modifier	Description
-52	Reduced Services
-53	Discontinued Procedure
-54	Surgical Care Only
-55	Postoperative Management Only
-56	Preoperative Management Only
-57	Decision for Surgery
-58	Staged or Related Procedure or Service by the Same Physician during the Postoperative Period
-59	Distinct Procedural Service
-62	Two Surgeons
-63	Procedure Performed on Infants Less than 4kg
-66	Surgical Team
-76	Repeat Procedure by Same Physician
-77	Repeat Procedure by Another Physician
-78	Unplanned Return to the Operating/Procedure Room by the Same Physician following Initial Procedure for a Related Procedure during the Postoperative Period
-79	Unrelated Procedure or Service by the Same Physician during the Postoperative Period
-80	Assistant Surgeon
-81	Minimum Assistant Surgeon
-82	Assistant Surgeon (when qualified resident surgeon not available)
-90	Reference (Outside) Laboratory
-91	Repeat Clinical Diagnostic Laboratory Test
-92	Alternative Laboratory Platform Testing
-99	Multiple Modifiers

Modifiers may be used to indicate to the recipient of a report that:

- A service or procedure has both a professional and technical component.
- A service or procedure was performed by more than one physician and/or in more than one location.
- A service or procedure has been increased or reduced.
- Only a part of a service was performed.
- An adjunctive service was performed.
- A **bilateral** procedure was performed.
- A service or procedure was provided more than once.
- Unusual events occurred.

Unlisted Procedure of Service

Some services and procedures performed by physicians are not found in the CPT manual. Therefore, a number of unlisted codes have been designated for reporting these procedures. When an unlisted procedure is used, the service or procedure should be described. Each of the unlisted procedural code numbers relates to a specific section of the book and is presented in the guidelines of that section. Unlisted Procedure codes are listed last in each section of the CPT manual and usually end with the digits "99" or "9."

Special Report

A service that is rarely provided, unusual, variable, or new may require a special report to determine the medical appropriateness of the service performed. Information that should be included is a precise description of the nature of, the extent of, and the necessity for the service or procedure. Included should be the time, effort, and equipment necessary to provide the service. Additional information should include the complexity of the symptoms, final diagnosis, physical findings, **concurrent** problems, diagnostic and therapeutic procedures, **prognosis,** and follow-up care.

Code Changes

If you are unsure when assigning a code, always refer to Appendix B, which contains a listing of additions, deletions, and revisions to codes in the CPT manual. New procedures numbers added to the CPT manual are identified throughout the manual with the symbol "●" placed before the code number. The symbol "▲" is used to indicate that the revision has resulted in a substantially altered procedure description. The symbols "► ◄" are used to indicate new and revised text other than the procedure descriptors. The "∅" symbol is used to identify a code that is exempt from the use of modifier 51 but has not been designated as a CPT add-on procedure or service. The symbol ⊘ is used to identify a code that includes moderate sedation (see Appendix G). The symbol "ζ" is used to identify a code for vaccines that are pending FDA approval (see Appendix K).

Listing of CPT Appendices: A–M

Appendix A: Modifiers

Appendix B: Summary of Additions, Deletions, and Revisions

Appendix C: Clinical Examples

Appendix D: Summary of CPT Add-On Codes

Appendix E: Summary of CPT Codes Exempt from Modifier 51

Appendix F: Summary of CPT Codes Exempt from Modifier 63

Appendix G: Summary of CPT Codes Which Include Moderate (Conscious) Sedation

Appendix H: Alphabetical Index of Performance Measures by Clinical Condition or Topic

Appendix I: Genetic Testing Code Modifiers

Appendix J: Electrodiagnostic Medicine Listing of Sensory, Motor, and Mixed Nerves

Appendix K: Product Pending FDA Approval

Appendix L: **Vascular** Families

Appendix M: Crosswalk to Deleted CPT Codes

APPLYING CODING THEORY TO PRACTICE

Please answer the following questions on the basis of the information provided to you in this chapter. (Please see Appendix A for answers and rationale.

1. Where will you find all the instructions necessary to properly code a procedure in the CPT code book?
   A. ❐ Appendix A
   B. ❐ Guidelines
   C. ❐ Index
   D. ❐ Unlisted Procedures

2. Why is it necessary for a medical coder to use a current editor of the AMA's CPT manual?
   A. ❐ It is the law
   B. ❐ For accurate coding
   C. ❐ Reimbursement will be less
   D. ❐ Reimbursement will be more

3. What is a two-digit modifier used for in CPT coding?
   A. ❐ Add-or code
   B. ❐ Conscious sedation
   C. ❐ Code changes
   D. ❐ Alteration of a procedure or service

4. Please list the three most important coding conventions, and identify them.

5. Please describe the difference between a "stand-alone" code, and an "unlisted procedure."

6. Please list the 8 sections of the CPT manual in order and their code ranges.
   1.
   2.
   3.
   4.
   5.
   6.
   7.
   8.

7. What is the significance of the semicolon?

8. What is an unlisted procedure, and where will it be found in the CPT manual?

9. Why would a medical coder refer to Appendix B?

10. What does the symbol "▲" stand for?
    A. ❐ Revision of a code
    B. ❐ Deletion of a code
    C. ❐ Add-on code
    D. ❐ New or revised text

11. What modifier would be assigned to an office consultation when the physician's care exceeded the criteria listed under code 99275?
    A. ❐ Modifier 22
    B. ❐ Modifier 53
    C. ❐ Modifier 21
    D. ❐ Modifier 25

12. What modifier would be assigned to an anterior packing of both nares for a nose bleed?
    A. ❐ Modifier 51
    B. ❐ Modifier 50
    C. ❐ Modifier 21
    D. ❐ Modifier 59

13. In what appendix would you find Add-Or Codes?
    A. ❐ Appendix F
    B. ❐ Appendix B
    C. ❐ Appendix D
    D. ❐ Appendix I

14. The symbol "◄ ►" is used to indicate:
    A. ❐ New and revised text
    B. ❐ Conscious sedation
    C. ❐ Special report indicated
    D. ❐ Modifier indicated

15. What section of the CPT manual includes the range of codes 90281-99607?
    A. ❐ Anesthesia
    B. ❐ Evaluation and Management
    C. ❐ Radiology
    D. ❐ Medicine

16. In what appendix would performance measures be found?
    A. ❐ Appendix B
    B. ❐ Appendix H
    C. ❐ Appendix M
    D. ❐ Appendix E

17. In which appendix would you search to find if the code 65820 has been deemed exempt from modifier 63?
    A. ❐ Appendix M
    B. ❐ Appendix A
    C. ❐ Appendix K
    D. ❐ Appendix F

18. In which part of the CPT manual would code 0016T be found?

A. ❏ Category II Codes

B. ❏ Medicine section

C. ❏ Category III codes

D. ❏ Anesthesia section

19. A service that is rarely provided, unusual, variable, or new may require a(n) _____ in determining medical appropriateness of the service.

A. ❏ Modifier

B. ❏ Add-on code

C. ❏ Special report

D. ❏ Unlisted procedure

20. Add-or codes indicate procedures that are always performed in addition to the primary services or procedures and must never be reported as stand-alone codes.

A. ❏ True

B. ❏ False

CHAPTER 5

Evaluation and Management Review

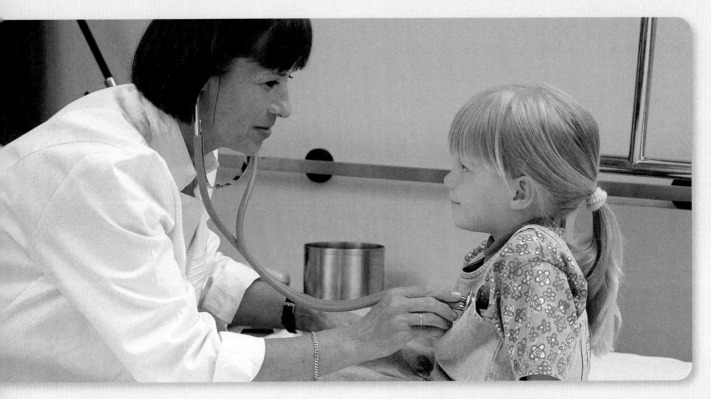

Learning Objectives

- The student will review all of the standards, guidelines, subsections, subheadings, and descriptors in the Evaluation and Management (E&M) section so that he or she can to assign codes accurately.

- The student will review and apply definitions of commonly used terms in the E&M section of the CPT manual.

- The student will review and apply all levels of service as they relate to each category.

- The student will review and apply clinical examples as they relate to each category.

Key terms

Adenopathy	Exacerbated
Comorbidities	Menses
Contusion	Morbidity
Correlate	Mortality
Dementia	Neonates
Domiciliary	Systemic

From the Author...

"E&M coding is a very large part of CPT coding and can sometimes be the most complex. The key to coding quickly and accurately is your understanding and level of knowledge of the E&M Service Guidelines. The E&M Service Guidelines break down the E&M code into the following components: history, examination, and decision making. Within these components, levels must be chosen to a degree of accuracy that conforms to the documentation presented. The degree of accuracy when choosing these levels is the key to success in coding evaluation and management services."

Classification of Evaluation and Management Services

The E&M section includes codes that pertain to the nature of physicians' work. The codes depend on type of service, patient status, and place where service was rendered. The E&M section is divided into broad categories such as office visits, hospital visits, and consultations. Most of the categories are divided into two or more subcategories of E&M services, which are further classified into levels of E&M services that are identified by specific codes. You can make many mistakes when assigning E&M codes. You need to study all of the subcategories carefully, be familiar with them, and review all of the levels before assigning a code.

The basic format of the levels of E&M services is basically the same for most categories. The format is as follows:

1. A unique code number is listed.
2. The place and type of service is specified.
3. The content of the service is defined.
4. The nature of the presenting problem(s) usually associated with a given level is (are) described.
5. Time is typically specified in the descriptor of the code.

New and Established Patients

A new patient is one who has not received any medical services within the last 3 years from the physician or another physician of the same specialty who belongs to the same group practice. An established patient is one who has received medical services within the last 3 years from the physician or another physician of the same specialty who belongs to

the same group practice. No distinction is made between new and established patients in the emergency department. E&M services in the emergency department category may be reported for any new or established patient who presents for treatment in the emergency department.

 Think Like A Coder 5.1

99215

(1) Office other outpatient visit is

(2) for the evaluation and management of an established patient, which requires at least two of these three key components:

(4) ❏ A comprehensive history

❏ A comprehensive examination

❏ Medical decision making of high complexity

(3) Counseling and/or coordination of care with other providers or agencies is/are provided consistent with the nature of the problem(s) and the patient's and/or family's needs.

(5) Usually, the presenting problems(s) is (are) of moderate to high severity. Physicians typically spend 40 minutes face to face with the patient and/or family.

Chief Complaint

The chief complaint is a brief statement describing the symptom, problem, diagnosis, or condition that is the reason a patient seeks medical care (see Figure 5.1).

MEDICAL RECORD	PROGRESS NOTES
DATE 1. x/x/xx	cc: pt complains of headache, blurred vision x 2 days
2. x/x/xx	cc: pt presents c̄ fever, red patches on skin & itching x 12 hours
3. x/x/xx	cc: pt complains of weight loss, chills, fever & anorexia x 2 weeks
4. x/x/xx	cc: pt presents c̄ abnormal bleeding from the rectum x 1 month

PATIENTS IDENTIFICATION (*For typed or written entries give Name—last, first, grade, rank; hospital or medical facility*)

Patient xxx xxxxx
xxx   xxxx

REGISTER NO.   WARD NO.

PROGRESS NOTES
STANDARD FORM 509

Figure 5.1
Example of Chief Complaints

Concurrent Care

Concurrent care is same-day service to one patient by more than one physician performing a similar procedure or service.

Counseling

Counseling is an interview with a patient and/or family concerning one of more of the following areas:

- Diagnostic results, impressions, and/or recommended diagnostic studies
- Prognosis
- Risks and benefits of management (treatment) options
- Instructions for management (treatment) and/or follow-up
- Importance of compliance with chosen management (treatment) options
- Risk factor reduction
- Patient and family education

Family History and History of Present Illness

Family history is a review of medical diseases or conditions in the patient's family that include significant information about:

- Diseases of family members that may be hereditary or place the patient at risk
- Specific disease related to problems identified in the Chief Complaint or History of Present Illness and/or System Review
- The health status or cause of death of parents, children, and siblings

Coding Alert!

New and Established Patients

When you are assigning E&M codes for a professional examination, make sure you re-read the assigned code to make sure that the correct heading (New Patient or Established Patient) has been chosen. Carelessness can cause an incorrect answer on the examination.

History of present illness is a chronological description of the development of the patient's present illness and the reason for seeking medical care from the first sign or symptom to the present day. This description should include the location, quality, context, severity, timing, and modifying factors that influence associated symptoms related to the present illness.

Levels of Service

The E&M service categories and subcategories include three to five levels of service codes. Seven components, applicable to all E&M services, must be considered before selecting a code. They are as follows:

- History
- Examination
- Medical Decision Making
- Counseling
- Coordination of Care
- Nature of Presenting Problem
- Time

Levels of E&M services are not interchangeable among the different categories or subcategories of service. The levels of E&M services include examinations, evaluations, treatments, conferences with or concerning patients, preventive pediatric and adult health supervision, and similar medical services, such as the determination of the need and/or location for appropriate care. Medical screening includes the history, examination, and medical decision making required to determine the need and/or location for appropriate care and treatment of the patient.

The first three components—history, examination, and medical decision making—are essential factors when you are considering what E&M service code to assign because they represent the amount of resources expended by the provider to render the service. The next three components—counseling, coordination of care, and the nature of presenting problem—are considered contributory factors in the majority of encounters. Even though these factors are important, the provision of these services is not required at every patient encounter.

Nature of Presenting Problem

The nature of the presenting problem is an illness, disease, condition, symptom, complaint, or finding with or without a diagnosis being established at the time of the service. The E&M codes include five types of presenting problems that are defined as follows:

- Minimal: A problem that may not require the presence of the physician, but service is provided under the physician's supervision.

Example

Initial visit for a 13-year-old female for the evaluation and management of a ***contusion*** *on the left elbow.*

- Self-limited or minor: A problem that runs a definite and prescribed course, is transient in nature, and is not likely to permanently alter health status or has a good prognosis with management or compliance.

Example

Office visit for an 11-year-old male established patient presenting with itching welts on the upper right leg.

- Low Severity: A problem with a low risk of **morbidity** without treatment, little or no risk of **mortality** without treatment, and expectation of full recovery without functional impairment.

Example

Office visit for a 45-year-old female with stable chronic asthma requiring regular drug therapy.

- Moderate Severity: A problem with a moderate risk of morbidity without treatment, a moderate risk of mortality without treatment, and an uncertain prognosis or increased probability of prolonged functional impairment.

Example

Office visit for a 22-year-old male, established patient, with diarrhea, regional enteritis, and a low-grade fever.

- High Severity: A problem with a high to extreme risk of morbidity without treatment, a moderate to high risk of mortality without treatment, or a high probability of severe, prolonged functional impairment.

Example

*Initial office visit for a 78-year-old female with **systemic** vasculitis and compromised circulation to the limbs.*

Coding Alert!

Nature of Presenting Problem

Memorizing the five types of presenting problems will allow for quicker, accurate coding decisions during the examination.

Past and Social History

A review of the patient's past medical history of illness or injury, including treatments and social habits, should include information about the patient's past history and social history.

Past History

- Prior major illnesses and injuries
- Prior operations
- Prior hospitalizations
- Current medications
- Allergies (food, drug)
- Age-appropriate immunizations status
- Age-appropriate dietary status

Social History

- Marital status and/or living arrangement
- Current employment
- Occupational history
- Use of drugs, alcohol, and tobacco
- Level of education
- Sexual history
- Other relevant social factors

Review of Systems

The Review of Systems is an inventory of body systems (refer to Chapter 2) obtained by the physician through a series of questions seeking to identify signs and symptoms the patient currently has or has experienced in the past. They are constitutional symptoms that are composed of:

- Eyes
- Ears, nose, mouth, and throat
- Cardiovascular
- Respiratory
- Gastrointestinal
- Genitourinary
- Musculoskeletal
- Integumentary
- Neurological
- Psychiatric
- Endocrine
- Hematological/lymphatic
- Allergic/immunological

The review of these systems helps the physician identify the problem and arrive at an accurate diagnosis.

Time

The inclusion of time as an explicit factor is done to assist physicians in selecting the most appropriate level of E&M services. It should be recognized that the specific times expressed in the visit code descriptors are averages and, therefore, represent a range of times that may be higher or lower depending on actual clinical circumstances. Time is not a descriptive component for the emergency department levels of E&M services because emergency department services are typically provided on a variable intensity basis, often involving multiple encounters with several patients over an extended period of time. Studies to establish levels of E&M services employed surveys of practicing physicians to obtain data on the amount of time and work associated with typical E&M services. Because "work" is not easily quantifiable, the codes must rely on objective, verifiable measures that **correlate** with physicians' estimates of the "work." It has been demonstrated that physicians' estimations of intraservice time, both within and across specialties, is a variable that is predictive of the "work" of E&M services.

Intraservice time, rather than total time, was chosen for inclusion with the codes because of its relative ease of measurement and because of its direct correlation with measurements of the total amount of time and work associated with typical E&M services. Intraservice times are defined as "face-to-face" time for office and other outpatient visits and as unit/floor time for hospital and other inpatient visits.

Face-to-Face Time

Face-to-face time is defined as the time the physician spends face to face with the patient and family. This includes the period during which the physician obtains a history (past, present, and family history), performs an examination, and counsels the patient. Face-to-face time associated with the services described by E&M codes is a valid estimate for the total work done before, during, and after the visit. Face-to-face time applies to the following categories and subcategories:

- Office and other outpatient visits
- Office consultations

Non-Face-to-Face Time

Physicians also spend time doing work before or after the face-to-face time with the patient, performing such tasks as reviewing records and tests, arranging further services, and communicating further with other professionals and the patient through written reports and telephone contact. Non–face-to-face time for office services, also called pre- and post-encounter time, is not included in the time component described in the E&M codes.

Unit/Floor Time

Unit/floor time is defined as the time the physician is present on the patient's hospital unit and rendering services for the patient at the bedside. This includes the period when the physician establishes and/or reviews the patient's health record, examines the patient, writes notes, and communicates about the patient with other professionals and the patient's family. Unit/floor time applies to the following categories and subcategories:

- Hospital observation services
- Inpatient hospital care
- Initial and follow-up hospital consultations
- Nursing facility

Unit/floor time associated with the services described by E&M codes is a valid estimate for the total work done before, during, and after the visit.

In the hospital, pre- and post-times do not include time spent off the patient's floor performing such tasks as reviewing pathology and radiology findings in another part of the hospital. Pre- and post-visit time is not included in the time component described in these codes. However, the work performed during the time spent off the patient's floor or unit was included in the calculation of the total work of typical services in physician surveys.

 Think Like A Coder 5.2

Face-to-Face Time

99203 Office or other outpatient visit for the evaluation and management of a new patient, which requires these three key components:

- A detailed history
- A detailed examination
- Medical decision making of low complexity

Counseling and/or coordination of care with other providers or agencies are provided consistent with the nature of the problem(s) and the patient's and/or family's needs.

Usually, the presenting problem(s) is (are) of moderate severity. Physicians typically spend 30 minutes face to face with the patient and/or family.

 Think Like A Coder 5.3

Initial office visit for an 18-year-old female presenting with irregular **menses** and painful urination. The physician spent 45 minutes face to face with the patient, and a comprehensive history and examination was performed.

- ❏ 99201
- ❏ 99215
- ❏ 99204
- ❏ 99205

Clinical Examples

Clinical examples of the codes for E&M services are provided to assist physicians in understanding the meaning of the descriptors and selecting the correct code. The clinical examples are listed in Appendix C. Please remember the same service or encounter may involve different amounts of work for physicians practicing in specialty areas. The appropriate level of encounter should be reported using the descriptor rather than the examples.

> ## Coding Alert!
>
> ### Clinical Examples
>
> Clinical examples can aid you in the understanding of various levels of the severity of conditions/diseases. However, never use these examples when assigning a code during an examination. Always use the E&M code descriptions when choosing a final coding assignment.

Review of Instructions for Selecting a Level of Evaluation and Management Service

When selecting a level of E&M service, you should do the following:

- Identify the category and subcategory of service.
- Review the reporting instructions for the selected category or subcategory.
- Review the Level of E&M service descriptors and examples in the selected category or subcategory.

The descriptors for the levels of E&M services recognize seven components, six of which are used in defining the levels of E&M services. These components as stated earlier in the chapter are:

- History
- Examination
- Medical decision making
- Counseling
- Coordination of care
- Nature of presenting problem
- Time

The first three listed components should be considered the key components in selecting the level of E&M services. The nature of the presenting problems and time are provided in some levels to assist the physician in determining the appropriate level of E&M service.

Determining Extent of History

The following types of histories are recognized. The level of complexity is based on the amount of information (number of elements) obtained by the physician (see Table 5.1).

- Problem focused: Limited to a chief complaint and a brief history of the present illness.

> ### Example
>
> *Patient: Complains of an earache, drainage, and decreased hearing in the left ear.*
>
> *Physician: Reviews with patient the history of chief complaint. Brief history includes the severity, duration, and symptoms of the earache. No PFSH (Past, Family or Social History) or ROS (Review of Systems) is needed.*

Table 5.1 Elements of a History

History of Present Illness	Review of Systems	Past, Family, Social History	History Type	Chief Complaint
Brief	N/A	N/A	Problem-focused	Chief complaint required
Brief	Problem pertinent	N/A	Expanded problem–focused	Chief complaint required
Extended	Extended	Pertinent	Detailed	Chief complaint required
Extended	Complete	Complete	Comprehensive	Chief complaint required

- Expanded problem focused: A chief complaint, brief history, and problem-pertinent system review.

Example

Patient: Complains of an earache, drainage and decreased hearing in the left ear.

Physician: Reviews with patient the history of chief complaint. Brief history includes the severity, duration, and symptoms of the earache. Physician also asks questions regarding the system involved, which in this case would be the respiratory system. No PFSH or ROS is needed.

- Detailed: Chief complaint; extended history of present illness; problem-pertinent system review extended to include a review of a limited number of additional systems; pertinent past, family, and/or social history directly related to the patient's problems.

Example

Patient: Complains of an earache, drainage and decreased hearing in the left ear.

Physician: Reviews with patient the history of chief complaint. An extevnded history of the chief complaint is obtained. An extended review of systems with positive and negative responses to related organ systems is conducted (respiratory, integumentary, cardiovascular, nervous, and endocrine systems). Finally, the physician asks questions regarding to pertinent past, family, and social history.

- Comprehensive: Chief complaint, extended history of present illness, and review of systems directly related to the problem(s) identified in the history of present illness, plus a review of all additional systems and complete past, family, and social history.

Example

Patient: Complains of an earache, drainage and decreased hearing in the left ear.

Physician: Reviews with patient the history chief complaint and obtains an extended history of the chief complaint. Next, he performs a complete review of systems that involves questions and comments about all body systems. Finally, the physician obtains (asks questions and receives responses) complete information regarding past, family, and social history of the patient.

Indexing Tip:

In the CPT index, you can access E&M codes quickly by finding keywords such as "Established Patient," or "New Patient." This will reduce the number of coding errors in problems involving "new" or "established" patients.

Extent of Examination Performed

The extent of the examination performed is dependent on clinical judgment and on the nature of the presenting problem(s). The levels of E&M services recognize four types of examination:

- Problem focused: a limited examination of the affected body area organ system.

Example

Patient: Complains of an earache, drainage, and decreased hearing in the left ear.

Physician: Examines the affected ear and possibly the respiratory system.

- Expanded problem focused: a limited examination of the affected body area or organ system and other symptomatic or related organ system(s).

Example

Patient: Complains of an earache, drainage, and decreased hearing in the left ear.

Physician: Conducts a limited examination of the affected ear, respiratory system, and possibly the nervous system.

- Detailed: an extended examination of the affected body area(s) and other symptomatic or related organ system(s).

Example

Patient: Complains of an earache, drainage, and decreased hearing in the left ear.

Physician: Conducts an extended examination of the affected ear and other body areas, such as nose, sinuses, head, neck, and heart and the respiratory, nervous, blood, endocrine, and sense organ systems of the body.

- Comprehensive: a general multisystem examination or a complete examination of a single organ system.

> ### Example
>
> *Patient: Complains of an earache, drainage and decreased hearing in the left ear.*
>
> *Physician: Conducts an extensive examination that encompasses either a complete work-up of the respiratory system or a complete multisystem examination that includes all of the body systems.*

For purposes of examination the following body areas are recognized:

- Head, including the face
- Neck
- Chest, including breasts and axilla
- Abdomen
- Genitalia, groin, buttocks
- Back
- Each extremity

For purposes of examination the following organ systems are recognized:

- Eyes
- Ears, nose, mouth, and throat
- Cardiovascular/blood
- Respiratory
- Gastrointestinal
- Genitourinary
- Musculoskeletal
- Skin
- Neurological
- Psychiatric
- Hematological/Lymphatic/Immunological

Level of Medical Decision Making

Determining the level of edical decision making can be difficult or tricky; you need to read carefully all of the levels that involve diagnoses, complexity, and risk. Medical decision making involves the complexity of establishing a diagnosis and/or selecting a management opinion or treatment plan as measured by the following:

- The number of possible diagnoses and/or the number of management options that must be considered.
- The amount and/or complexity of medical records, diagnostic tests, and/or other information that must be obtained, reviewed, and analyzed.
- The risk of significant complications, morbidity, and/or mortality, as well as **comorbidities,** associated with the patient's presenting problem(s), the diagnostic procedure(s), and/or the possible management options.

Four types of medical decision making are recognized:

- Straightforward
- Low complexity
- Moderate complexity
- High complexity

To qualify for a given type of decision making, two of the three elements in the Table 5.2.must be met or exceeded.

Table 5.2 Complexity

Number of Diagnoses or Management Options	Amount and/or Complexity of Data to be Reviewed	Risk of Complications and/or Morbidity or Mortality	Type of Decision Making
Minimal	Minimal or none	Minimal	Straightforward
Limited	Limited	Low	Low complexity
Multiple	Moderate	Moderate	Moderate complexity
Extensive	Extensive	High	High complexity

Appropriate Level of E&M Services

To better prepare yourself for a professional coding examination, remember that it is crucial to choose the correct level of E&M service code for accurate answers. The following are steps that should be taken when selecting a level of E&M service:

1. Identify the category or subcategory of service, for example, Initial or regular office visit; new or established patient; newborn care; comprehensive nursing care versus subsequent nursing care.
2. Review all notes that fall under categories and subcategories for special reporting of services.
3. Review all of the code descriptions within the categories and subcategories, and choose the most accurate code or level of service.
4. Use Table 5.1 to help determine the level of history when determining E&M service codes.
5. Determine the extent of examination performed by reviewing the operative note on the examination, and use the lists found under "Determine the Extent of Examination Performed." Using the four types of examinations, body areas, and organ systems, choose the correct level of service.
6. Using Table 5.2, determine the complexity of medical decision making.

Think Like A Coder 5.4

Evaluation and Management Code Assignment

Problem: The physician provides preventive medicine services to a 45-year-old female established patient who is in relative good health. The physician obtains a history inclusive of a complete HPI, (history of present illness) complete ROS and PFSH, along with an examination that entails all body systems and body areas. The physician counsels the patient on exercise and proper diet.
Correct code assignment: 99396
Rationale: **Category:** Preventive Medicine Services **Subcategory:** Established Patient **History:** Comprehensive **Examination:** Comprehensive **Age:** 40-64 yrs.

Coding Alert!

Assigning E&M codes quickly and accurately calls for practice! Memorize Tables 5.1 and 5.2 and examination criteria, then practice coding and watch your accuracy and speed increase. You will be on your way to passing the national coding examination.

7. Elect and verify the appropriate level of E&M services on the basis of Table 5.3 and the information provided in this chapter.

Office or Other Outpatient Services

Office or Other Outpatient Services is the subsection used to report E&M services provided in the physician's office or in an outpatient or ambulatory facility. This subsection contains two categories: New Patient and Established Patient.

Indexing Tip:

Remember: All E&M codes begin with the numerals "99."

Think Like A Coder 5.5

Initial office visit of a 24-year-old female who presents with symptoms of an upper respiratory infection that has progressed to unilateral nasal discharge and discomfort in the maxillary sinus. A detailed examination was performed by the physician.

- ❑ 99202
- ❑ 99201
- ❑ 99203
- ❑ 99204

Coding Alert!

It is imperative that you read each E&M descriptor to ascertain if the code requires two of the three key components or three of the three key components. Many codes have been assigned incorrectly because of lack of attention to this part of the descriptor.

Two or Three of the Three Key Components:

99204: Office of other outpatient visit for the evaluation and management of a new patient, which requires *three* key components.

- ❑ A comprehensive history
- ❑ A comprehensive examination
- ❑ Medical decision making of moderate complexity

99214: Office or other outpatient visit for the evaluation and management of an established patient, which requires at least *two* of the three key components.

- ❑ A comprehensive history
- ❑ A comprehensive examination
- ❑ Medical decision making of moderate complexity

Table 5.3 Selection of Level of Service

New Patient: (All three key components must meet or exceed the stated requirements to qualify for a particular level of E&M service code)	Established Patient (Two of three key components must meet or exceed the stated requirements to qualify for a particular level of E&M services code)	Time
• Office or other outpatient services	Office or other outpatient services Subsequent hospital care	When counseling and/or coordination of care dominates, more than 50% of the face-to-face physician-patient encounter, time is considered the key factor to qualify for a particular level of E&M services code.
• Initial observation care	Follow-up inpatient consultations	
• Office or other outpatient consultations	Subsequent nursing facility care	
	Domiciliary, rest home, or custodial care	
• Initial inpatient consultations	Home services	
• Confirmatory consultations		
• Emergency department services		
• Comprehensive nursing facility assessments		
• Domiciliary, rest home, or custodial care		
• Home services		

Hospital Observation Services

Hospital observation services codes are used to report E&M services provided to patients designated/admitted as "observation status" in a hospital. It is not necessary for the patient to be located in an observation area designated by the hospital. However, if an area in the hospital exists as a separate unit, these codes should be used if the patient is placed in such an area. Times have not been established for these services to date.

Indexing Tip:

You can find Hospital Observation Services in the index under "Hospital Services." To save time, you can also just refer to the E&M section of the CPT manual and look for subsection "Hospital Observation Services."

Think Like A Coder 5.6

1. Initial observation for a 12-year-old male who was hit with a baseball bat during a little league baseball game. Information gathered by family members was that the boy was hit directly in the forehead, at full contact, and began to get up, stagger, and pass out. The patient has no history of other head injuries and is negative for neurological deficits. The patient was unconscious for about 5 minutes and was brought to consciousness by smelling salts. Examination revealed: Vital signs unstable: T (temperature) 98.8, P (pulse) thready at 98, B/P (blood pressure) 80/48, R (respiration) 12. HEENT (head, ears, eyes, nose and throat): Normocephalic. Pupils: Unequal. Neck: Supple without **adenopathy.** Throat: Clear. Chest: Clear to P&A. Heart: Tachycardia noted. Back: Unremarkable. Extremities: No deformities noted. Physician admitted the patient for 24 hours of observation for concussion and to rule out subdural hematoma. The medical decision making was of moderate complexity.

   ☐ 99219
   ☐ 99217
   ☐ 99220
   ☐ 99218

2. In the coding scenario in question 1, if the history was comprehensive in nature, what E&M code would you now assign?

   ☐ 99220
   ☐ 99263
   ☐ 99219
   ☐ 99218

Hospital Inpatient Services

Hospital inpatient services codes are used to report E&M services provided to individuals who are admitted to the hospital. Hospital inpatient services include those services provided to patients in a partial hospital setting. There are two categories to this subsection of the E&M section: Initial Hospital Care and Subsequent Hospital Care, which includes Observation or Inpatient Care Services and Hospital Discharge Services.

Coding Alert!

E&M Services on the same date provided at sites that are related to the admission "observation status" should NOT be reported separately.

Think Like A Coder 5.7

For patients admitted to initial observation or initial hospital care and discharged on a different date, what range of codes should be used?

☐ 99234-99236 and 99221-99223
☐ 99218-99220 and 99221-99223
☐ 99218-99220 and 99231-99233

Indexing Tip:

All consultations in the E&M section can be found in the index under "Consultation."

Consultations

Consultation is defined as a type of service provided by a physician whose opinion or advice regarding evaluation and/or management of a specific problem is requested by another physician or other appropriate source. A physician consultant may initiate diagnostic and/or therapeutic services at the same or subsequent visit. The written or verbal request for a consult may be made by a physician or other appropriate source and documented in the patient's medical record. The consultant's opinion and any services that were ordered or performed must also be documented in the patient's medical record and communicated by written report to the requesting physician or other appropriate source.

Coding Alert!

Consultations

When you are coding any type of consultation with the exception of "Confirmatory Consultations," the element of time is always indicated. The element of time makes coding assignment easier and quicker.

A consultation initiated by a patient and/or family and not requested by a physician is not reported using the initial consultation codes but may be reported using the codes for confirmatory consultation or office visits, as appropriate. If a confirmatory consultant is required by a third-party payer, modifier 32 should also be reported. Any specifically identifiable procedure performed on or subsequent to the date of the initial consultation should be reported separately. If subsequent to the completion of a consultation, the consultant assumes responsibility for management of a portion or all of the patient's condition(s), the follow-up consultation codes should not be used. In the hospital setting, the consulting physician should use the appropriate inpatient hospital consultation code for the initial encounter and then the subsequent hospital care codes. In the office setting, the appropriate established patient code should be used.

There are four subcategories in the Consultation section of the CPT manual: Office, Initial Inpatient, Follow-up Inpatient, and Confirmatory Consultations. Make sure to read all of the subcategory reporting instructions before assigning a code.

 Think Like A Coder 5.8

Follow-up inpatient consultation for an 83-year-old female in a skilled nursing facility. Patient presents with a history of hypertension, myocardial infarction, and diabetes. Her symptoms have **exacerbated** over the last 24 hours, and she now has fever and chills, with a gangrenous elbow ulcer; rhonchi; and dyspnea and appears lethargic and tachypneic. Physician performs a comprehensive history and a comprehensive examination and spends approximately 90 minutes on the unit.

- ❑ 99255
- ❑ 99245
- ❑ 99327
- ❑ 99254

Emergency Department Services

Emergency department service codes are used to report E&M services provided in the emergency department of a hospital. Remember, no distinction is made between new and established patients in the emergency department. An emergency department is defined as an organized hospital-based facility for the provision of unscheduled episodic services to patients who present for immediate medical care. The facility must be available 24 hours a day.

 Indexing Tip:

When looking for Emergency Department Services in the index, it will refer you to "Critical Care." Make sure you read the emergency department notes in each category for accurate coding.

Note: There is a difference between "Critical Care" and "Intensive Care."

Critical Care Services

Critical care is the direct delivery by a physician of medical care for a critically ill or critically injured patient. A critical illness or injury acutely impairs one or more vital organ systems such that there is a high probability of imminent or life-threatening deterioration in the patient's condition. Critical care involves high-complexity decision making to assess, manipulate, and support vital system functions; to treat single or multiple vital organ system failure; and/or to prevent further life-threatening deterioration of the patient's condition. Critical care may be provided on multiple days, even if no changes are made in the treatment rendered to the patient, provided that the patient's condition continues to require the level care described previously. Time is the essential element when assigning these codes.

Inpatient critical care services provided to infants 29 days through 24 months of age are reported with pediatric critical care codes. The pediatric critical care codes are reported as long as the infant or young child is younger than 24 months of age and qualifies for critical care services during the hospital stay. Inpatient critical care services provided to **neonates,** 28 days of age or less, are reported with the neonatal critical care codes. The reporting of pediatric and neonatal critical care services is not based on time or the type of unit and is not dependent upon the type of provider delivering the care. To report critical care services provided in the outpatient setting for neonates and pediatric patients up through 24 months of age, see the hourly Critical Care codes. For any given period of time spent providing critical care services, the physician must devote his or her full attention to the patient and cannot provide services to any other patient during the same period of time.

Time spent with the individual patient should be recorded in the patient's record. The time that can be reported as critical care is the time spent engaged in work directly related to the individual's patients' care whether that time was spent at the immediate bedside or elsewhere on the floor or unit. Time spent in activities that occur outside of the unit or off the floor—for example, telephone calls—may not be reported as critical care since the physician is not immediately available to the patient.

Code 99291 is used to report the first 30 to 74 minutes of critical care on a given date. It should be used only once per date even if the time spent by the physician is not continuous on that date. Critical care of less than 30 minutes total duration on a given date should be reported with the appropriate E&M code. Code 99292 is used to report additional block(s) of time, up to 30 minutes each beyond the first 74 minutes.

Think Like A Coder 5.9

A 15-year-old male presents in critical condition. He is in a comatose state after a drinking and driving accident and is admitted to critical care unit for 2 hours and 45 minutes.

❑ 99291, 99292 × 3

❑ 99291, 99292 × 4

❑ 99291, 99292 × 2

❑ No code from this section should be used.

Inpatient Neonatal and Pediatric Critical Care Intensive Services

Codes 99293-99296 are used to report services provided by a physician directing the inpatient care of a critically ill neonate/infant. The initial-day neonatal critical care code (99295) can be used in addition to codes 99360, 99436, or 99440 as appropriate; when the physician is present for the delivery, 99360 or 00436; and when newborn resuscitation, 99440, is required.

Codes 99295 and 99296 are used to report services provided by a physician directing the inpatient care of a critically ill neonate through the first 28 days of life. They represent care starting with the date of admission, 99295, and subsequent day(s), 99296, and may be reported only once per day, per patient. Codes 99293 and 99294 are used to report services provided by a physician directing the inpatient care of a critically ill infant or young child from 29 days of postnatal age through 24 months of age.

When a neonate or infant is not critically ill but requires intensive observation, frequent interventions, and other intensive care services, the following codes should be used. The Continuing Intensive Care Services codes 99298- 99300 should be used to report services for those neonates/infants with present body weight of 5000 grams or less. When the present body weight of the neonate/infants exceeds 5000 grams, the Subsequent Hospital Care Services codes 99231-99233 should be used.

To report critical care services provided in the outpatient setting for neonates and pediatric patients 24 months of age or younger, use the hourly Critical Care Codes 99291 and 99292. If the same physician provides critical care services for a neonatal or pediatric patient in both the outpatient and inpatient settings on the same day, report

Indexing Tip:

You may index Pediatric Critical Care by either "Pediatric Critical Care," or "Critical Care, Pediatrics."

only the appropriate Neonatal or Pediatric Critical Care code, 99293-99296, for all critical care services provided on that day.

Nursing Facility Services

Nursing facility services codes are used to report E&M services to patients in nursing facilities, formerly known as skilled nursing facilities, intermediate care facilities, or long-term care facilities. These codes should also be used to report E&M services provided to a patient in a psychiatric residential treatment center. If procedures such as medical psychotherapy are provided in addition to E&M services, these should be reported in addition to the E&M services. Two subcategories of nursing facilities are recognized: Initial Nursing Facility Care and Subsequent Nursing Facility Care. Both subcategories apply to new or established patients.

Domiciliary, Rest Home, or Custodial Care Services codes are used to report E&M services in a facility that provides room, board, and other personal assistance services, generally on a long-term basis. They also are used to report E&M services in an assisted living facility. The facility's services do not include a medical component.

Indexing Tip:

You can index nursing facilities by using the term "Domiciliary Services," or "Nursing Facility Services." If you index "Rest Home," you will be directed to "Domiciliary Services."

Coding Alert!

Nursing Facility Services

Nursing facilities were formerly referred to as skilled nursing facilities, intermediate care facilities, or long-term care facilities.

Think Like A Coder 5.10

The coordination of care is performed on a 72-year-old male resident of a rest home. The patient, an insulin-dependent diabetic amputee with hearing and visual impairments and possible **dementia** is currently experiencing respiratory problems. The physician performs a detailed history and examination, and the medical decision making is of high complexity.

❑ 99310

❑ 99328

❑ 99232

❑ 99343

Indexing Tip:

To index home services, look in the index under "Home Services." "House Call" and "Home Visit" are the same services with the same E&M codes and fall under Home Services.

Home Services, Prolonged Services

Home service codes are used to report E&M services provided in a private residence. On your coding examination, do not confuse this subcategory with Nursing Facility Services. These codes are broken down into two categories: new and established patient.

Prolonged service codes are used when a physician provides prolonged service involving direct, face-to-face patient contact that is beyond the usual service in either the inpatient or outpatient setting. This service is reported in addition to other physician services, including E&M services at any level. Appropriate codes should be selected for supplies provided or procedures performed in the care of the patient during this period.

Coding Alert!

Home Services

For quick and accurate coding assignment, remember that all Home Services codes include a time element in the descriptor of the code.

Case Management Services, Care Plan Oversight Services

Case management services are services provided by a physician who is responsible for direct care of a patient and for coordinating and controlling access to or initiating and/or supervising other health care services needed by patient.

Care plan oversight services are reported separately from codes for office/outpatient, hospital, home, nursing facility, or domiciliary services or non–face-to-face services. Care plan oversight services differ from case management services in that a physician must be responsible for the direct care of the patient when using codes under Case Management Services. When using codes for Care Plan Oversight Services, the physician is acting in a predominantly supervisory role, or indirect care, during a 30-day period with the patient. The complexity and approximate physician time of the care plan oversight services provided within a 30-day period determine code selection. Only one physician may report services for a given period of time, to reflect that physician's sole or predominant supervisory role with a particular patient. These codes should not be reported for

supervision of patients in nursing facilities or under the care of home health agencies unless they require recurrent supervision of therapy.

Indexing Tip:

To find case management codes, index "Case Management." For Care Plan Oversight Services, the index refers you to "Physician Services."

Think Like A Coder 5.11

A medical team conference was held for 60 minutes face-to-face for the care plan and coordination for a 6-year-old refugee from Taiwan with multiple heart defects, cerebral palsy, and juvenile diabetes with signs of retinal neuropathy.

- ❑ 99354, 99355
- ❑ 99367
- ❑ 99374
- ❑ 99366

Preventive Medicine Services and Newborn Care

Preventive medicine services codes are codes used to report the preventive medicine E&M of infants, children, adolescents, and adults. The extent and focus of the services will largely depend on the age of the patient. If an abnormality is encountered or a preexisting problem is addressed in the process of performing this preventive medicine E&M service, and if the problem or abnormality is significant enough to require additional work to perform the key components of a problem-oriented E&M service, then the appropriate Office/Outpatient code 99201-99215 should also be reported. The comprehensive nature of the preventive medicine service codes 99381-99397 reflects an age- and gender-appropriate history/exam and is not synonymous with the comprehensive examination required in E&M codes 99201-99350.

Newborn care codes are used to report services provided to newborns in several different settings. For newborn hospital discharge services provided on a date subsequent to the admission date of the newborn, use 00238. For discharge services provided to newborns admitted and discharged on the same date, use code 99435.

Indexing Tip:

To find Preventive Medicine Services in the index simply look under "Preventive Medicine."

Coding Alert!

Preventive Medicine Services

Immunizations and ancillary studies involving laboratory or radiology procedures, other procedures, or screening tests identified with a specific CPT code are reported separately.

Indexing Tip:

If you feel familiar enough with the E&M section of the CPT manual, try not to use the index while coding the following problems. Try to quickly find the subsections, categories, and subcategories in the E&M section of the manual and choose the appropriate coding assignment.

 Think Like A Coder 5.12

Physician provided individual counseling/intervention for a 19-year-old male who has a history of opioid addiction, alcohol abuse, and promiscuous sexual activity. Time spent with patient was 45 minutes.

- ☐ 99411, 99412
- ☐ 99401, 99403
- ☐ 99403
- ☐ 99395

Select the most appropriate code assignment for each coding scenario. (Please see Appendix A for answers and rationale.)

1. Inpatient admission of a 27-year-old female who delivered a male infant weighing 10 lb., 9 oz. four days earlier. Patient presented with a third-degree perineal laceration that was subsequently repaired. The physician performed an expanded problem-focused history of the mother's delivery and a problem-focused examination. The physician indicated that the baby was "large for dates," causing the perineal laceration.
   A. ❐ 99252
   B. ❐ 99232
   C. ❐ 99231
   D. ❐ 99282

2. A 57-year-old established female patient presented at an immediate care facility with complaints of vaginal itching × 2 days. The physician performed an expanded problem-focused history and examination. No diagnosis was reached, and the patient was provided with a prescription. Later that evening, the patient presented again at the immediate care facility for a possible sprained wrist while playing racquet ball. The sprain did not require casting or strapping. The history and examination performed were problem focused, and the medical decision making was straightforward.
   A. ❐ 99213, 99212
   B. ❐ 99213, 99212–25
   C. ❐ 99202, 99212
   D. ❐ 99202, 99213

3. A 32-year-old male patient presented with symptoms of prostatitis, and his family physician referred him to a urologist. The urologist performed a detailed history and examination for this new patient during this consultation. The urologist prescribed medication, a kidneys, ureter, and bladder follow-up visit in 10 days.
   A. ❐ 99203
   B. ❐ 99241
   C. ❐ 99202
   D. ❐ 99253

4. What code would be assigned for the physician direction of emergency medical systems emergency care via helicopter transport for advanced life support for a critically injured 8-month-old male infant? Time spent face to face during the transport included 90 minutes.
   A. ❐ 99288
   B. ❐ 99293
   C. ❐ 99294
   D. ❐ 99291, 99292

5. A 43-year-old female was seen in the emergency department for jitteriness and severe anxiety experienced as a result of an accidental overdose of Solumedrol that had been prescribed for her asthma, which is currently under control. Impression: Accidental overdose of Solumedrol because of acute asthma attack. The presenting problems were of low to moderate severity in nature.
   A. ❐ 99282
   B. ❐ 99283
   C. ❐ 99251
   D. ❐ 99341

6. What modifier would be used to identify a significant, separately identifiable E&M service by the same physician on the same day of the procedure or other service?
   A. ❐ -21
   B. ❐ -24
   C. ❐ -25
   D. ❐ -51

7. A 48-year-old male established patient is seen in the office for complaints of left-upper quadrant pain × 2 months. History of present illness: Recently, the pain has exacerbated and the patient can no longer work as a result. The patient describes the pain as severe, recurring, and sharp. The patient had a sonogram × 4 months ago that was positive for gallstones. No fever or chills are present, and the patient has no history of jaundice, dark urine or dark-colored stool. Past history: Surgeries: Appendectomy and T&A; exercise-induced asthma periodically. Social history: Patient denies using tobacco and drinks alcohol occasionally; married with two grown children. Family history: Mother and father still living and in good health; only child. Review of systems: Negative. Physical examination: Physical examination reveals a normal healthy male in physical distress because of severe pain in left-upper quadrant. HEENT: Normocephalic and atraumatic. Rectal: Guaiac is negative with no masses. Abdomen: Soft and slightly tender to palpation in the left upper quadrant. Plan: Patient to be admitted to the hospital for further evaluation for possible cholecystectomy.
   A. ❐ 99203
   B. ❐ 99213
   C. ❐ 99214
   D. ❐ 99214–25

8. Physician performed a well-baby physical examination on a well-developed, healthy 9-month-old male new patient. The examination included the ordering of appropriate immunizations, nutritional guidance for the baby to the mother, history of the infant, and complete physical examination.
   A. ❐ 99391
   B. ❐ 99381
   C. ❐ 99382
   D. ❐ 99392

9. A physician performs a home visit on an 83-year-old female established patient who is homebound. The patient has hypopituitarism secondary to radiation therapy for

brain tumor 15 months ago. Physician notes protein-calorie malnutrition. History of present illness: Patient says she was feeling fine up until 2 days ago when she became confused and disoriented. Physical examination: Patient is a pleasant 83-year-old female who currently resides by herself. Vital signs: T 98.8, P 66, B/P 112/72, R 22. HEENT: Normocephalic and PERLA. Neck: Supple with good range of motion. Chest: Revealed few crackling rales bilaterally. Heart: PMI not felt. Extremities: Good range of motion. Abdomen: No organomegaly and was soft with no masses. Neurological: Revealed confusion, not oriented. Physician spends 40 minutes face to face with patient. Plan: Patient to be admitted to hospital for observation and CAT scan.

A. ❐ 99343

B. ❐ 99318

C. ❐ 99349

D. ❐ 99325

10. What code would be assigned to a history and examination of a newborn infant who was delivered in the hospital just 30 minutes earlier?

A. ❐ 99432

B. ❐ 99431

C. ❐ 99381

D. ❐ 99391

11. A patient is seen for complaints of shortness of breath and productive cough. The physician orders an injection of penicillin. The patient goes into anaphylactic shock with acute respiratory failure. Cardiopulmonary resuscitation is administered, and the patient is transported by ambulance to emergency services. The physician at the receiving hospital provides two-way voice communication with the ambulance personnel while en route to the hospital. The patient is admitted to the critical care unit and is monitored for 3 hours before release. Code the emergency services and critical care services.

A. ❐ 99291, 99292 × 2

B. ❐ 99285, 99292 × 4

C. ❐ 99289, 99290 × 4

D. ❐ 99284, 99291, 99292 × 4

12. Physician performs a rest home visit for a 72-year-old established male patient in a long-term nursing facility because of the increased creatinine levels diagnosed during a routine postoperative visit. The patient is 6 months post kidney transplant. A biopsy was ordered and performed which revealed chronic rejection syndrome. The patient is responding inadequately to the transplant and has developed a complication that with medication would be considered minor.

A. ❐ 99324

B. ❐ 99334

C. ❐ 99304

D. ❐ 99342

13. Critical care services were provided to a 5-day-old female infant whose blanket caught on fire after mother fell asleep while smoking a cigarette. The infant suffered first- and second-degree burns of all extremities and back and required respiratory support. She was placed in neonatal critical care for 6 days before being moved to intensive care.

A. ❐ 99296 × 5

B. ❐ 99293 − 21

C. ❐ 99295 × 5

D. ❐ 99298 × 5

14. What code would be assigned to a service provided by a physician standing by during a high-risk multiple birth delivery that lasted 70 minutes?

A. ❐ 99358, 99359

B. ❐ 99360 × 2

C. ❐ 99358, 99359 × 2

D. ❐ 99355

15. Individual counseling was performed for a 58-year-old male who was drinking heavily when he slipped on the floor and dislocated his shoulder. He is a known chronic alcoholic with cirrhosis of the liver and hepatitis D. Preventive medicine counseling was provided to him regarding his alcohol abuse, and options and prognosis if he continued to drink heavily were discussed. Total encounter was 60 minutes in length.

A. ❐ 99412

B. ❐ 99401, 99404

C. ❐ 99368

D. ❐ 99404

16. Date of admission: November 13, 2007. Date of Discharge: November 18, 2007. Admitting diagnosis: Pneumonia, hypertension, history of congestive heart failure, cervical carcinoma insitu. Brief history: A 54-year-old female with a complaint of chest tightness and severe pain who was seen at Immediate Care was found to have bilateral pneumonia, hypertension, and hypoxemia. The patient was subsequently transferred to a local hospital for admission. Hospital course: The patient was admitted and placed on antibiotics and oxygen supplement. The patient improved, showing gradual resolution of hypoxemia. The patient was discharged in stable condition. Prognosis: Good. Discharged on medications for pneumonia and hypertension. The patient was to follow up with family physician in 1 week. The discharge encounter last 40 minutes.

A. ❐ 99235

B. ❐ 99239

C. ❐ 99217

D. ❐ 99238, 99239

17. A 38-year-old male was placed on hospital observation for complaints of insomnia, weakness, and shortness of breath × 2 days. Physical examination revealed B/P 144/80,

P 102 and regular. Neck: Distention and 45-degree elevation, rales at both lung bases. Cardiac examination revealed an enlarged heart with PMI pacemaker implantation felt at the midclavicular line. Systolic murmur was noted. Assessment: Calcified aortic stenosis, congestive heart failure. Plan: Admit for treatment of sodium restriction and diuretic. The presenting problems were of high severity.

A. ❏ 99233

B. ❏ 99236

C. ❏ 99223

D. ❏ 99236–25

18. What code would be assigned to a very-low-birthweight 27-day-old male infant whose weight was 1400 grams during a subsequent intensive care stay of 2 days?

A. ❏ 99298 × 2

B. ❏ 99295 × 2

C. ❏ 99296 × 2

D. ❏ 99293 × 2

19. Modifier -24 is assigned for:

A. ❏ Prolonged E&M services

B. ❏ Significant, separately identifiable E&M service by the same physician on the same day of the procedure of other service.

C. ❏ Unrelated E&M service by the same physician during a postoperative period.

D. ❏ Multiple services

20. What code would be assigned to a care plan oversight service performed by a physician in 45 minutes?

A. ❏ 99358

B. ❏ 99375

C. ❏ 99326

D. ❏ 99380

21. What code would be assigned to anticoagulant management for an outpatient taking warfarin for 180 days with physician review and interpretation of INR (international normalized ratios) testing?

A. ❏ 99450

B. ❏ 99363, 99364

C. ❏ 99444

D. ❏ 99363, 99364 × 2

22. The E&M of a 94-year-old patient admitted to nursing care facility is performed after a hospital admission for evaluation of abdominal distention and left lower abdominal pain. Physician performs a detailed interval history. History of present illness: The patient has a 24-hour history of increasing abdominal tenderness and distention with loose bowel movements in the colostomy bag; she is status post a diverting transverse colostomy in December of 2004 for sigmoid phlegmon, secondary to tic disease. Past medical history: Past history reveals Parkinson's syndrome, congestive heart failure, prior

left hip fracture, Alzheimer's mixed type, colostomy, and chronic obstructive pulmonary disease.

Social history: Patient lives alone at home with home health aid, and denies tobacco and alcohol use. Patient is ambulatory with the aid of a walker; however, her ability to ambulate has been more difficult lately. Physical examination: Patient is an elderly 94 year-old female who, at present, is ambulatory with some difficulty. Vital signs: T 101.2, P 62, B/P 98/62, R 12. HEENT: Unremarkable. Anicteric. Poor respiratory excursion without rales or wheezes. Heart: S1, S2. Abdomen: Softly distended with minimal diffuse tenderness without guarding or rigidity. Bowel sounds present. Rectal: Brown liquid stool. Extremities: Negative. Abdominal x-ray shows no air fluids and no free air under the diaphragm. Neurological: No deficits noted. Chest: Clear to P&A.

Plan: Patient can no longer live at home during this current illness. IV antibiotic therapy is administered. Occupational therapy will be discussed. Medical decision making is of moderate complexity.

A. ❏ 99309

B. ❏ 99301

C. ❏ 99313

D. ❏ 99303

23. A 30-year-old female patient gave birth to a 6 lb., 4 oz. male infant with apgars of 8 and 10. The pediatrician in attendance, who was requested by delivering physician, performed the initial stabilization of the newborn and preliminary physical examination.

A. ❏ 99435

B. ❏ 99433

C. ❏ 99436

D. ❏ 99295

24. A 38-year-old male was placed on hospital observation for complaints of insomnia, weakness, and shortness of breath × 2 days. Physical examination revealed B/P 144/80, P 102 and regular. Neck: Distention and 45-degree elevation, rales at both lung bases. Cardiac examination revealed an enlarged heart with PMI felt at the midclavicular line. Systolic murmur was noted. Assessment: Calcified aortic stenosis, congestive heart failure. Plan: Admit for treatment of sodium restriction and diruretic. The presenting problems were of high severity.

A. ❏ 99233

B. ❏ 99236

C. ❏ 99223

D. ❏ 99236–25

25. Date of admission: November 13, 2007. Date of Discharge: November 18, 2007. Admitting diagnosis: Pneumonia, hypertension, history of congestive heart failure, cervical carcinoma in situ. Brief history: A 54-year-old female with a complaint of chest tightness and severe pain was

seen at local Prompt Care and found to have bilateral pneumonia, hypertension, and hypoxemia. The patient was subsequently transferred to a local hospital for admission. Hospital course: The patient was admitted and placed on antibiotics and oxygen supplement. The patient improved, showing gradual resolution of hypoxemia. The patient was discharged in stable condition. Prognosis: Good. Discharged on medications for pneumonia and hypertension. The patient was to follow up with family physician in 1 week. The discharge encounter last 40 minutes.

A. ❑ 99235
B. ❑ 99239
C. ❑ 99217
D. ❑ 99238, 99239

CHAPTER 6

Anesthesia Review

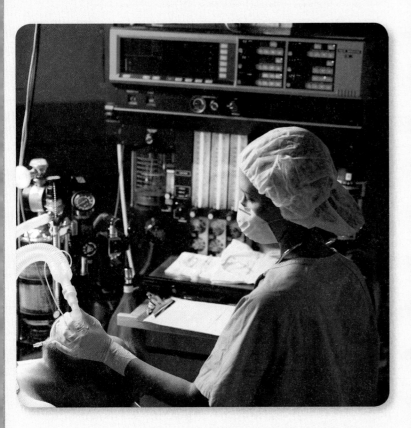

From the Author...

"The Anesthesia section of the CPT manual is the smallest section of the manual and fairly easy to code from. By indexing the term "anesthesia" and searching for the anatomical site, you can usually find an anesthesia code with a fair amount of ease. However, when you are presented with coding anesthesia for a procedure that you are unfamiliar with, knowing anatomy, physiology, and medical terminology comes in handy. After reading the procedure, you will have to decide the anatomical site where the procedure is taking place on the basis of the context of the material. Once you have decided on the anatomical site, finding the code is relatively quick and accurate."

Key terms

Intravenous
Iridectomy
Laminectomy
Moribund
Thoracotomy

Learning Objectives

- The student will review all of the standards, guidelines, subsections, subheadings, and descriptors in the Anesthesia section of the CPT manual so that he or she can assign codes accurately and with ease.

- The student will review and apply all of the Physical Status Modifiers as appropriate.

- The student will review and apply Qualifying Circumstances as appropriate.

- The student will review and understand the importance of Time Reporting.

Services that involve the administration of anesthesia are reported by the use of CPT codes 00100-01999 and by the use of modifiers. They are reported only by the anesthesiologist who is administering the anesthesia, meaning only the anesthesiologist performing the act of administering anesthesia can request payment for this procedure, and only if that anesthesiologist is not performing the surgery. Anesthesia codes are assigned on the basis of the body site being operated on and are not based on the type of anesthesia administered. The reporting of anesthesia services is appropriate by or under the responsible supervision of an anesthesiologist, meaning that if the anesthesiologist does not administer the anesthesia and a nurse anesthetist does, payment can be requested for this procedure by using a nurse anesthetist who was supervised by an anesthesiologist. These services may include but are not limited to general anesthesia, regional anesthesia, and supplementation of local anesthesia. These services include the usual preoperative and postoperative visits, the anesthesia care during the procedure, the administration of fluids and/or blood, and the usual monitoring services. Unusual forms of monitoring such as intra-arterial, central venous, and Swan-Ganz are not included.

To report moderate conscious sedation provided by an anesthesiologist also performing the service for which the sedation is being provided, see codes 99143-99145. To report regional or general anesthesia provided by an anesthesiologist also performing the services for which the anesthesia is being provided, see modifier -47 in Appendix A.

Indexing Tip:

Remember all anesthesia codes begin with the numeral "0".

Time Reporting

Remember that time for anesthesia procedures may be reported as is customary in the local area. Anesthesia time begins when the anesthesiologist begins to prepare the patient for the induction of anesthesia in the operating room or in an equivalent area and ends when the anesthesiologist is no longer in personal attendance or when the patient may be safely placed under postoperative supervision.

Physician's Services and Materials Supplied by Physician

Physician's services rendered in the office, home, or hospital; consultation; and other medical services are listed in the Evaluation and Management section of the CPT manual. Supplies and materials provided by the physician over and above those usually included with the office visit or other services rendered may be listed separately. List drugs, tray supplies, and materials provided, and identify with code 99070.

Special Report

A service that is rarely provided, unusual, variable, or new may require a special report in order to determine medical appropriateness of the service. Pertinent information should include an adequate definition or description of the nature, extent, and need for the procedure and the time, effort, and equipment necessary to provide the service. Additional items which may be included are:

- Complexity of symptoms
- Final diagnosis
- Pertinent physical findings
- Diagnostic and therapeutic procedures
- Concurrent problems
- Follow-up care

Think Like A Coder 6.1

An anesthesiologist administers anesthesia in a hospital setting to a patient who is extremely anxious when undergoing a dental procedure. This dental procedure is usually performed with the administration of a local anesthetic provided by a dentist in the office.

A Special Report would need to be filed because of the unusual circumstances surrounding the administration of anesthesia. Occasionally, a procedure which usually requires either no anesthesia or local anesthesia, because of unusual circumstances must be done under general anesthesia. This circumstance may be reported by adding modifier -23 to the procedure code of the basic service

Anesthesia Modifiers

Modifiers frequently used in conjunction with anesthesia codes (00100-01999) are:

Increased Procedural Services: When the work required to provide a service is substantially greater than typically required, it may be identified by adding the modifier -22 to the usual procedure code. Documentation must support the substantial additional work and the reason for the additional work.

Unusual Anesthesia: Occasionally, a procedure, which usually requires either no anesthesia or local anesthesia, because of unusual circumstances must be performed under general anesthesia. This circumstance may be reported by adding modifier -23 to the procedure code of the basic service.

Anesthesia by Surgeon: Regional or general anesthesia provided by the surgeon may be reported by adding modifier -47 to the basic service. This does not include local anesthesia.

Indexing Tip:

When indexing an anesthesia coding problem, remember to always look up the word "anesthesia" in the index and search by procedure or body part.

Example: Hip Replacement

Index: Anesthesia, Replacement, Hip code(s) 01212-01215

Think Like A Coder 6.2

An anesthesiologist administers general anesthesia to a 52-year-old male and performs a cervical **laminectomy** with decompression of the spinal cord involving two segments.

Code: 63015, 00604, –47

Think Like A Coder 6.3

A 58-year-old male who was not expected to live without the procedure underwent a repair for an atrial septal defect with cardiopulmonary bypass.

- ❏ P1
- ❏ P3
- ❏ P5
- ❏ P6

Physical Status Modifiers

A physical status modifier in the Anesthesia section is used to indicate a patient's condition at the time of service when anesthesia is administered. The physical status modifier also identifies the complexity of the anesthesia administered based on physical symptoms of the patient. Table 6.1 outlines the physical status modifiers and their alphanumerical codes.

The levels of these modifiers are consistent with the American Society of Anesthesiologists ranking of patient physical status. Physical status is included in the CPT manual to distinguish among various levels of complexity of the anesthesia service provided.

Qualifying Circumstances

Qualifying circumstance codes are used only when anesthesia is provided under difficult circumstances because of the patient's condition, unusual risk factors, or operative conditions. More than one qualifying circumstance can be assigned. Remember the following when assigning qualifying circumstance codes:

- They are never reported alone.
- These codes can be found in the Medicine section of the CPT manual.
- More than one code can be used.
- The codes are sequenced after the anesthesia code.

Table 6.2 is a list of the qualifying circumstance codes.

Table 6.1 Physical Status Modifiers

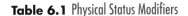

Physical Status Modifier	Definition
P1	Normal healthy patient
P2	Patient with mild systemic disease
P3	Patient with severe systemic disease
P4	Patient with severe systemic disease that is a constant threat to life
P5	**Moribund** patient who is not expected to survive without the operation
P6	Patient who has been declared brain dead and whose organs are being removed for donor purposes

Table 6.2 Qualifying Circumstance Codes

Qualifying Circumstance Code	Description
99100	Anesihesia for patient of extreme age, under 1 year and over 70 years
99116	Anesthesia complicated by use of total body hypothermia
99135	Anesthesia complicated by use of controlled hypotension
99140	Anesthesia complicated by emergency conditions

💡 Think Like A Coder 6.4

Choose the correct Qualifying Circumstance code for the problem below.

A 41-year-old female was prepped and underwent surgery for an acute onset of chest pain compatible with a pulmonary embolus. The patient's blood pressure was unusually low and was difficult to control during surgery.

- ☐ 99100
- ☐ 99116
- ☐ 99135
- ☐ 99140

Coding Alert!

Conscious Sedation

Conscious sedation is when a patient is in a minimally depressed state of consciousness during which the patient has the ability to maintain an airway and respond to physical or verbal commands. In the CPT manual conscious sedation is identified by the symbol "⊙", a darkened period with a circle around the perimeter, in front of the code. The following is an example:

Code 33010

⊙ 33010 Pericardiocentesis; initial

Types of Anesthesia

Anesthesia is referred to as a partial or complete loss of sensation, with or without the loss of consciousness. Table 6.3 outlines the types of anesthesia used in surgical practice.

How to Locate Anesthesia Codes

It is imperative to have a strong understanding of anatomy and physiology in order to code quickly and accurately in the anesthesia section of the CPT manual. The most efficient way to locate anesthesia codes is to index "Anesthesia"

Table 6.3 Types of Anesthesia

Anesthesia Type	Definition of Type
General anesthesia (see Figure 6.1)	Anesthesia that is complete and affects the entire body with loss of consciousness when the anesthetic agent acts on the brain. This type of anesthesia is usually administered by inhalation or **intravenous** method.
Local anesthesia	Anesthesia that affects a local area only, acting upon nerves or nerve tracts. Local anesthesia is administered by the placement of a needle in the skin and injecting an anesthetic agent.
Regional anesthesia	Anesthesia that is a nerve or field blocking, causing insensibility over a particular area of the body.

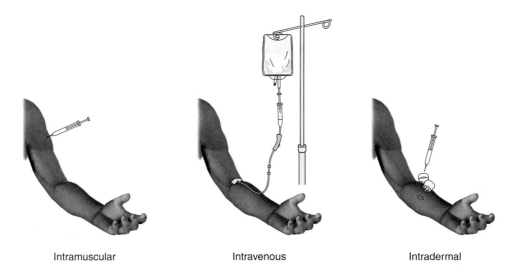

Intramuscular   Intravenous   Intradermal

Figure 6.1

Anesthesia Administration – General anesthesia is typically administered through intravenous infusion. Local anesthetics can be administered by an intradermal or intramuscular injection.

From N. Thierer and L. Breitbard, *Medial Terminology, Language for He\alth Care,* 2e. Copyright © 2006 The McGraw-Hill Companies, Inc. Reprinted with permission.

as your usual practice. When you locate "Anesthesia" in the index, you will notice the indentations are composed of procedures and body parts listed in alphabetical order. To find the anesthesia code for **iridectomy,** you will find the "i's" under "Anesthesia" and search through them (code 00147). To find the body part tibia you will find the "t's" under "Anesthesia" and search through them (codes 01390-01392, 01484).

At times you may not find the anesthesia code by procedure or by body part. If you cannot locate the anesthesia code under "Anesthesia" by procedure or body part, go directly to the Anesthesia section and page through until you find the correct subsection and then locate your code. This method of locating codes is not recommended for all sections of the CPT manual; however, the Anesthesia section is very small and can be paged through quickly.

 Think Like A Coder 6.5

Locating Anesthesia Codes

By Procedure

Problem: Lumbar sympathectomy

Locate in index: Anesthesia > sympathectomy > lumbar > 00632

By Body Part

Problem: Needle biopsy of pleura

Locate in index: Anesthesia > Pleura > Needle biopsy > 00522

 Think Like A Coder 6.6

Locating Anesthesia Codes

By Procedure

Problem: Total thymectomy with transcervical approach

Locate in Index: Anesthesia > cannot find thymectomy or thymus

Go directly to Anesthesia section of the CPT manual.

Thymus is located in the mediastinum.

Begin to page through the Anesthesia section.

Find "Intrathoracic" > locate code 00540: Anesthesia for **thoracotomy** procedures involving lungs, pleura, diaphragm, and mediastinum; not otherwise specified.

APPLYING CODING THEORY TO PRACTICE

Choose the correct anesthesia coding assignment (code for anesthesia only). (Please see Appendix A for answers and rationale).

1. Anesthesiologist provided and monitored anesthesia for a complete adrenalectomy with excision of adjacent retroperitoneal tumor.
   A. ❏ 60545
   B. ❏ 00864
   C. ❏ 00866
   D. ❏ 60540

2. Anesthesiologist provided and monitored anesthesia for a heart-lung transplant with recipient cardiectomy-pneumonectomy for a patient who would not survive the day without the procedure.
   A. ❏ 33935
   B. ❏ 00580, P5
   C. ❏ 00560, P5
   D. ❏ 33935, 33940

3. Anesthesiologist provided and monitored anesthesia for a morbidly obese patient for the surgical placement of adjustable gastric band and subcutaneous port components.
   A. ❏ 00740
   B. ❏ 43770-52
   C. ❏ 43770-52, 43771
   D. ❏ 00797

4. Anesthesiologist provided and monitored anesthesia for a craniectomy for the evacuation of a subdural intracerebellar hematoma in a 76-year-old female.
   A. ❏ 00212, 99100
   B. ❏ 61312, 61313, 99100
   C. ❏ 61312, 99100
   D. ❏ 00210, 99100

5. Surgeon repaired a 6.3-cm complex wound on a 10-year-old boy's forehead after administering medication for conscious sedation because of the anxiety the patient was experiencing. The procedure lasted 25 minutes with a trained observer present.
   A. ❏ 13132, 13133, 99144
   B. ❏ 13132, 99144
   C. ❏ 00190
   D. ❏ 00210

6. Surgeon performed a cesarean section on a 26-year-old female while the anesthesiologist administered a regional anesthetic to the patient, who suffers from a mild systemic disease.
   A. ❏ 01962, P3
   B. ❏ 00880, P2
   C. ❏ 01961, P2
   D. ❏ 00940, P2

7. Surgeon performed the initial debridement and dressing of partial thickness burns over 2% of total body surface for a 74-year-old male patient.
   A. ❏ 16020
   B. ❏ 15922, 15610
   C. ❏ 16020, 01951
   D. ❏ 01951

8. Surgeon performed an arthoscopically aided treatment of a tuberosity fracture of the knee with manipulation on a 14-year-old male athlete.
   A. ❏ 29850, 29851
   B. ❏ 01400, 99100
   C. ❏ 01400, P2
   D. ❏ 01400

9. Anesthesiologist provided and monitored anesthesia for a left lobectomy in a 77-year-old female patient with lung cancer, severe COPD, and emphysema.
   A. ❏ 00540, P3, 99100
   B. ❏ 00546, 99100
   C. ❏ 00540, 00546, P3
   D. ❏ 00546, P3

10. Patient who suffers from severe anxiety underwent general anesthesia for the intermediate repair of a 5.4-cm wound on the left foot.
    A. ❏ 01462-26
    B. ❏ 12042-26
    C. ❏ 01462-23
    D. ❏ 12042, P2

11. Surgeon performed a bilateral vasectomy on a 34-year-old male.
    A. ❏ 00920
    B. ❏ 00800
    C. ❏ 00921
    D. ❏ 00865

12. The code for the daily hospital management of a continuous epidural for a 57-year-old cancer patient with intractable pain is:
    A. ❏ 01992
    B. ❏ 01991
    C. ❏ 01999
    D. ❏ 01996

13. ABSTRACT:

PATIENT: 63-year-old female

PREOPERATIVE DIAGNOSIS: Left breast cancer

OPERATION: Left simple mastectomy

ANESTHESIA: General endotracheal

PROCEDURE: Patient was placed on operating table in the supine position. General anesthesia was induced, and the patient was prepped and draped in the usual manner. A transverse incision was made around the left breast to the level of the anterior ancillary line. Skin flaps were raised with sharp dissection, and the breast was then taken off the pectoralis muscles and fascia. Hemostasis was achieved with 3-0 and 4-0 chromic sutures. Drains were placed beneath the skin flaps and were then anchored to the chest wall. The edges of the skin of the left breast were then approximated with 4-0 vicryl sutures. A sterile, dry dressing was placed. The patient tolerated the procedure well and was taken to the recovery room.

    A. ❑ 00404

    B. ❑ 00402

    C. ❑ 01610

    D. ❑ 00402, 99116

14. A 16-year-old female underwent surgery for brain biopsy in which burr holes were used along with ventriculography.

    A. ❑ 61140, 61150

    B. ❑ 00190

    C. ❑ 00214

    D. ❑ 61120

15. A 37-year-old female underwent a total laryngectomy with radical neck dissection.

    A. ❑ 00326

    B. ❑ 31360, 31365

    C. ❑ 31365

    D. ❑ 00320

CHAPTER 7

Surgery Review

Learning Objectives

- The student will review all of the standards, guidelines, subsections, subheadings, and descriptors in the Surgery section of the CPT manual so that he or she can assign codes accurately by the use of reinforcers.
- The student will review and apply all of the modifiers that are appropriate to this section.
- The student will review and apply the CPT Surgical Package definition while assigning codes.
- The student will review and utilize subsection information to create a more in-depth understanding of surgery coding assignments.
- The student will review the steps to assigning codes in the Surgery section.

From the Author...

"The Surgery section of the CPT is the largest section in the manual and is the heart of CPT. This is where your knowledge of anatomy and physiology and its accompanying body systems comes into play. The Surgery section is broken down into the body systems beginning with the integumentary system and ending with the auditory system. As with any section in the CPT manual, you must first become a pro at understanding the guidelines that precede the codes and their descriptors. In both coding examinations, you will be challenged with assigning codes for procedures in all of the subsections. The key to successful mastery of the Surgery section is to be very familiar with their distinct subsections and accompanying notes.

For example, the cardiovascular subsection contains 25 subsection notes that must be read and understood in order to assign codes appropriately. This is quite an undertaking! Read and re-read these notes as you practice your coding assignments, and your understanding of each subsection will increase, providing you a greater chance of success. Indexing plays an equally important role in your success when coding from all of the subsections in the Surgery section. Remember you can index in various ways to find a code: by body part, by condition, by main term, and by the use of synonyms and acronyms. Make sure you have memorized ALL modifiers to ensure accurate coding assignment. Practice combined with understanding and knowledge of each subsection will be the key to passing this portion your national certification."

Key terms

Adjuvant	Infiltration
Anastomosis	Lesion
Arthrodesis	Percutaneous Skeletal Fixation
Bifurcated	
Capsulotomy	Procurement
Cranioplasty	Sigmoidoscopy
Currettement	Subcutaneous
Hyperkeratotic	Urodynamics

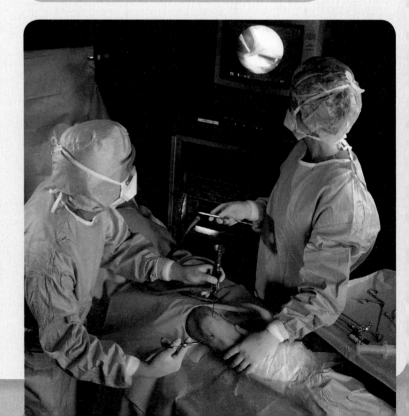

Surgery

The surgery section of the CPT manual is divided into the following subsections:

- Integumentary System
- Musculoskeletal System
- Respiratory System
- Cardiovascular System
- Digestive System
- Urinary System
- Male/Female Genital System
- Nervous System
- Ocular/Auditory System

Several of the subheadings and subsections have special needs or instructions unique to that section. It is imperative to remember to read all "Notes" carefully in order to assign codes and modifiers correctly.

CPT Surgical Package Definition

The services provided by the physician to any patient by their very nature are variable. The CPT codes that represent a readily identifiable surgical procedure therefore include a variety of procedures. The following services are always included in a given CPT code in addition to the operation performed:

- Local **infiltration,** metacarpal/metatarsal/digital block or topical anesthesia.

- Related E&M encounter on the date immediately before or on the date of procedure.
- Immediate postoperative care, including dictating operative notes and talking with the family and other physicians.
- Writing orders.
- Evaluating the patient in the postanesthesia recovery area.
- Typical postoperative follow-up care.

Coding Alert!

Reading "Notes" in the subsection information can make the difference between assigning the right and wrong code and getting a correct answer on your coding examination!

Commonly Used Modifiers in the Surgery Section

Modifiers are designed to give Medicare and commercial payers the additional information needed to process and adjudicate a claim. A modifier is the way a physician or medical facility can indicate that the service has been altered by a special circumstance. The following modifiers are commonly used in conjunction with CPT codes found in the surgery section. (see Table 7.1).

Table 7.1 Modifiers Commonly Used in the Surgery Section

Modifier	Description of Modifier Use
-22 Increased Procedural Services	When the work required to provide a service is substantially greater than typically required, it may be identified by adding the modifier -22 to the usual procedure code. Documentation must support the substantial additional work and the reason for the additional work.
-32 Mandated Services	Services related to mandated consultation and/or related services (PPO – Preferred Provider Organization – third-party payer) may be identified by adding modifier -32 to the basic procedure code.
-47 Anesthesia by Surgeon	Regional or general anesthesia provided by the surgeon may be reported by adding modifier -47 to the basic service.
-50 Bilateral Procedure	Unless otherwise identified in the listing, bilateral procedures that are performed at the same operative session should be identified by adding modifier -50 to the appropriate five-digit code.

(continued)

Table 7.1 Continued

Modifier	Description of Modifier Use
-51 Multiple Procedures	When multiple procedures, other than E&M services, physical medicine and rehabilitation services, or provision of supplies are performed at the same session by the same provider, the primary procedure or service may be reported as listed. The additional procedure(s) or service(s) may be identified by appending -51 modifier to the primary procedure or service code(s).
-52 Reduced Services	Under certain circumstances, a service or procedure is partially reduced or eliminated at the physician's discretion. Under these circumstances, the service provided can be identified by its usual procedure number and the addition of modifier -52, signifying that the service is reduced. This provides means of reporting reduced services without disturbing the identification of the basic service.
-53 Discontinued Procedure	Under certain circumstances, the physician may elect to terminate a surgical or diagnostic procedure because extenuating circumstances or those that threaten the well-being of a patient. Under these circumstances, the modifier -53 indicates that a surgical or diagnostic procedure was started but then discontinued.
-54 Surgical Care Only	When one physician performs a surgical procedure and another provides pre-operative and/or postoperative management, surgical services may be identified by adding modifier -54 to the usual procedure number.
-55 Postoperative Management Only	When one physician performs the postoperative management and another physician performs the surgical procedure, the postoperative component may be identified by adding modifier -55 to the usual procedure number.
-56 Preoperative Management Only	When one physician performs the preoperative care and evaluation and another physician performs the surgical procedure, the preoperative component may be identified by adding modifier -56 to the usual procedure number.
-57 Decision for Surgery	An E&M service that results in the initial decision to perform the surgery may be identified by adding the modifier -57 to the appropriate level of E&M service.
-58 Staged or Related Procedure or Service by the Same Physician during the Postoperative Period	The physician may need to indicate that the performance of a procedure or service during the postoperative period was (a) planned prospectively at the time of the original procedure (staged), (b) more extensive than the original procedure, or (c) for therapy following a diagnostic surgical procedure. This circumstance may be reported by adding modifier -58 to the staged or related procedure.
-59 Distinct Procedural Service	Under certain circumstances, the physician may need to indicate that a procedure or service was distinct or independent from other services performed on the same day. This circumstance may be reported by adding modifier -59 to the staged or related procedure.
-62 Two Surgeons	When two surgeons work together as primary surgeons performing distinct part(s) of a procedure, each surgeon should report his/her distinct operative work by adding modifier -62 to the procedure code and any associated add-on code(s) for that procedure as long as both surgeons continue to work together as primary surgeons. Each surgeon should report the co-surgery once using the same procedure code.
-76 Repeat Procedure by the Same Physician	The physician may need to indicate that a procedure or service was repeated subsequent to the original procedure or service. This circumstance may be reported by adding modifier -76 to the repeated service or procedure.

(continued)

Table 7.1 Continued

Modifier	Description of Modifier Use
-77 Repeat Procedure by Another Physician	The physician may need to indicate that a basic procedure or service performed by another physician had to be repeated. This situation may be reported by adding modifier -77 to the repeated procedure or service.
-78 Return to the Operating Room/ Procedure Room by the Same Physician Following Initial Procedure for a Related Procedure during the Postoperative Period	The physician may need to indicate that another procedure was performed during the postoperative period of the initial procedure (unplanned procedure following initial procedure). When this procedure is related to the first and requires the use of an operating or procedure room, it may be reported by adding modifier -78 to the related procedure.
-79 Unrelated Procedure or Service by the Same Physician during the Postoperative Period	The physician may need to indicate that the performance of a procedure or service during the postoperative period was unrelated to the original procedure. This circumstance may be reported by using modifier -79.

Separate Procedures

Separate procedures are commonly performed as an integral component of a total service or procedure. When you encounter "separate procedure" listed in parenthesis ( ) beside the procedure, you should bill only for the major procedure. On your coding examination, do not be "tricked" by choosing an answer that involves separate procedures when there is one major procedure that should be assigned. The procedure identified as separate procedure should NOT be billed. Separate procedures are often improperly reported as related procedures. Remember, related procedures are performed for the same diagnosis and within the same operative area. A separate procedure can be a component of, or incidental to, a larger, related procedure.

 Think Like A Coder 7.1

Read the following example.

28260   **Capsulotomy,** midfoot; medial release only (separate procedure)

28262   with tendon lengthening

Is code 28262 considered a separate procedure?

❑ yes

❑ no

❑ depends on the procedure

❑ not enough information

Materials Supplied by a Physician

Do not report supplies that are commonly included in surgical packages, such as gauze, and sponges. Surgical services do not include the supply of sterile trays or drugs. Remember to list the specific supply code as necessary.

Reporting More Than One Procedure/Service

When reporting more than one service or procedure on the same date, in the same session, or during a postoperative period (keeping in mind the "surgical package" concept), several CPT modifiers may apply.

Modifiers:

-51 - Multiple procedures.

-78 - Unplanned return to the operating/procedure room by the same physician following initial procedure for a related procedure during the postoperative period.

-79 - Unrelated procedure or service by the same physician during the postoperative period.

-24 - Unrelated E@M service by the same physician during a postoperative period.

-25 - Significant, separately identifiable E&M service by the same physician on the same day of the procedure or other service.

-58 - Staged or related procedure or service by the sam physician during the postoperative period.

Special Report

A "special report" must always be attached when a procedure or service is rarely provided, unusual, or new to help determine medical appropriateness. Important information should include a detailed description of the nature, extent, and need for the procedure or service and the time, effort, and equipment necessary to provide the service to the patient. The following is a list of additional items that may be included for special reports.

•   Complexity of symptoms presented

•   Final diagnosis

•   Pertinent physical findings such as size, locations, and number of lesions

- Diagnostic and therapeutic procedures including major and supplementary surgical procedures
- Concurrent problems
- Follow-up care

Unlisted Service or Procedure

An unlisted procedure and service codes are assigned when no specific code accurately describes the procedure or service performed. When reporting such a service, the appropriate Unlisted Procedure code may be used to indicate the service, which is identified by submission of a Special Report.

Unlisted procedures are typically found at the end of every section or subsection.

Coding Alert!

Unlisted Service or Procedure

A service or procedure may be provided in any subsection of the Sugery Section of the CPT manual that is not listed in the specific edition of the CPT codebook you are using. When reporting such a service, the appropriate Unlisted Procedure code may be used to indicate service, identifying it by "Special Report" as discussed previously in this chapter. Always remember that Unlisted Procedures are placed at the end of each section in the CPT manual.

Quick and Accurate Coding

To code surgeries quickly and accurately, you must ask yourself three things (see Figure 7.1):

1. What body system is involved?
2. What anatomical site is involved?
3. What form of procedure is involved?

Carefully read the coding problem and ascertain what body system is presented, what anatomical site (body area) is involved, and what surgical approach is taken.

Think Like A Coder 7.2

Problem: Open treatment of a tibial fracture, unicondylar, proximal with internal fixation.

Index: What body system   Musculoskeletal
is involved?
Form of procedure   Fracture
Anatomical site   Tibia
Procedure descriptor   Open Treatment 27535

Code Assignment: 27535

Figure 7.1

Coding Quickly and Accurately – Body System: Musculoskeletal; Form of Procedures: Fracture; Anatomic Site: Tibia; Code: 27535

Source: *Current Procedural Terminology*, American Medical Association, 2008.

Think Like A Coder 7.3

Using the "three questions," code the following problem quickly and accurately.

Procedure: Excision of malignant lesion measuring 3.8 cm of the female genitalia.

- 11604
- 11624
- 11424
- 11420, 11424

Index tip: Excision > Skin > Malignant

Add-On Codes

Please remember that add-on codes are reported for procedures and services performed in addition to a primary procedure performed. These additional or supplemental procedures are designated as "add-on" codes and are identified in the CPT manual with a "+" in front of the code number. All add-on codes found in the CPT manual are exempt from the use of modifier -51 (multiple procedures) because these procedures are not reported as stand-alone codes.

> **Example**
>
> Code 44139 appears as:
>
> +44139   Mobilization (take-down) of
>   splenic flexure performed in
>   conjunction with partial colec-
>   tomy. (List separately in addition
>   to primary procedure.)

Integumentary System

Integumentary System subsection in the Surgery section is broken down into the following subsections:

- Skin, **Subcutaneous,** and Accessory Structures
- Nails
- Pilonidal Cyst
- Introduction
- Repair
- Destruction
- Breast

Skin, Subcutaneous, and Accessory Structures

Biopsy

Biopsied tissue can either be benign (noncancerous) or malignant (cancerous). During certain surgical procedures in the integumentary system, such as excision, destruction, or shave removals, the specimen is routinely submitted for pathological examination in order to ascertain malignancy or nonmalignancy. Biopsy codes 11000-11101 are used to report skin biopsies for each lesion that is biopsied. With code 11101, each separate or additional lesion must be listed separately in addition to the primary procedure code 11100. Only use a separate code for a biopsy when the procedure is provided separately from any other procedure or service. Tissue removed during excision such as shaving, and submitted to pathology is not reported seperately as a biopsy, it's included in the code for the excision. Don't use modifier -51.

Excision, Benign Lesion/Excision, Malignant Lesion

Excision of a benign lesion (noncancerous) or a malignant (cancerous) lesion of the skin (see Figure 7.2) includes local anesthetic. Excision in the CPT manual is defined as full-thickness (through the dermis) removal of a lesion including margins and simple closure when performed. Pay close attention to the size of the lesion while choosing the correct coding assignment. Coding assignment is determined by measuring the greatest clinical diameter of the **lesion** plus the "margin" required to remove the lesion. The term "margin" refers to the narrowest margin required to adequately excise the lesion, based on the physician's medical judgment. The measurement of lesion plus margin is always made before performing the procedure.

Repair

The codes in this section are used to define wound closure with steri-strips, staples, or sutures. Table 7.2 defines the classification of wound repairs found in the CPT manual.

Multiple Wound Repair

For multiple wound repair, please remember that you must add together the lengths of wounds in the same classification. The same classification involves all of the anatomical sites in a particular code with the same wound repair classification. An example of this would be code 12041, which involves intermediate wound repair of the neck, hands, feet, and external genitalia. You must add all of the repairs in the primary coding descriptor and use the sum as the correct clinical diameter. However, when repairs include more than one classification of wound (simple and intermediate, for example), list the more complicated (intermediate) as the primary procedure and the less complicated as the secondary procedure and attach the -51 modifier.

Table 7.2 Wound Repair Classifications

Simple Wound Repair Codes 12001-2021	Simple repair is used when the wound is superficial, involving the epidermis, dermis, and subcutaneous tissues without involving deeper structures, and requires only simple, one-layer closures.
Intermediate Wound Repair Codes 12031-2057	Intermediate repair is used when the wound meets simple repair guidelines as well as requiring layered closure of one or more of the deeper layers of subcutaneous tissue and superficial fascia. Single-layered closure of heavily contaminated wounds that have required extensive cleaning or removal of particulate matter also constitute intermediate repair.
Complex Wound Repair Codes 13100-3160	Complex repair of wounds includes more than layered closure, such as scar revision, debridement, stents, or retention sutures. Complex wound repair does not include excision of benign or malignant lesions.

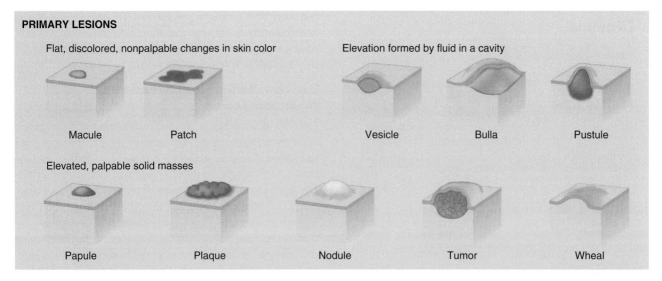

PRIMARY LESIONS

Flat, discolored, nonpalpable changes in skin color

Macule   Patch

Elevation formed by fluid in a cavity

Vesicle   Bulla   Pustule

Elevated, palpable solid masses

Papule   Plaque   Nodule   Tumor   Wheal

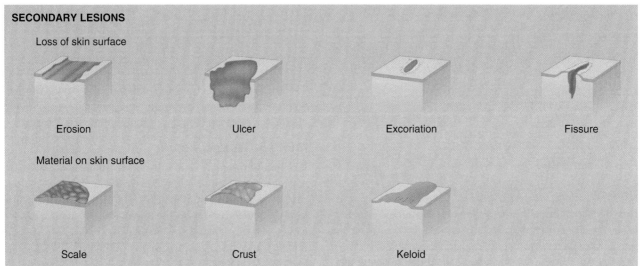

SECONDARY LESIONS

Loss of skin surface

Erosion   Ulcer   Excoriation   Fissure

Material on skin surface

Scale   Crust   Keloid

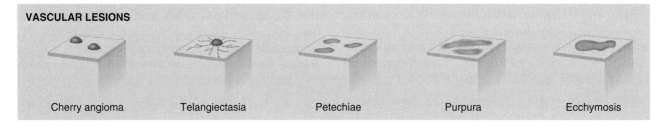

VASCULAR LESIONS

Cherry angioma   Telangiectasia   Petechiae   Purpura   Ecchymosis

Figure 7.2
Various Types of Skin Lesions

From N. Thierer and L. Breitbard, *Medial Terminology, Language for Health Care,* 2e. Copyright © 2006 The McGraw-Hill Companies, Inc. Reprinted with permission.

Indexing Tip:

When quickly looking for the correct code in the index for wound repair, always index "repair" > skin > wound.

Destruction and Excision, Breast

Destruction

Do not confuse "destruction" for "excision"; destruction is the ablation of benign, premalignant, or malignant tissue by ANY method, including procedures such as cryosurgery, electrosurgery, chemical and laser treatments, with or without **curettement,** and use of local anesthesia that usually does not require closure procedure.

Excision, Breast

Excisional breast surgery includes particular biopsy procedures, the removal of cysts, and the excision of other benign or malignant tumors or lesions. For quick reference in this surgery area, note the following:

- Breast biopsies are reported using codes 19100-19103.
- Mastectomy procedures are reported using codes 19300-19307.

Think Like A Coder 7.4

Choose the correct codes for the following problems.

1. A physician performed simple repairs of the following wounds on a 17-year-old male: a 4.5-cm wound on the face, a 3.2-cm wound of the lip, and a 1.4-cm wound of the hand.

   ☐ 12015

   ☐ 12054

   ☐ 12015, 12001-51

   ☐ 12015, 12002-51

2. A physician performed the paring of five **hyperkeratotic** lesions from the left index finger.

   ☐ 11200

   ☐ 11055, 11056-51

   ☐ 11055 × 5

   ☐ 11057

Musculoskeletal System

Musculoskeletal System subsection in the Surgery section is broken down into the following subsections:

- General
- Head
- Neck (Soft Tissues) and Thorax
- Spine (Vertebral Column)
- Shoulder
- Humerus (Upper Arm) and Elbow
- Forearm and Wrist
- Hand and Fingers
- Pelvis and Hip Joint
- Femur (Thigh Region) and Knee Joint
- Leg (Tibia and Fibula) and Ankle Joint
- Foot and Toes
- Application of Casts and Strapping
- Endoscopy/Arthroscopy

Fractures

Three different types of treatment procedures are commonly used to repair fractures. You will need to review Table 7.3 closely in order to distinguish between closed, open, and percutaneous treatments. Figure 7.3 provides an illustration of the different types of fractures that can occur and the categories of fracture treatments into which they fall. Memorizing Table 7.3 will allow you to code more quickly and accurately when taking your coding examination.

Spine (Vertebral Column)

Within the Spine subsection, bone grafting procedure codes are separate and in addition to **arthrodesis.** Pay close attention to bone grafting codes in other musculoskeletal sections; see specific codes, descriptors, and accompanying guidelines in order to assign the correct code. To report bone grafts performed after arthrodesis, see codes 20930-20938; these codes show that they are -51 modifier exempt (Ø). Hence, bone graft codes are reported without modifier -51.

Table 7.3 Fracture Treatments

Closed treatment	A closed treatment is defined as treatment in which a fracture site is not surgically opened and thus is not exposed to the external environment and directly visualized.
Open treatment	An open treatment is defined as treatment in which a fractured bone is either (a) surgical opened (exposed to the external environment) and the fracture visualized, with possible internal fixation or (b) opened in an area remote from the fracture site in order to insert an intramedullary nail across the fracture site.
Percutaneous Skeletal fixation	Percutaneous skeletal fixation is defined as a fracture treatment that is neither open or closed. With this treatment, the fracture fragments are not visualized, but fixation (pins) is performed across the fracture site with the aid of x-ray imaging.

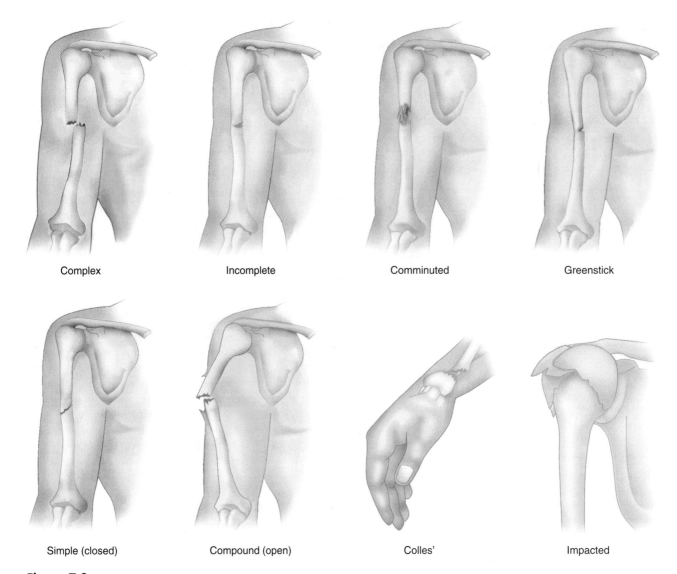

Complex   Incomplete   Comminuted   Greenstick

Simple (closed)   Compound (open)   Colles'   Impacted

Figure 7.3
Various Types of Fractures

From N. Thierer and L. Breitbard, *Medial Terminology, Language for Health Care,* 2e. Copyright © 2006 The McGraw-Hill Companies, Inc. Reprinted with permission.

For spinal procedures, instrumentation is reported separately. To report instrumentation procedures performed with definitive vertebral procedure(s), see 22840-22855. Instrumentation procedure codes 22840-22848 and 22851 are reported in addition to the definitive procedure(s). Modifier -62 may not be appended to the definitive or add-on spinal instrumentation procedure code(s) 22840-22848 and 22850-22852. Modifier -62 is assigned when two surgeons work together as primary surgeons performing distinct parts

 Indexing Tip:

Always read the subsection notes and their specific "examples" in order to make sure your coding assignment is correct. Professional examinations will intentionally create a coding problem around subsection notes.

Table 7.4 Spinal Segments Used in Reporting Codes

Spinal Segment Abbreviation	Spinal Segment	Spinal Interspaces
T1-T2	Thoracic vertebra 1 and 2	One interspace between T1 and T2
L1-L4	Lumbar vertebra, 1, 2, 3, 4	Two interspaces between L2 and L3
C1-C3	Cervical vertebra 1, 2, 3	Two interspaces between C1 and C2, C2 and C3

of a procedure and each surgeon should report his or her distinct operative work by adding -62. In the case of codes 22840-22848 and 22850- 22852 these codes are not distinct part of a primary procedure that both surgeons are performing separate work on for one procedure. When arthrodesis is performed in addition to another procedure, the arthrodesis should be reported in addition to the original procedure with modifier -51.

Arthrodesis

Arthrodesis is the surgical fixation or fusion of a joint. It may be performed independently of other procedures, but when it is combined with another definitive procedure such as osteotomy, fracture care, etc., modifier -51 is appropriate for assignment. However, arthrodesis codes 22585, 22614 and 22632 are considered add-on codes (+) and should not be used with modifier -51. Code 22585 can be reported when additional interspaces are involved in the surgical procedure. Code 22614 can be reported when additional vertebral segments are involved in the surgical procedure. And, code 22632 can be reported when additional interspaces are involved in the surgical procedure.

Application of Casts and Strapping

Casting and strapping codes apply when the cast application or strapping is a replacement procedure used during or after the period follow-up care and also when the cast application or strapping is an initial service performed without a restorative treatment or procedure to stabilize or protect a fracture, injury, or dislocation and to afford comfort to a patient. Restorative treatment or procedures rendered

Think Like A Coder 7.5

Choose the correct codes for the following problems.
1. A 56-year-old male underwent arthrodesis by posterior interbody technique and laminectomy to prepare two lumber interspaces.

❏ 22612 × 2

❏ 22808

❏ 22630, 22632

❏ 22808

2. A 10-year-old male's cast was removed after partial melting during an accident. After evaluation, the physician who initially placed the cast reapplied the cast again from elbow to finger with fiberglass.

❏ No charges would be applied

❏ 29065

❏ 29260

❏ 29075

❏ 29705

by another physician following the application of the initial cast/splint/strap may be reported with a treatment of fracture and dislocation code. A physician who applies the initial cast, strap, or splint and also assumes all of the subsequent fracture, dislocation, or injury care cannot use the application of casts and strapping codes as an initial service because the first cast/splint/or strap application is included in the treatment of the fracture.

> ### Coding Alert!
> Codes for **cast removals** should be used only for casts applied by another physician.

Respiratory System

Respiratory System subsection in the Surgical section is broken down into the following subsections:

- Nose
- Accessory Sinuses
- Larynx
- Trachea and Bronchi
- Lungs and Pleura

Endoscopy

Surgical sinus endoscopy codes in the Respiratory System subsection typically classify procedures as unilateral unless the code description specifies otherwise. Diagnostic endoscopy codes 31231-31235 include an inspection of the interior of the nasal cavity, the middle and superior meatus, the turbinates, and the sphenoethmoid recess. Please make sure that, when a diagnostic evaluation is performed in all these areas during one session, a separate code is not reported for each area—this would be considered unbundling. Code full extent of endoscopic procedure performed from beginning to end.

Lung Transplantation

Lung allotransplants include the following distinct components, and a separate code is assigned to each individual physician who performs the specified component:

1. Cadaver donor pneumonectomy: Harvesting the allograft (transplant tissue from a member of one's species) and the cold preservation of the allograft by perfusing with cold preservation solution and cold maintenance.
2. Backbench work: The preparation of a cadaver donor lung allograft before lung transplantation and dissecting the allograft from surrounding soft tissues to prepare the pulmonary venous/atrial cuff, pulmonary artery, and bronchus unilaterally.
3. Recipient lung allotransplantation: The transplantation of a single or double lung allograft and care of the patient recipient.

Indexing Tip:

When searching for a code for an endoscopy procedure, refer immediately in your index to "endoscopy" and find the anatomical site for quick and accurate coding assignment.

Think Like A Coder 7.6

Choose the correct codes for the following problems.

1. A physician performed a flexible bronchoscopy with laser destruction of a 1.6-cm tumor and placed a catheter for intracavitary radiation treatment.

   - ❑ 31641, 31643-51
   - ❑ 31643
   - ❑ 31785
   - ❑ 31641, 77761-51

2. A physician performed a sinus endoscopy with total anterior and posterior ethmoidectomy with maxillary antrostomy on a 53-year-old female.

   - ❑ 31233, 31256-51
   - ❑ 31267
   - ❑ 31255, 31256-51
   - ❑ 31231, 31256-51

Cardiovascular System

Cardiovascular System subsection in the Surgery section is broken down into the following subsections:

- Heart and Pericardium
- Arteries and Veins
- Hemic and Lymphatic Systems
- General
- Lymph Nodes and Lymphatic Channels
- Mediastinum and Diaphragm

Cardiovascular System is one of the largest subsections in the Surgery section of the CPT manual. It contains numerous "notes" that contain pertinent information on how the medical coder should proceed with assigning the correct cardiovascular procedure codes. Table 7.5 outlines the subheadings in the cardiovascular subsection that contain "notes" and the codes that affect them.

Pacemaker or Pacing Cardioverter-Defibrillator

Know what type of pacemaker you are coding for before assigning a code. Review these four items before choosing a pacemaker code:

1. Single or dual chamber pacemaker
2. Initial, repair, replacement, or upgrade of a pacemaker
3. Entire pacemaker system or just electrodes
4. Fluoroscopic guidance or no fluoroscopic guidance

Table 7.5 Cardiovascular System Notes

Subheading Note	Codes That Are Included in Notes
Pacemaker or Pacing Cardioverter-Defibrillator	33202-33249
Electrophysiologic Operative Procedures	33250-33266
Venous Grafting Only for Coronary Artery Bypass	33510-33516
Combined Arterial-Venous Grafting for Coronary Bypass	33517-33530
Arterial Grafting for Coronary Artery Bypass	33533-33548
Endovascular Repair of Descending Thoracic Aorta	33880-33891
Heart-Lung Transplantation	33930-33945
Arteries and Veins	34001-34530
Endovascular Repair of Abdominal Aortic Aneurysm	34800-34834
Endovascular Repair of Iliac Aneurysm	34900

(continued)

Table 7.5 Continued

Subheading Note	Codes That Are Included in Notes
Bypass Graft—Vein	35500-35671
Composite Graft	35681-35683
Adjuvant Techniques	35685-35686
Vascular Injection Procedures	36000-36522
Central Venous Access Procedures	36555-36598
Transcatheter Procedures	37184-37216
Intravascular Ultrasound Services	37250-37251
Bone Marrow or Stem Cell Services/Procedures	38204-38242

Now you are ready to choose the pacemaker coding assignment.

A pacing cardioverter-defibrillator, like a pacemaker system, includes a pulse generator and electrodes although pacing cardioverter-defibrillators may require multiple leads, even when only a single chamber is being placed. A pacing cardioverter-defibrillator system may be inserted in a single chamber or in dual chambers.

Pacemaker and cardio-defibrillators differentiate between temporary and permanent devices and also between one-chamber versus dual chamber. Divided by where pacer is placed, approach (epicardial/tranvenous), and type of service. Patient record must indicate revision or replacement. Pacemaker

pulse generator is also called a battery. Pacemaker leads are also called electrodes. Usual follow up is 90 days (global period).

Electrophysiological Operative Procedures

Codes for electrophysiological operative procedures describe the surgical treatment of supraventricular dysrhythmias. Dysrhythmias, which are typically found and mapped on an electrocardiogram print-out, help physicians diagnose heart disorders and disease (see Figure 7.4). Tissue ablation and reconstruction can be accomplished by various methods such as surgical incision, radiofrequency,

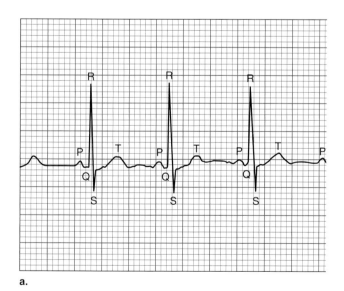

a.

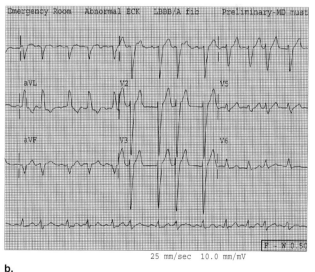

25 mm/sec   10.0 mm/mV

b.

Figure 7.4

Electrocardiogram – a. Normal Electrocardiogram. b. Abnormal Electrocardiogram that results in diagnoses of heart disease and disorders.

cryotherapy, ultrasound, microwave, and laser. The following are definitions of operative ablations:

1. Limited operative ablation and reconstruction include surgical isolation of triggers of supraventricular dysrhythmias by operative ablation that isolates the pulmonary veins or other anatomically defined triggers in the left or right atrium.

2. Extensive operative ablation and reconstruction include all of the services in "limited" and additional ablation of atrial tissue to eliminate sustained supraventricular dysrhythmias.

Venous Grafting Only for Coronary Artery Bypass

Codes used to report coronary artery bypass procedures using venous grafts only should not be used to report the performance of coronary artery bypass procedures using arterial grafts and venous grafts during the same procedure. See 33517-33523 and 33533-33536 for reporting combined arterial venous grafts.

Procurement of the saphenous vein graft is included in the description of the work for 33510-33516 and should not be reported as a separate service or co-surgery. To report harvesting of an upper extremity vein, use 35500 in addition to the bypass procedure. To report harvesting of a femoropopliteal vein segment, report 35572 in addition to the bypass procedure. When a surgical assistant performs graft procurement, add modifier -80 to 33510-33516.

> ### Example
>
> #### Coronary Artery Bypass for Venous Graft Only
>
> **Problem:** A 74-year-old female patient underwent the procurement of the saphenous vein graft for a coronary artery bypass that included four coronary venous grafts. A surgical assistant performed the graft procurement.
>
> **Coding Assignment:** 33513-80
>
> **Rationale:** Code 33513 indicates coronary artery bypass for four coronary venous (only) grafts. Procurement of the saphenous vein graft is included in the description of the work for codes 33510-33516, so an additional code is not required.

Combined Arterial-Venous Grafting for Coronary Bypass

Codes used to report coronary artery bypass procedures using venous graft and arterial grafts during the same procedure may not be used alone. To report combined arterial-venous grafts, you must report two codes: (1) the appropriate combined arterial-venous graft code, 33517-33523, and (2) the appropriate arterial graft code, 33533-33536.

Procurement of the saphenous vein graft is included in the description of the work for 33517-33523 and should not be reported as a separate service or co-surgery. Procurement of

the artery for grafting is included in the description of the work for 33533-33536 and should not be reported as a separate service or co-surgery, except when an upper extremity artery is procured. To report harvesting of an upper extremity artery, use 35600 in addition to the bypass procedure. To report harvesting of an upper extremity vein, use 35500 in addition to the bypass procedure. To report harvesting of a femoropopliteal vein segment, report 35572 in addition to the bypass procedure.

Arterial Grafting for Coronary Artery Bypass

Codes 33533-33548 are used to report coronary artery bypass procedures using either arterial grafts only or a combination of arterial-venous grafts. The codes include the use of the internal mammary artery, the gastroepiploic artery, the epigastric artery, the radial artery, and arterial conduits procured from other sites. Procurement of the artery for grafting is included in the description of the work for 33533-33536 and should not be reported as a separate service or co-surgery, except when an upper extremity artery is procured.

> ### Example
>
> #### Combined Arterial-Venous Grafting for Coronary Bypass
>
> **Problem:** A 46-year-old male patient underwent a coronary artery bypass using three venous grafts and two coronary arterial grafts. Procurement of the veins and arteries was performed by the primary surgeon.
>
> **Coding Assignment:** 33519, 33534
>
> **Rationale:** Code 33519 indicates the coronary artery bypass using venous and arterial grafts. Code 33519 also indicates that three venous grafts are used. The coder is instructed to use 33519 in conjunction with codes 33533-33536. Code 33534 is assigned to indicate the coronary artery bypass using two coronary arterial grafts. Modifier -80 would not be assigned since the primary physician procured the harvesting of the veins and grafts. The procurement of the harvested veins and grafts are included in both codes descriptions.

 ## Indexing Tip:

Keywords to use when indexing cardiovascular procedures include veins, arteries, repair, bypass graft, blood vessels, grafts, and vascular.

Endovascular Repair of Descending Thoracic Aorta

Codes 33880-33891 represent a family of procedures to report placement of an endovascular graft for the repair of the descending thoracic aorta. These codes include all device introduction, manipulation, positioning, and deployment. Balloon angioplasty and/or stent deployment within the target treatment zone for the endoprosthesis, either before or after endograft deployment, should not be reported separately. Open arterial exposure and associated closure of the arteriotomy sites, introduction of guidewires and catheters, and extensive repair or replacement of an artery should be additionally reported.

Heart/Lung Transplant

Heart allotransplantation with or without lung allotransplantation involves three distinct components of physician work:

1. Cadaver donor cardiectomy with or without pneumonectomy: Harvesting the allograft and cold preservation of the allograft.

2. Backbench work: Preparation of a cadaver donor heart and lung allograft before transplantation, including dissection of the allograft from surrounding soft tissues to prepare the aorta, superior vena cava, inferior vena cave, inferior vena cava, and trachea for implantation, or preparation of a cadaver donor heart allograft before transplantation, including dissection of the allograft from surrounding soft tissues to prepare aorta, superior vena cava, inferior vena cava, pulmonary artery, and left atrium for implantation.

3. Recipient heart allotransplantation with or without lung allotransplantation:, Transplantation of allograft and care of the recipient.

> ## Example
>
> ### Endovascular Repair of Abdominal Aortic Aneurysm
>
> **Problem:** A physician performed cardiovascular repair of infrarenal abdominal aortic aneurysm for a 31-year-old Down's syndrome male patient, using initial third-order selective catheter placement and modular bifurcated prosthesis with one docking limb.
>
> **Coding Assignment:** 34802, 36247
>
> **Rationale:** Code 34802 is assigned to indicate the endovascular repair of infrarenal abdominal aortic aneurysm with modular **bifurcated** prosthesis (one docking limb). Code 36247 is assigned to indicate that an initial third-order selective catheter placement was performed. The "Note" under Endovascular Repair of Abdominal Aortic Aneurysm instructs the coder to use additional codes 36200 and 36245-36248 for placement of guidewires or catheters.

Vascular Injection Procedures

Listed services for injection procedures include necessary local anesthesia, introduction of needles or catheter, injection of contrast media with or without automatic power injection, and/or necessary pre- and postinjection care specifically related to the injection procedure. Catheters, drugs, and contrast media are not included in the listed service for the injection procedure.

Selective vascular catheterization should be coded to include introduction and all lesser order selective catheterization used in the approach. Additional second- and/or third-order arterial catheterization within the same family of arteries or veins supplied by a single first-order vessel should be expressed by 36012, 36218, or 36248.

Central Venous Access Procedures

In order to use "central venous access procedure" codes, the tip of the catheter or device must terminate in the subclavian, brachiocephalic, or iliac veins; superior or inferior vena cava; or the right atrium. Table 7.6 outlines the procedures that involve these types of devices.

>
> ## Think Like A Coder 7.7
>
> Choose the correct codes for the following problems.
>
> 1. A surgical assistant performed a coronary artery bypass graft and two coronary venous grafts with endoscopic harvesting of saphenous vein on a 50-year-old male.
>
>   ❑ 33511, 33508-80
>   ❑ 33534, 33508-51
>   ❑ 33534, 33508-80
>   ❑ 33518
>
> 2. A physician performed a subsequent percutaneous transluminal mechanical arterial thrombectomy on a 47-year-old post-menopausal female with fluoroscopic guidance and intraprocedural pharmacological thrombolytic injections.
>
>   ❑ 37188, 76000
>   ❑ 37185
>   ❑ 37185, 76000
>   ❑ 37187

Table 7.6 Central Venous Access Procedures

Procedure	Device Explanation
Insertion	Catheter placed through a newly established venous access
Repair	Fixing a device without replacement of either catheter or port/pump
Partial replacement	Only the catheter component associated with port/pump device, but not entire device
Complete replacement	The entire device, by the same venous access site
Removal	Removal of the entire device

Digestive System

Digestive System in the Surgery section is broken down into the following subsections:

- Lips
- Vestibule of Mouth
- Tongue and Floor of Mouth
- Dentoalveolar Structure
- Palate and Uvula
- Salivary Gland and Ducts
- Pharynx, Adenoids, and Tonsils
- Esophagus
- Stomach
- Intestines (Except Rectum)
- Meckel's Diverticulum and the Mesentery
- Anus
- Liver
- Biliary Tract
- Pancreas
- Abdomen, Peritoneum, and Omentum

Endoscopy/Laparoscopy

Endoscopy is the examination of the interior of a canal or hollow viscus by means of a special instrument called an endoscope. In the digestive system types of examinations used with endoscopes are as follows:

1. Proctosigmoidoscopy: The examination of the rectum and sigmoid colon.

2. **Sigmoidoscopy:** The examination of the entire rectum and sigmoid colon, possibly including the examination of a portion of the descending colon.

3. Colonoscopy: The examination of the entire colon, from the rectum to the cecum, possibly including the examination of the terminal ileum.

Surgical laparoscopy always includes diagnostic laparoscopy. To report a diagnostic laparoscopy, peritonoscopy (separate procedure), use code 49320.

Intestines

Excision

Intestinal allotransplantation involves three distinct components of physician work.

1. Cadaver donor enterectomy: Harvesting the intestine graft and cold preservation of the graft. Living donor enterectomy includes harvesting the intestine graft, cold preservation of the graft, and care of the donor.

2. Backbench work: Standard preparation of an intestine allograft before transplantation, including mobilization and fashioning of the superior mesenteric artery and vein. Additional reconstruction of an intestine allograft before transplantation may include venous and/or arterial anastomosis.

3. Recipient intestinal allotransplantation with or without recipient enterectomy: Transplantation of allograft and care of the recipient.

> ## Coding Alert!
>
> The digestive system notes include codes for transplantations of the intestines, liver, and pancreas. All these codes include notes involving specifications of cadaver donor, backbench work, and recipient allotransplantation.

Example

Laparoscopy

Problem: A physician performed a diagnostic laparoscopy on a morbidly obese patient with varying degrees of symptoms and comorbidities. The physician then went on to perform a surgical laparoscopy for gastric restrictive procedure with gastric bypass and small intestine reconstruction to limit absorption.

Coding Assignment: 43645 Surgical laparoscopy

Rationale: Code 43645 is assigned to indicate the diagnostic laparoscopy that was performed on the patient led to the gastric bypass and small intestine reconstruction by laparoscope. The surgical laparoscopy always includes the diagnostic laparoscopy so no additional code is required.

Repair of Hernia

Repair of hernia codes are categorized by type of hernia, such as femoral, inguinal, or incisional. Please pay close attention to the category that describes whether the hernia repair is either "initial" or "recurrent." Also, additional parameters include the age of the patient for the hernia repair and the clinical presentation, such as a reducible versus incarcerated or strangulated hernia. With the exception of the incisional hernia repairs, codes 49560-49566, the use of mesh or another prosthesis is not separately reported. The excision/repair of strangulated organs or structures such as testicle(s), intestine, or ovaries are reported by using the appropriate code for the excision/repair in addition to the appropriate code for the repair of the strangulated hernia.

Urinary System

Urinary System subsection in the Surgery section is broken down into the following subsections:

- Kidney
- Ureter
- Bladder
- Urethra

Renal Transplantation

Renal autotransplantation (kidney transferred by grafting into a new position in the body of the same individual) includes reimplantation of the autograft as the primary procedure, along with secondary extracorporeal procedures such as nephrectomy and nephrolithotomy, which should be reported with modifier -51. As with all transplants coded in the Surgery section the following three components apply to renal transplantations:

1. Cadaver donor: Harvesting the graft
2. Backbench work: Standard preparation of cadaver and donor and reconstruction
3. Recipient allotransplantation: Transplantation of the allograft

Urodynamics

When multiple procedures are performed in the same investigative session, modifier -51 should be used. All procedures listed in the Urodynamics subsection imply that these services are performed by or are under the direct supervision of, a physician and that all instruments, equipment, fluids, gases, probes, etc., are provided by the physician. When a physician only interprets the results or operates the equipment of any urodynamics, modifier -26 should be used to identify physician services. Please remember that all procedures in **urodynamics** imply that the services rendered are performed by or are under the direct supervision of a physician.

Endoscopy: Cystoscopy, Urethroscopy, Cystourethroscopy

Endoscopic descriptions are listed so that the main procedure can be identified without having to list all the minor related functions performed at the same time, for example, ureteral catheterization following extraction of ureteral calculus. When the secondary procedure requires significant additional time and effort, it may be identified by the assignment of modifier -22. Insertion of a temporary indwelling bladder catheter, such as a Foley (see Figure 7.5) is a common procedure to code.

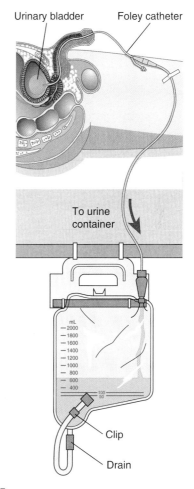

Figure 7.5

Temporary Indwelling Bladder Catheter

From N. Thierer and L. Breitbard, *Medial Terminology, Language for Health Care*, 2e. Copyright © 2006 The McGraw-Hill Companies, Inc. Reprinted with permission.

Indexing Tip:

Keywords to index for quick and accurate coding assignment for the urinary system include, kidney, laparoscopy, urethra, *and* bladder.

Think Like A Coder 7.9

Choose the correct codes for the following problem.

A physician performed an ureteroneocystostomy: bilateral **anastomosis** of ureter to contralateral ureter.

- ☐ 50800-50
- ☐ 50782
- ☐ 50780-50
- ☐ 50947

Male and Female Genital System

Male and Female Genital System subsection in the Surgery section is broken down as shown in Table 7.7.

Table 7.7 Male and Female Genital System

Male	Female
Penis	Vulva, Perineum, and Introitus
Testis	Vagina
Epididymis	Cervix Uteri
Tunica Vaginalis	Corpus Uteri
Scrotum	Oviduct/Ovary
Vas Deferens	Ovary
Spermatic Cord	In Vitro Fertilization
Seminal Vesicles	Maternity Care and Delivery
Prostate	
Intersex Surgery	

Female Genital System

Vulva, Perineum, and Introitus

A vulvectomy is either partial, complete, or radical excision of the vulva. Table 7.8 identifies the descriptions pertinent to the vulvectomy codes.

Maternity Care and Delivery

The subsection Maternity Care and Delivery is broken down into three major areas: antepartum services (before delivery), delivery (cesarean and vaginal), and postpartum care (cesarean and vaginal). Antepartum services include the initial and subsequent history, physical examination, recording of weight, blood pressure, fetal heart tones, routine urinalysis, and monthly visits. Delivery services include admission, history and physical, management of uncomplicated labor, and vaginal or cesarean delivery. Postpartum services include hospital and office visits following delivery by cesarean or vaginal birth.

If a patient has a successful vaginal delivery (see Figure 7.6) after a previous cesarean delivery use codes 59610-59622. Code descriptors for codes 59610-59622 include the phrase, "after previous cesarean delivery." If the attempt is unsuccessful and another cesarean delivery is carried out, use codes 58618-59622. To report elective cesarean deliveries, use code 59510, 59514, or 59515.

Coding Alert!

Remember: A surgical laparoscopy always includes diagnostic laparoscopy. To report only a diagnostic laparoscopy, use code 49320.

Table 7.8 Vulvectomy Descriptions

Procedure	Definition
Simple vulvectomy	The removal of skin and superficial subcutaneous tissue
Radical vulvectomy	The removal of skin and deep subcutaneous tissue
Partial vulvectomy	The removal of less than 80% of the vulvar area
Complete vulvectomy	The removal of more than 80% of the vulvar area

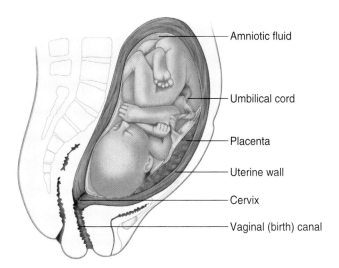

Figure 7.6

vaginal delivery – A full-term fetus that is positioned "head-down" for a vaginal delivery.

Labels on figure:
- Amniotic fluid
- Umbilical cord
- Placenta
- Uterine wall
- Cervix
- Vaginal (birth) canal

From D. Shier et al., Hole's *Human Anatomy & Physiology*, 11e. Copyright © 2007 The McGraw-Hill Companies. Reprinted with permission.

Male Genital System

The male genital subsection is divided into anatomic sub-headings. The break down the anatomy of the male in this subsection are as follows: penis, testis, epididymis, tunica vaginalis, scrotum, vas deferens, spermatic cord, seminal vesicles, and prostate. This subsection is very small and the coding assignments are determined by either the reason for the surgery or the approach.

Example

Reason for the Surgery

Repair

54304   Plastic operation on penis for correction of chordee or for first stage hypospadias repair with or without transplantation of prepuce and/or skin flaps.

Approach

The approach procedures include subheadings such as incision, destruction, introduction, excision and laparoscopy.

Incision

54700   Incision and drainage of epididymis, testis and/or scrotal space.

Introduction

54231   Dynamic cavernosometry, including intra-cavernosal injection of vasoactive drugs.

Think Like A Coder 7.10

Choose the correct codes for the following problems.

1. A physician performed a diagnostic laparoscopy on a 27-year-old male followed by a surgical orchiectomy. The same physician also performed a needle biopsy of the patient's epididymis during the same operative session.

   ❑ 49320, 54690, 54800-51
   ❑ 54520, 54800-51
   ❑ 54690, 54800-51
   ❑ 49320, 54800-51

2. A physician performed a nonlaparoscopic vaginal hysterectomy on a 32-year-female with a 310-g uterus. Physician also removed the left fallopian tube and left ovary and performed a repair of an enterocele.

   ❑ 58554
   ❑ 58544
   ❑ 58180
   ❑ 58292

Nervous and Endocrine Systems

Endocrine System subsection in the Surgery section is broken down into the following subsections:

- Parathyroid
- Thymus
- Adrenal Glands
- Pancreas
- Carotid Body

The nervous system subsection is broken down into the following subsections:

- Skull, Meninges, and Brain
- Spine and Spinal Cord
- Extracranial Nerves, Peripheral Nerves, and Autonomic Nervous System

Surgery of Skull Base

The surgical management of lesions involving the skull base often requires the skills of several surgeons of different surgical specialties working together or in tandem during the operative session. These operations are usually not staged because of the need for definitive closure of dura, subcutaneous tissues, and skin to avoid serious infections such as osteomyelitis and/or meningitis. The procedures are

Table 7.9 Skull Base Surgery Procedures

Procedure	Definition
Approach procedure	The approach procedure is described according to anatomical area involved, such as anterior cranial fossa, middle cranial fossa, posterior cranial fossa, and brainstem or upper spinal cord.
Definitive procedure	The definitive procedure describes the repair, biopsy, resection, or excision of various lesions of the skull base and, when appropriate, primary closure of the dura, mucous membranes, and skin.
Repair/reconstruction procedures	The repair/reconstruction procedures are reported separately if extensive dural grafting, **cranioplasty,** local or regional myocutaneous pedicle flaps, or extensive skin grafts are required.

categorized according to approach procedure, definitive procedure, and repair/reconstruction. Table 7.9 demonstrates the categories of the procedures used during skull base surgery so the coder can assign quick and accurate codes.

Example

Skull Base Surgery

Approach Procedure: Anterior Cranial Fossa

61580: Craniofacial approach to anterior cranial fossa; extradural, including lateral rhinotomy, ethmoidectomy, sphenoidectomy, with maxillectomy or orbital exenteration.

Definitive Procedure: 61600: Resection or excision of neoplastic, vascular or infectious lesion of base of anterior cranial fossa; extradural

Repair and/or Reconstruction of Surgical Defect of Skull Base: 61618: Secondary repair of dura for cerebrospinal fluid leak in the anterior, middle, or posterior cranial fossa following surgery of the skull base; by free tissue graft

These operations are usually not staged and are completed during one operative session by multiple surgeons. If one surgeon performs more than one procedure, then both codes are reported by using modifier -51.

Injection, Drianage, or Aspiration

Injection of contrast during fluoroscopic guidance and localization is an inclusive component of codes 62263-62264, 62270-62273, 62280-62282, 62310-62319, and 0027T. Fluoroscopic guidance and localization is reported by code 77003 unless a formal contrast study is performed, in which case the use of fluoroscopy is included in the supervision and interpretation codes. For radiological supervision and interpretation of epidurography, use 72275. Code 72275 should be used only when an epidurogram is performed, images documented, and a formal radiological report is issued.

Code 62264 describes multiple adhesiolysis treatment sessions performed on the same day. Adhesions or scarring may be lysed by injections or neurolytic agent(s). If required, adhesions or scarring may also by lysed mechanically by using a percutaneously-deployed catheter. Codes 62263 and 62264 include the procedure of injections of contrast for epidurography, 72275, and fluoroscopic guidance and localization, 77003, during initial or subsequent sessions.

Please keep in mind that the assigning codes for procedures performed on nervous system can be difficult and sometimes confusing. In order for you to avoid mistakes on this section in your coding examination, please read ALL notes that follow categories and subcategories.

Example

Surgery Section > Nervous System > Anterior or Anterolateral Approach for Extradural Exploration/Decompression

For the following codes, when two surgeons work together as primary surgeons performing distinct part(s) of a spinal cord exploration/decompression operation, each surgeon should report his/her distinct operative work by appending modifier -62 to the procedure code (and any associated add-on codes for that procedure code as long as both surgeons continue to work together as primary surgeons). In this situation, modifier -62 may be appended to the definitive procedure code(s) 63075, 63077, 63081, 63085, 63087, and/or 63090 and, as appropriate, to associated additional interspace add-on code(s) 63076, 63078, 63082, 63086, 63088, and/or 63091 as long as both surgeons continue to work together as primary surgeons.

Without reading and comprehending this note, which follows the subcategory "Anterior or Anterolateral Approach for Extradural Exploration/Decompression," you may not realize that these procedures more than likely involve two surgeons. Read the operative note very carefully. Failure to read the operative note could cause an error when you are assigning and choosing codes during your coding examination!

Indexing Tip:

When indexing for procedures in the nervous system, index using the procedure performed. Example: "skull base surgery," "craniectomy," "injection," "decompression," "neuroplasty," etc.

Coding Alert!

In many instances with nervous system codes, two surgeons will work together as both primary surgeons. In this case, always use modifier -62 to indicate two surgeons working together as primary surgeons performing distinct parts of a procedure.

Think Like A Coder 7.11

Choose the correct code for the following problem.

A surgeon performed a skull base procedure that included an infratemporal pre-auricular approach to the middle cranial fossa, with disarticulation of the mandible and a craniotomy, on a 12-year-old male child. The same surgeon, during the primary procedure, excised an infectious lesion of the infratemporal fossa. Immediately following the skull base surgery, a surgeon specializing in reconstruction performed a secondary repair of dura for cerebrospinal fluid leak in the middle cranial fossa.

- ❐ Physician 1: 61591, 61607-51; Physician 2: 61618-62
- ❐ Physician 1: 61591, 61605-51; Physician 2: No code is reported
- ❐ Physician 1: 61590, primary procedure not reported; Physician 2: 61618-62
- ❐ Physician 1: 61590, 61605-51; Physician 2: 61618

Eye, Ocular Adnexa, and Auditory System

Eye and Ocular Adnexa subsection in the Surgery section is broken down into the following subsections:

- Eyeball
- Anterior Segment
- Posterior Segment
- Ocular Adnexa
- Conjunctiva

The Auditory System subsection is broken down into the following subsections:

- External Ear
- Middle Ear
- Inner Ear
- Temporal Bone, Middle Fossa Approach
- Operating Microscope

Eye and Ocular Adnexa subsection notes are very limited and do not include instructions with most procedure codes. Table 7.10 outlines specific procedures pertinent to each subsection in the Eye and Ocular Adnexa and Auditory System.

Think Like A Coder 7.12

Choose the correct codes for the following problems.

1. A physician performed strabismus surgery on one vertical muscle of the left eye of a 4-year-old female and placed one adjustable suture to finalize the surgery.

   - ❐ 67314, 67335
   - ❐ 67318
   - ❐ 67331, 67335
   - ❐ 67311, 67335

2. A physician performed a tympanoplasty with mastoidectomy on a 62-year-old male with reconstructed canal wall and ossicular chain reconstruction.

   - ❐ 69643
   - ❐ 69636
   - ❐ 69644
   - ❐ 69632

Table 7.10 Subsection Procedures for Eye and Ocular Adnexa and Auditory System

Subsections	Subsection Procedures
Eyeball	Removal of eye, secondary implants, removal of foreign body, and repair of laceration
Anterior Segment	Cornea, anterior chamber, anterior sclera, iris, ciliary body, lens: excision, removal or destruction, and repair or revision
Posterior Segment	Vitreous, Retina or Choroid: repair and destruction
Ocular Adnexa	Orbit: exploration; Eyelids: incision, destruction, repair, and reconstruction
Conjunctiva	Conjunctiva: incision and drainage, excision and destruction, injection, and conjunctivoplasty; Lacrimal System: incision, excision, repair, and probing
External Ear	External Ear: Incision, excision, removal, and repair (see Figure 7.7)
Middle Ear	Middle Ear: introduction, incision, excision, repair, and other procedures (see Figure 7.7)
Inner Ear	Inner Ear: incision and destruction, excision, introduction, and other procedures (see Figure 7.7)
Temporal Bone, Middle Fossa Approach	N/A
Operating Microscope	Used for techniques of microsurgery in this subsection

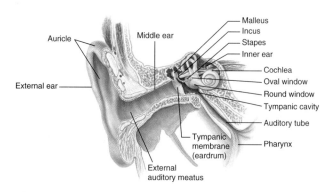

Figure 7.7

The Anatomy of the Ear — The organ of hearing showing the external ear, middle ear, and inner ear.

From N. Thierer and L. Breitbard, *Medial Terminology, Language for Health Care*, 2e. Copyright © 2006 The McGraw-Hill Companies, Inc. Reprinted with permission.

APPLYING CODING THEORY TO PRACTICE

Choose the correct surgery coding assignment. (Please see Appendix A for answers and rationale.)

1. A physician performed an intermediate repair of two wounds, one located on the trunk, measuring 12.4 cm, the other located on the right leg, measuring 6.1 cm. There was also a complex repair of the left eyelid, measuring 3.5 cm, for a 22-year-old female car accident victim.
   A. ❒ 12035, 13152-51
   B. ❒ 12045, 13132-51
   C. ❒ 12005, 13152
   D. ❒ 12031, 12035, 13152-51

2. A patient fractured his left tibia and fibula. She had an open treatment of her shaft fractures with cerclage and multiple screws placed by intramedullary implant.
   A. ❒ 27758
   B. ❒ 27832
   C. ❒ 27759
   D. ❒ 27784

3. A chest x-ray revealed a suspicious mass on right lung of 47-year-old male smoker. A diagnostic, rigid bronchoscopy with fluoroscopic guidance was performed, involving a single bronchial biopsy. The pathology report came back positive for cancer, and a single lobectomy was performed.
   A. ❒ 31641, 32484-51
   B. ❒ 31625, 32480-51
   C. ❒ 31628, 32484-51
   D. ❒ 31625

4. A surgeon removed the single pacemaker pulse generator from a 79-year-old male and immediately replaced it with a single-chamber pacemaker pulse generator. The same physician did not place the epicardial leads to the permanent pacemaker.
   A. ❒ 33225
   B. ❒ 33234, 33212
   C. ❒ 33234, 33213
   D. ❒ 33233, 33212

5. A surgeon performed biopsies of the right and left breasts on a 37-year-old female who presented with numerous breast lumps bilaterally. The biopsies were performed by using fine needle aspirations and imaging guidance. Also, code for the imaging guidance by computed tomography.
   A. ❒ 77031
   B. ❒ 10022, Radiology: 77012
   C. ❒ 10022, Radiology: 76942
   D. ❒ 19100, Radiology: 76942

6. A surgeon removed the bilateral ventilating tube from an 8-year-old male patient, requiring general anesthesia.
   A. ❒ 31500
   B. ❒ 69424, 00120
   C. ❒ 43760
   D. ❒ 69424-50

7. A surgeon performed a bilateral vasectomy on a 36-year-old male and two postoperative semen examinations.
   A. ❒ 55250
   B. ❒ 55250 × 2
   C. ❒ 55400-50, 55250 × 2
   D. ❒ 55200

8. A surgeon performed a laminectomy with exploration and decompression of the cauda equine without discectomy on three thoracic segments. In the same operative session, a laminotomy with decompression and excision of one cervical disc was performed.
   A. ❒ 63015, 63035
   B. ❒ 63016, 63030-51
   C. ❒ 63016, 63020-51
   D. ❒ 63001, 63020-51

9. A 63-year-old female returned to the operating room during her post-operative period from a hip replacement. A repair was made on the hip, including the graft of a tendon extension from the external oblique muscle to the greater trochanter.
   A. ❒ 27132
   B. ❒ 27100-78
   C. ❒ 27134
   D. ❒ 27105-78

10. A 53-year-old male was prepped and draped in the usual manner as a physician performed an anterovertical hemilaryngectomy. Halfway through the procedure, the patient began to show signs of respiratory and cardiac distress. The anesthesiologist and the physician decided to discontinue the procedure until the patient's vital signs were stable.
    A. ❒ 31370-52
    B. ❒ 31380-52
    C. ❒ 31380-53
    D. ❒ 31577-53

11. Mohs micrographic surgery requires a single physician (1) to act in two integrated but separate and distinct capacities: surgeon and pathologist. If either of these responsibilities is delegated to another physician (2), who reports these services separately, who can report these codes?
    A. ❒ Physician 2
    B. ❒ Physician 1 and 2
    C. ❒ Physician 2 if he or she performed the procedures
    D. ❒ Pathologist

12. A surgeon performed a removal and replacement of an internally dwelling bilateral ureteral stent on an 81-year-old female, using percutaneous approach. Radiological supervision and interpretation was included.
    A. ❒ 50382-50
    B. ❒ 50384-50
    C. ❒ 50387-50
    D. ❒ 50387-50, 72170

13. A surgeon repaired an iliac aneurysm on a 59-year-old male by performing a endovascular graft placement of the iliac with radiological supervision and interpretation. Physician also placed an extension prosthesis during the repair.

   A. ❑ 34900, 34825-51, 75954
   B. ❑ 34900, 75954
   C. ❑ 34825, 75954
   D. ❑ 34900, 34825-51

14. If a procedure is staged for multiple operative sessions and is performed by the same physician during the same postoperative period, what modifier would be reported along with the primary procedure code?

   A. ❑ -59
   B. ❑ -52
   C. ❑ -58
   D. ❑ -78

15. A 37-year-old female, 33 weeks gestation, presented with measurements showing fetal age of over 35 weeks gestation. Physician performed a therapeutic amniocentesis for the reduction of amniotic fluid, which had increased because of fluid retention. Patient did not present with pre-eclamptic symptoms.

   A. ❑ 59001, 59025-51
   B. ❑ 59001
   C. ❑ 59074
   D. ❑ 59012, 59025-51

16. A surgeon performed a corneal incision on an 81-year-old male who had had previous eye surgery that resulted in a surgically induced astigmatism.

   A. ❑ 65435
   B. ❑ 65772
   C. ❑ 65775
   D. ❑ 65865

17. A surgeon performed a bilateral insertion of pressure equalization tubes for a 5-year-old male, using general anesthesia.

   A. ❑ 69436-50, 00320
   B. ❑ 69433-50, 00120
   C. ❑ 69436-50, 00120
   D. ❑ 69436-50

18. A 74-year-old female with a visually significant cataract of left eye was seen preoperatively by her primary care physician. The patient was cleared for local anesthetic. The patient was brought into the ambulatory surgical unit and underwent an uncomplicated phacoemulsification and posterior intraocular lens implant of the left eye using topical anesthetic. She was taken to the recovery room in good condition.

   A. ❑ 66983
   B. ❑ 66984
   C. ❑ 66984-50
   D. ❑ 66830

19. OPERATIVE REPORT

Patient Name: XXXX XXXXX

Date: May 2, XXXX

Preoperative Diagnosis: Bilateral upper eyelid dermatochalasis

Postoperative Diagnosis: Same

Procedure: Bilateral upper lid blepharoplasty

Surgeon: XXXX XXXXX

Indications:

Patient is a 47-year-old female who complained of the above symptoms and elected to have this surgery. The procedure, its alternatives, and risks were discussed with the patient, and she gave consent.

Procedure:

The patient was brought into the operating room and placed in the supine position on the operating table. The patient was intubated, and general anesthesia was induced. A cuffed tube was used to minimize the risk of aspiration. The excess and redundant skin of the upper lids producing redundancy and impairment of lateral vision was carefully measured, and the incisions were marked for fusiform excision with a marking pen. The surgical calipers were used to measure the supratarsal incisions so that the incision was symmetrical from the ciliary margin bilaterally. The upper eyelid areas were bilaterally injected with 1% lidocaine with 1:100,000. The face was prepped and draped in the usual sterile manner. Previously outlined excessive skin, weighing down both lids of both the right and left upper eyelid, was excised with blunt dissection. Hemostasis was obtained with a bipolar cautery. A thin strip of orbicularis oculi muscle was excised in order to expose the orbital septum on the right. The defect in the orbital septum was identified, and herniated orbital fat was exposed. The abnormally protruding positions in the medial pocket were carefully excised and the stalk meticulously cauterized with the bipolar cautery unit. A similar procedure was performed exposing a herniated portion of the nasal pocket. The lateral aspects of the upper eyelid incisions were closed with a couple of interrupted 4-0 Vicryl sutures. The patient was extubated and sent to the recovery room in stable condition, having tolerated the procedure well.

   A. ❑ 15822
   B. ❑ 15823-50
   C. ❑ 15820, 15821-50
   D. ❑ 15822, 15823

20. OPERATIVE REPORT

Patient Name: XXXX XXXXX

Date: August 27, XXXX

Preoperative Diagnosis: Squamous cell carcinoma of the scalp

Postoperative Diagnosis: Same

Operation Performed: Excision of malignant lesion of the scalp, advancement flap closure, with a total area of 13 centimeters by 17 centimeters.

Surgeon: XXXX XXXXX

Indications: Patient was a 49-year-old male with a 6-cm lesion of the anterior midline scalp which was biopsy-positive for skin malignancy, specifically, squamous cell carcinoma. This appeared to be affixed to the underlying scalp. The procedure, its alternatives and risks, were discussed with the patient, and he gave consent.

Procedure: The patient was taken to the operating room and was placed supine on the operating room table. The area was prepped with Hibiclens. The area around the face and scalp was anesthesized with 1% lidocaine with epinephrine 1:100,000. The head was prepped and draped in the usual sterile fashion. A supraperiosteal radical resection was performed. The tumor was located at the deep margin measuring 6 cm and involving the periosteum. The edges were marked along the four quadrants and were sent for frozen section evaluation. Frozen section revealed positive margins at one end of the resection. Therefore, an additional circumferential resection was performed, and the final margins were all negative. The circumferential periosteal margins were noted to be negative. Advancement flaps were created, both on the left and the right side of the scalp, with the total undermined area being approximately 18 cm by 16 cm. The galea was incised in multiple areas, to provide for additional mobilization of the tissue. The tissue was closed under tension with 3-0 Vicryl suture deep in the galea and surgical staples superficially.

The patient was taken to the recovery room in stable condition.

DISPOSITION: The patient was discharged to home. A bulky pressure dressing of gauze and paper tape was applied to the scalp and forehead. Written wound care instructions were reviewed in detail with the patient. A follow-up visit was scheduled for the patient.

    A. ❏ 11644, 14041

    B. ❏ 11626, 14021

    C. ❏ 11606, 12034

    D. ❏ 11644, 12044

CHAPTER 8

Radiology Review

Learning Objectives

- The student will review all of the standards and guidelines organization, format and content of the CPT Radiology section.

- The student will review and interpret CPT radiology notes/reports and assign codes accordingly.

- The student will review and assign all modifiers that are pertinent in the Radiology section.

- The student will review the difference between technical components and supervision and interpretation as it relates to radiology.

Remember to use all appropriate modifiers such as -26, the modifier for professional component, and you will be ready to ace this part of your examination."

Key terms

Arthrography
Dosimetry
Intravascularly
Pathology
Tangential

From the Author...

"Mastery of the Radiology section depends on understanding how this section is arranged. The section begins with Diagnostic Radiology, which is arranged by anatomical sites beginning with the head and neck and continuing down the body. Following Diagnostic Radiology is a series of subsections that contain specific notes on each radiological intervention. Again, please read all notes carefully before assigning codes, especially the notes that accompany nuclear medicine.

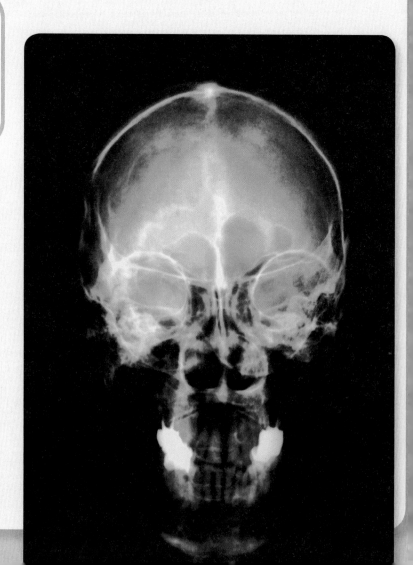

The Radiology section of the CPT manual includes the following subsections:

- Diagnostic Radiology (Diagnostic Imaging)
- Diagnostic Ultrasound
- Radiological Guidance
- Breast, Mammography
- Bone/Joint Studies
- Radiation Oncology
- Nuclear Medicine

Supervision and Interpretation

As you know, many codes in the Radiology section of the CPT manual include the phrase "radiological supervision and interpretation" in the code descriptor. These codes are used to describe the radiological component of a procedure that most often two physicians perform. When a physician both performs the procedure and provides imaging supervision and interpretation, a combination of procedure codes outside of the 70000 series are to be reported. Please remember (read your notes) that the radiological supervision and interpretation codes do not apply to the radiation oncology subsection.

Coding Alert!

Example of a "complete" procedure:
Injection procedure for shoulder *arthrography*
The physician is allowed to submit codes 23350, 73040
Code 23350 is for the injection procedure, and code 73040 is for the radiological supervision and interpretation of the results.

Modifiers in the Radiology Section

The modifiers most commonly used in the Radiology section are outlined in Table 8.1.

Table 8.1 Commonly Used Modifiers in the Radiology Section

Modifier	Description
-22 Increased Procedural Services	When the work required to provide a service is substantially greater than typically required, it may be identified by adding the modifier -22 to the usual procedure code. Documentation must support the substantial additional work and the reason for the additional work.
-26 Professional Component	Certain procedures are a combination of a physician component and a technical component. When the physician component is reported separately, the service may be identified by adding modifier -26 tothe usual procedure number.
-51 Multiple Procedures	When multiple procedures, other than E&M services, physical medicine and rehabilitation services, or provision of supplies, are performed at the same session by the same provider, the primary procedure or service may be reported as listed. The additional procedure (s) or service(s) may be identified by appending modifier -51 to the additional procedure or service code(s).
-52 Reduced Services	Under certain circumstances a service or procedure is reduced or eliminated at the physician's discretion. Under these circumstances, the service provided can be identified by its usual procedure number and the addition of modifier -52, signifying that the service is reduced. This provides means of reporting reduced services without disturbing the identification of the basic service.
-53 Discontinued Procedure	Under certain circumstances, the physician may elect to terminate a surgical or diagnostic procedure because of extenuating circumstances or those that threaten the well being of a patient. Under these circumstances, modifier -53 indicates that a surgical or diagnostic procedure was started but then discontinued.
-59 Distinct Procedural Service	Under certain circumstances, the physician may need to indicate that a procedure or service was distinct or independent from other services performed on the same day. This service can be identified by modifier -59.
-TC Technical component	This modifier is added if the radiologist or the provider performs the radiologic procedure.

Think Like A Coder 8.1

Choose the correct answer for the following problem. The phrase "with contrast" used in the codes for procedures performed with contrast for imaging enhancement represents contrast material administered:

intrathecally

intra-articularly

intravascularly

intrathecally, intra-articularly, and intravascularly

Professional Versus Technical Component

When coding for radiology services, the codes must accompany the appropriate modifiers if applicable. Radiological procedures include both a technical component and a professional component. The modifier for technical component for a radiology code is TC and the modifier for a professional component is -26. If the physician performs both components of the radiological procedure, it is considered a "global procedure" for which only the radiology code is assigned.

Example:

Code 73719 appears as:

73719   Magnetic resonance imaging, lower extremity other than joint; with contrast material(s)

To code for the technical component only, the assignment would be:

73719TC

To code for the professional component only, the assignment would be:

73719-26

To code for the global procedure in which one physician performed both components, the assignment would be:

73719

Special Report

To help determine medical appropriateness, a "special report" must always be attached when a procedure or service is rarely provided, unusual, or new. Important information should include a detailed description of the nature, extent, and the need for the procedure or service and the time, effort, and equipment necessary to provide the service to the patient. Additional items that may be included for special reports are as follows:

- Complexity of symptoms presented
- Final diagnosis
- Pertinent physical findings such as size, locations, and number of lesions
- Diagnostic and therapeutic procedures, including major and supplementary surgical procedures
- Concurrent problems
- Follow-up care

Administration of Contrast Materials

The phrase "with contrast" used in the codes for procedures performed with contrast for imaging enhancement represents contrast material administered intravascularly, intra-articularly or intrathecally. For intra-articular injection, use the appropriate joint injection code. If radiographic arthrography is performed, also use the arthrography supervision and interpretation code for the appropriate joint. If computer tomography (CT) or magnetic resonance (MR) arthrography is performed without radiographic arthrography, use the appropriate joint injection code, the appropriate CT or MR, code, and the appropriate imaging guidance code for needle placement for contrast injection. For spine examinations using CT, MR imaging (MRI), or MR angiography, "with contrast" includes intrathecal or intravascular injection. For intrathecal injection, use also code 61055 or 62284.

Injection of intravascular contrast material is part of the "with contrast" CT, CT angiography, MRI, and MR angiography procedures. Oral and/or rectal contrast administration alone does not qualify as a study "with contrast."

Radiology System Coding Notes for Review

Aorta and Arteries

Diagnostic angiography, description of the blood vessels, and radiological supervision and interpretation codes should not be used with the interventional procedures for:

- Contrast injections, angiography, roadmapping, and/or fluoroscopic guidance for intervention.

- Vessel measurement.
- Postangioplasty/stent angiography.

Diagnostic angiography (see Figure 8.1) performed at the time of an interventional procedure is separately reportable if:

- No prior catheter-based angiographic study is available and a full diagnostic study is performed, and the decision to intervene is based on the diagnostic study.
- The prior study is available, but as documented in the medical record:
  - The patient's condition with respect to the clinical indication has changed since the prior study.

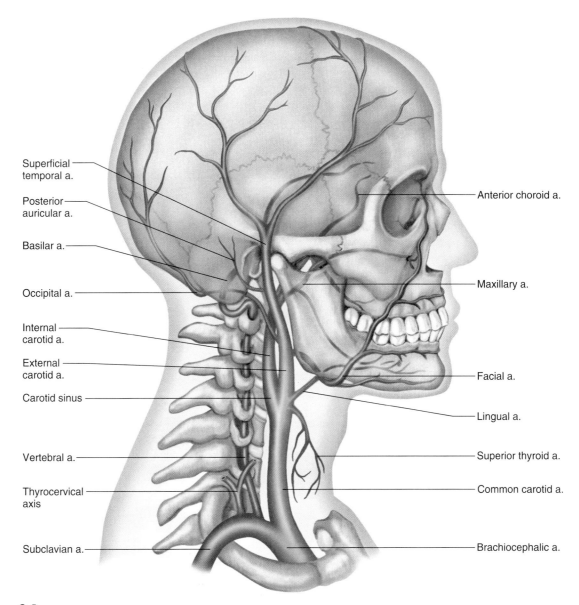

Superficial temporal a.
Posterior auricular a.
Basilar a.
Occipital a.
Internal carotid a.
External carotid a.
Carotid sinus
Vertebral a.
Thyrocervical axis
Subclavian a.

Anterior choroid a.
Maxillary a.
Facial a.
Lingual a.
Superior thyroid a.
Common carotid a.
Brachiocephalic a.

Figure 8.1

Diagnostic Angiography – Main arteries of the head and neck. An angiogram is a radiographic record of the size, shape, and location of blood vessels. This figure shows the arteries associated with the head.

From D. Shier et al., Hole's *Human Anatomy & Physiology*, 11e. Copyright © 2007 The McGraw-Hill Companies. Reprinted with permission.

- There is inadequate visualization of the anatomy and/or **pathology.**
- There is a clinical change during the procedure that requires new evaluation.

Please be advised that diagnostic angiography performed alone in a separate setting and is not included as part of the interventional procedure is separately reported. Diagnostic angiography performed at the time of an interventional procedure is not reported separately, as it is part of the procedure and its descriptor.

Example

Code: +75774 Angiography, selective, each additional vessel studies after basic examination, and radiological supervision, and interpretation. (List separately in addition to code for primary procedure).

Veins and Lymphatics

Veins and Lymphatics have important notes that you must be careful to take into consideration while assigning from this subsection. Diagnostic venography (radiological supervision and interpretation) codes should not be used with interventional procedures for:

- Contrast injections, venography, roadmapping, and/or fluoroscopic guidance for the intervention.
- Vessel measurement.
- Postangioplasty/stent venography.

This work is captured in the radiological supervision and interpretation codes. Diagnostic venography performed at the time of an interventional procedure is separately reportable if:

- No prior catheter-based venography study is available and a full diagnostic study is performed, and the decision to intervene is based on the diagnostic study.
- A prior study is available, but as documented in the medical record:

    - The patient's condition with respect to the clinical indication has changed since the prior study.
    - There is inadequate visualization of the anatomy and/or pathology.
    - There is a clinical change during the procedure that requires new evaluation outside the target area of intervention.

Please be advised that diagnostic venography performed in a separate setting from an interventional procedure is separately reported unless it is part of the interventional procedure and then it is not reported and is specifically included in the interventional code.

Coding Alert!

Diagnostic venography and diagnostic angiography performed in a separate setting from an interventional procedure is separately reported.

Indexing Tip:

For procedures that include fluoroscopic guidance, you can index the term "fluoroscopy" and see listing by anatomical site.

Diagnostic Ultrasound

When clinically indicated, diagnostic ultrasound examinations require permanently recorded images with measurements and a final, written report issued for the patient's medical record. Ultrasound procedures also require permanently recorded images of the site (abdomen, retroperitoneum, pelvis, etc.) to be localized, as well as documented description of the localization process, either separately or within the report itself. Table 8.2 outlines the four types of diagnostic ultrasounds.

Table 8.2 Diagnostic Ultrasound Types

Ultrasound Type	Definition
A-Mode	One-dimensional ultrasonic measurement
M-Mode	One-dimensional ultrasonic measurement with movement of the trace to record amplitude and velocity of moving echo-producing structures
B-scan	Two-dimensional ultrasonic scanning with a two-dimensional display
Real-time scan	Two-dimensional ultrasonic scanning with display of both two-dimensional structure and motion and time
Doppler Ultrasound	Evaluates movement by measuring changes in the frequency of echoes reflected from moving structures.

Indexing Tip:

The quickest and most accurate way to find diagnostic ultrasound codes is by indexing "ultrasound" or "echography," then indexing by anatomical site.

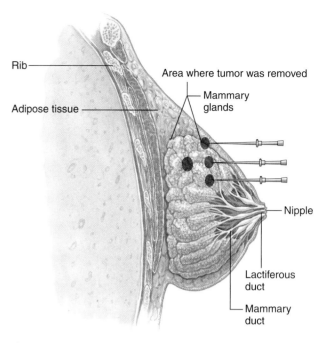

Figure 8.2

Radiation Oncology: The brachytherapy procedure involves placing tiny flexible, plastic catheters into the breast that deliver a concentrated radiation dose. The procedure usually takes 4 to 7 days instead of weeks.

From N. Thierer and L. Breitbard, *Medial Terminology, Language for Health Care*, 2e. Copyright © 2006 The McGraw-Hill Companies, Inc. Reprinted with permission.

Radiation Oncology

Radiation oncology is designed for the therapeutic use of shrinking or eliminating neoplastic tumors. Types of radiation include electromagnetic radiation, which is composed of x-rays and gamma rays. The delivery method used for therapeutic radiation treatment can be internal or external. Internal radiation, or brachytherapy, is applied by placing the radioactive material inside the patient in close proximity to the tumor or lesion (see Figure 8.2). External radiation is applied by targeting a beam of radiation through the patient's skin toward the area of the tumor. In the listings for radiation oncology, codes for teletherapy and brachytherapy include initial consultation, clinical treatment planning, simulation, medical radiation, physics, **dosimetry,** treatment devices, special services, and clinical treatment management procedures. Codes from the CPT Evaluation and Management Section, Surgery or Medicine Sections are reported by the radiation oncologists who provides:

1. Preliminary consultation services.
2. Evaluates a patient prior to the decision to treat.
3. Delivers full medical care in addition to the treatment management.

They include normal follow-up care during course of treatment and for three months following its completion.

Clinical Treatment Planning

Clinical treatment planning is complex and comprise various services such as:

- Interpretation of special testing
- Treatment volume determination
- Treatment time and dosage determination
- Choice of treatment modality

 Indexing Tip:

For codes used in Radiation Oncology (77280–77799), index the term "radiation therapy" for quick and accurate coding assignment.

Coding Alert!

Radiologists provide consultations before beginning a treatment plan. These treatment planning consultations should be coded along with the appropriate surgical, medicine, or evaluation and management code.

- Tumor localization
- Determination of number and size of treatment ports

Three levels of service describe clinical treatment planning for radiation therapy: simple, intermediate, and complex. The clinical management of therapeutic radiology simulation-aided setting is described in Table 8.3.

Radiation Treatment Management

Radiation treatment management is reported in units of treatments sessions or fractions regardless of the actual

Table 8.3 Clinical Treatment Planning Management

Treatment Level of Planning Management	Definition
Simple	Simulation of a single treatment area with either a single port or parallel opposed ports and simple or no blocking.
Intermediate	Simulation of three or more converging ports, two separate treatment areas, and multiple blocks.
Complex	Simulation of **tangential** portals, three or more treatment areas, rotation or arc therapy, complex blocking, custom shielding blocks, brachytherapy source verification, hyperthermia probe verification, and any use of contrast materials.
Three-dimensional	Three-dimensional (3D) computer-generated reconstruction of tumor volume and surrounding critical normal tissue structures from direct CT scans and/or MRI data in preparation for non-coplanar or coplanar therapy. The simulation uses documented 3D beam's eye view of volume-dose displays or multiple or moving beams. Documentation with 3D volume reconstruction and dose distribution is required.

time period in which the services are furnished. These services do not have to be furnished on consecutive days; however, there must be a distinct break in the therapy session for multiple fractions representing two or more treatment sessions furnished on the same day. The professional services furnished during treatment management consist of:

- Review of port films
- Review of dosimetry, dose delivery, and treatment parameters
- Review of patient treatment set-up
- Examination of patient for medical evaluation and management

Proton Beam Treatment Delivery

Proton beam treatment delivery concentrates the radiation in a much smaller area than radiation treatment, releasing most of its energy in and directly around the tumor. In Table 8.4, the levels of complexity of proton beam treatment delivery are defined.

Clinical Brachytherapy

Clinical brachytherapy consists of natural or man-made radioactive elements that are internally applied to the affected area or in close proximity to the affected area (see Figure 8.2). There are three levels of intracavitary placements for brachytherapy:

- A *simple* application has one to four sources or ribbons.
- An *intermediate* application has 5 to 10 sources or ribbons.
- A *complex* application has more than 10 sources or ribbons.

The "sources" described refer to the intracavitary placement or permanent interstitial placement. The "ribbons" refer to temporary interstitial placement.

Indexing Tip:

Under "Brachytherapy," code descriptors consist of phrases such as "infusion" or "installation of radio-element." Unless you know that this specifically refers to brachytherapy, you may index > application > radioelement, for quick and accurate coding assignment.

Table 8.4 Levels of Proton Beam Delivery

Proton Beam Level of Complexity	Definition
Simple	Proton treatment delivery to a single treatment area by a single non-**tangential**/oblique port, with custom block with compensation
Intermediate	Proton treatment delivery to one or more treatment areas by two or more ports or one or more tangential/oblique ports, with custom blocks and compensators
Complex	Proton treatment delivery to one or more treatment areas by two or more ports per treatment area with matching or patching fields and/or multiple isocenters, with custom blocks and compensators

APPLYING CODING THEORY TO PRACTICE

Choose the correct radiology coding assignment. (Please see Appendix A for answers and rationale).

1. A radiologist performed a CT scan on a 12-year-old male's inner ear without contrast material, followed by CT with contrast material on the inner ear and further sections of the ear.
   A. ❏ 70488
   B. ❏ 70482
   C. ❏ 70481
   D. ❏ 70120

2. A physician performed a postoperative biliary duct calculi removal by use of Burhenne technique and provided the radiological supervision and interpretation.
   A. ❏ 74327
   B. ❏ 47554, 74363
   C. ❏ 47630, 74327
   D. ❏ 47554, 75982

3. A physician performed a renal scan with vascular flow and a function study on a 77-year-old diabetic female without pharmacological intervention.
   A. ❏ 78709
   B. ❏ 78700, 78709
   C. ❏ 78707
   D. ❏ 78701

4. A physician performed a positron emission tomography scan for whole body tumor imaging for a 51-year-old male. The scan was interrupted by the occurrence of petit mal seizures in the patient, and the procedure took 45 minutes longer than usual to complete.
   A. ❏ 78802-26
   B. ❏ 78813-22
   C. ❏ 78814-22
   D. ❏ 78813-59

5. RADIOLOGY REPORT: UPPER GI SERIES, KUB WITH DELAYED
   FILMS, HIGH-DENSITY BARIUM
   An upper gastrointestinal series and kidney, ureter, and bladder study reveals a moderate amount of fecal matter present in the colon. Barium reveals normal esophagus, and the stomach is transverse in type. Present is a small sliding hiatal hernia; the stomach empties well, and the duodenal bulb fills moderately with ulceration.
   IMPRESSION: Small sliding hiatal hernia
   A. ❏ 74235
   B. ❏ 74241-26
   C. ❏ 74246-26
   D. ❏ 74247

6. A physician performed angiography on a left external carotid, selective, on a 62-year-old male, including supervision and interpretation.
   A. ❏ 75662
   B. ❏ 75665
   C. ❏ 75660
   D. ❏ 75680

7. A physician performed the supervision and interpretation only for a radiological examination, six views of the mandible, on a 22-year-old male who was the victim of a gang fight.
   A. ❏ 70110-26
   B. ❏ 70110-52
   C. ❏ 70150-26
   D. ❏ 70330-26

8. RADIOLOGY REPORT: CHEST X-RAY
   A 46-year-old female presented to the emergency department with a six day history of wheezing, coughing, and blood in sputum. The patient was given albuterol and arterial blood gases were taken. A chest radiological examination consisting of two frontal and lateral views and oblique projections was given. Past medical history revealed previous history of emergency services for asthma and pneumonia. The patient was placed on prednisone, 40 mg b.i.d. The chest x-ray was positive for infiltrates, and the report was sent to the oncology department.
   IMPRESSION: Rule out malignant neoplasm
   A. ❏ 99283, 71022
   B. ❏ 99282, 71030
   C. ❏ 99283, 71023
   D. ❏ 99283, 71035

9. A physician performed a static-only spleen imaging with vascular flow as well as a liver study for a 37-year-old male with suspected cirrhosis of the liver.
   A. ❏ 78185, 78202
   B. ❏ 78185, 78206
   C. ❏ 78185, 78216
   D. ❏ 78216

10. A physician performed myocardial perfusion imaging, single study during exercise, for a 39-year-old male, with quantification. A cardiovascular stress test using maximal bicycle exercise with continuous electrocardiographic monitoring was performed along with physician supervision, interpretation, and report.
    A. ❏ 93017
    B. ❏ 78461, 93015
    C. ❏ 78460, 93015
    D. ❏ 78459, 93015

11. A physician created a complex brachytherapy isodose plan involving 11 ribbons, volume implant calculations, and over 13 sources for remote afterloading.
    A. ❏ 77290, 77327
    B. ❏ 77328
    C. ❏ 77315
    D. ❏ 77784

12. A 27-year-old male was referred to an oncologist after a diagnosis oral cancer. The physician prescribed radiopharmaceutical therapy by oral administration.
    A. ❏ 77402
    B. ❏ 77373
    C. ❏ 79005
    D. ❏ 70328

129

13. A physician performed a flexible, diagnostic esophagoscopy with removal of a foreign body and collection of a specimen by washing. A different physician provided radiological supervision and interpretation for the procedure.

A. ❑ 74235, 43200

B. ❑ 74235-26

C. ❑ 43215

D. ❑ 43215, 74235

14. Physician "A" performed a percutaneous placement of an inferior vena cava filter. Physician "B" provided radiological supervision and interpretation for the procedure.

A. ❑ Physician A: 77761 Physician B: 31643

B. ❑ Physician A: 75945 Physician B: No code would be reported

C. ❑ Physician A: 75940 Physician B: 37620

D. ❑ Physician A: 75940 Physician B: No code would be reported

15. A physician performed a CT scan of the soft tissue neck with contrast material and a report of 3D rendering, interpretation, and report requiring image post-processing on an independent workstation, for a 16-year-old female.

A. ❑ 70487, 76376

B. ❑ 70360, 76377

C. ❑ 70491

D. ❑ 70491, 76377

16. RADIOLOGY REPORT: AP & Lateral of Left Foot
Views of the left foot on a 37-year-old male injured during football practice reveal a line of translucency in the proximal shaft in the fourth toe proximal to PIP, proximal interphalangeal. Soft tissue swelling is also noted.
IMPRESSION: Nondisplaced fracture of the shaft of the fourth proximal phalanx.

A. ❑ 73630

B. ❑ 73620

C. ❑ 73718

D. ❑ 73719

17. A 51-year-old male underwent a percutaneous transcatheter introduction of vascular stent, external iliac artery. Code for the technical component only.

A. ❑ 75961-TC

B. ❑ 75960-26

C. ❑ 75960-TC

D. ❑ 75896

18. A 36-year-old female, car accident victim, underwent the following x-rays: Neck, six views including oblique and flexion, and thoracic spine two views. Code for supervision and interpretation only.

A. ❑ 72080-26, 72070-TC

B. ❑ 70360-26, 72070-26

C. ❑ 72052-TC, 72070-26

D. ❑ 72052-26, 72070-26

19. During a routine hip replacement surgery on a 71-year-old female, the physician opted to have an x-ray taken of the patient's hip. After the interpretation of the x-ray was completed, the physician continued with the surgery, which resulted in a successful left hip replacement. Code for the global procedure.

A. ❑ 73500

B. ❑ 73530

C. ❑ 73525-26

D. ❑ 73525-TC

20. A physician provided the supervision and interpretation of a cardiac MRI for morphology and function without contrast material with velocity quantification and stress.

A. ❑ 75560-26

B. ❑ 75558

C. ❑ 75558-26

D. ❑ 75564-26

CHAPTER 9

Pathology and Laboratory Review

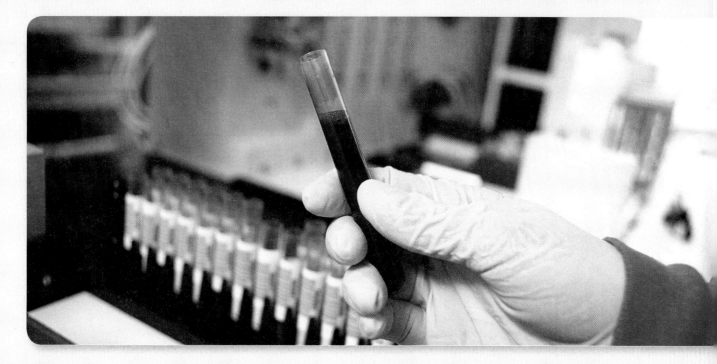

Learning Objectives

- The student will review all of the standards and guidelines organization, format, and content of the Pathology and Laboratory section.

- The student will review and interpret CPT Pathology and Laboratory notes and assign codes accordingly.

- The student will review and assign all modifiers that are pertinent in the Pathology and Laboratory section.

- The student will review the difference between quantitative and qualitative testing.

- The student will review the different levels of surgical pathology.

Key terms

Acronyms	Infusions
Antibodies	Morphology
Antigens	Prothrombin
Enucleation	Quantitative
Evocative	Qualitative
Immunoglobulin	

From the Author...

"The Pathology and Laboratory section of the CPT manual is unique compared with all of the other sections in the manual. It covers chemicals, compounds, drugs, **antigens, antibodies,** tissues, cells, and anatomical parts. The diversity of this section makes it difficult to understand all of the testing and the **acronyms** that accompany the descriptors. To code successfully and accurately in this section, the key is to index with precision. For example, to find the code for TSI, you can index either TSI or thyroid stimulating immune globulins. Be precise when you index and when you read the descriptors. The descriptors can become confusing, as many of them have "look alikes" with very similar spelling. Read carefully and assign with precision!"

The Pathology and Laboratory section of the CPT manual includes the following subsections:

- Organ-oriented or Disease-Oriented Panels
- Drug Testing
- Therapeutic Drug Assays
- Evocative/Suppression Testing
- Consultations (Clinical Pathology)
- Urinalysis
- Chemistry
- Hematology and Coagulation
- Immunology
- Tissue Typing
- Transfusion Medicine
- Microbiology
- Anatomic Pathology
- Cytopathology
- Cytogenic Studies
- Surgical Pathology
- Transcutaneous Procedures
- Other Procedures
- Reproductive Medicine Procedures

The Pathology and Laboratory section of the CPT manual includes services by a physician or technologists under the responsible supervision of a physician. These codes are used for diagnostic studies, drug testing and assays, consultations, toxicology, chemistry, hematology, immunology, and surgical and anatomic pathology. Under a physician's orders, medical technologists or other qualified allied health professionals perform a range of highly specialized tests by examining body specimens, body fluids, tissues, and cells. Medical laboratory professionals prepare the specimens for gross or microscopic examination and test interpretation and analyze chemical components of submitted specimens. Test results are then reported to the physician who ordered the test for interpretation and possible diagnosis.

> **Coding Alert!**
>
> It is appropriate to designate multiple procedures in the Pathology and Laboratory section that are rendered on the same date by separate entities.

Qualitative and Quantitative Tests

The Pathology and Laboratory section of the CPT manual includes many codes that refer to the procedures or test as "**quantitative**" or "**qualitative.**" Qualitative screening refers to tests that detect the presence of a particular substance and the quality or condition of the substance. Quantitative screening refers to test results that express numerical amounts of the substance being tested. Quantitative studies typically follow qualitative studies because the presence of the substance has been established.

Table 9.1 Commonly Used Modifiers in the Pathology and Laboratory Section

Modifier	Description
-22 Unusual Procedural Services	When the service(s) provided is (are) greater than that usually required for the listed procedure, it may be identified by adding modifier -22 to the usual procedure number. A report may also be appropriate.
-26 Professional Component	Certain circumstances in pathology and laboratory require a combination of physician component and a technical component. When the physician component is reported separately from the technical component, the service may be identified by adding modifier -26 to the usual procedure number.
-32 Multiple Procedures	Services related to mandated consultation and/or related services such as a third-party payer or governmental agency may be identified by using modifier -32.
-52 Reduced Services	Under certain circumstances, a service or procedure may be reduced or eliminated at the physician's discretion. Under these circumstances, the service provided can be identified by its usual procedure number and the addition of modifier -52, signifying that the service is reduced.
-53 Discontinued Procedure	Under certain circumstances, the physician may elect to terminate a surgical or diagnostic procedure because of extenuating circumstances or those that threaten the well being of the patient. This circumstance may be reported by adding modifier -53 to the code. This modifier is not used to report the discontinuance of a procedure based on a patient's decision to do so.

(Continued)

Table 9.1 Continued

Modifier	Description
-59 Distinct Procedural Service	Under certain circumstances, the physician may need to indicate that a procedure or service was distinct or independent from other services performed on the same day. Modifier-59 is used to identify procedures/services that are not normally reported together but are appropriate under the circumstances. This may represent a different session or patient encounter.
-90 Reference (Outside) Laboratory	When laboratory procedures are performed by a party other than the treating or reporting physician, the procedure may be identified by adding modifier -90 to the usual procedure number.
-91 Repeat Clinical Diagnostic Laboratory Test	In the course of treatment of the patient, it may be necessary to repeat the same laboratory test on the same day to obtain subsequent (multiple) test results. Under these circumstances, the laboratory test performed can be identified by its usual procedure number and the addition of modifier -91.

Pathology and Laboratory Notes for Review

Organ or Disease-Oriented Panels

Disease-oriented panels are laboratory tests in which more than one procedure is typically performed from just one blood sample of a patient. These panels include basic metabolic panels, general health panels, thyroid stimulating hormone panel, obstetric panel, lipid panel, renal function panel, hepatitis panel, and hepatic function panel. For an example of an organ or disease-oriented panel, see Figure 9.1. These panel components are not intended to limit the performance of other tests. If a test is performed in addition to those specifically indicated for a specific panel, those tests should be reported separately in addition to the disease-oriented panel code. The most commonly used panels are the general health panel, obstetric panel, and basic metabolic panel. If a panel isn't complete, the coder must code each substance separately. Remember to not use modifier -52 for reduced service if a panel isn't complete.

> ### Example – 80076
>
> **Hepatic Function Panel**
> *This panel must include the following:*
> Albumin (82040)
> Bilirubin, total (82247)
> Bilirubin, direct (82248)
> Phosphatase, alkaline (84075)
> Protein, total (84155)
> Transferase, alanine amino (AST) (SGOT) (84450)

Drug Testing

Code the number of procedures not the number of drugs tested. Please keep in mind that qualitative analysis does not identify the amount of the drug present, just that the

80047   Basic metabolic panel (calcium, ionized)

This panel must include the following:

Calcium, ionized (82330)

Carbon dioxide (82374)

Chloride (82435)

Creatinine (82565)

Glucose (82947)

Potassium (84132)

Sodium (84295)

Urea Nitrogen (BUN) (84520)

80055   Obstetric panel

This panel must include the following:

Blood count, complete (CBC), automated and automated differential WBC count (85025 or 85027 and 85004)

OR

Blood count, complete (CBC), automated (85027) and appropriate manual differential WBC count (85007 or 85009)

Hepatitis B surface antigen (HBsAg) (87340)

Antibody, rubella (86762)

Syphilis test, qualitative (eg, VDRL, RPR, ART) (86592)

Antibody screen, RBC, each serum technique (86850)

Blood typing, ABO (86900) AND

Blood typing, Rh (D) (86901)

Figure 9.1

Basic Metabolic and Obstetrical Panels – Two of the most commonly used panels in medical coding.

Source: *Current Procedural Terminology,* American Medical Association, 2008.

drug or substance is present. The following is a list of drugs or classes of drugs that are commonly assayed (the analysis of a substance) by qualitative screen, followed by confirmation with a second method:

- Alcohols
- Amphetamines
- Barbiturates
- Benzodiazepines
- Cocaine and metabolites
- Methadones
- Methaqualones
- Opiates
- Phencyclidines
- Phenothiazines
- Propoxyphenes
- Tetrahydrocannabinoids
- Tricyclic antidepressants

Confirmed drugs may also be quantitated. Use 80100 for each multiple drug class chromatographic procedure. Use 80102 for each procedure necessary for confirmation. For chromatography, each combination of stationary and mobile phase should be counted as one procedure. If multiple drugs can be detected by using a single analysis, use 80100 only once.

Example

Code: *80102*

A drug confirmation test was conducted on 15-year-old male who tested positive for alcohol and cocaine.

Code Assignment: *80102 × 2*

Evocative/Suppression Testing

Evocative refers to a substance that a patient must take because of the body's inability to produce it naturally. Evocative and suppression testing allows the physician to determine a baseline of the chemical being tested and the effects on the body after evocation. Test panel codes 80400-80440, should be used for the reporting of the laboratory component of the overall testing protocol. You will use codes

---

Coding Alert!

Please note that the descriptors for each panel with evocative/suppression testing identifies the type of test included in that panel and the number of times the test must be performed.
Example: 80408 Aldosterone suppression evaluation panel
This panel must include the following:
Aldosterone (82088 × 2)
Renin (84244 × 2)

90760, 90761, 90722-90744, 90755 for the physician's administration of the evocative and suppression agents and 99070 for supplies and drugs. Use the proper evaluation and management code to report attendance and monitoring during the testing. Prolonged physician care codes are not reported separately when these tests involve prolonged **infusions** reported with codes 90760-90761.

Urinalysis

The Urinalysis subsection includes codes for several methods of urinalysis. Codes 81000-81099 are assigned for the analysis of one or more components of the urine. The reported code is based on the method by which the urine is tested, (tablet reagent, dipstick), the element being tested (protein, bacteria), and the purpose for the urinalysis (e.g., vaginitis, pregnancy). The most basic service for urinalysis is the dipstick, which is a small strip of plastic that contains a chemical that reacts to products in the urine, if they are present, by changing colors. Automated urinalysis requires less medical decision-making for the physician and is a less complex method. An automated urinalysis is performed with the help of automated medical equipment, and manual is performed by a pathologist/physician without the help of automated medical equipment. If it is not specified in the medical record whether the urinalysis was automated or manual, the coder should assume that the automated method was used.

This section not only distinguishes urinalysis codes by automated versus manual but also with microscopy versus without microscopy. "With microscopy" indicates the urine was further assessed by the physician using a microscope to view for bacteria and other elements to aid in diagnosis. "Without microscopy" indicates the diagnosis is made by viewing the urine without the aid of a microscope.

Example

Urinalysis; non-automated, without microscopy

Code: *81002 Urinalysis, by dipstick or tablet reagent for bilirubin, glucose hemoglobin, ketones, leukocytes, intrite, pH, protein, specific gravity, urobilinogen, any number of these constituents; nonautomated, without microscopy.*

Chemistry

Chemistry codes are used to report individual chemistry tests for such substances as aluminum, ammonia, and amino acids. The material for examination may be from any source unless the code descriptor indicates otherwise. All of these codes refer to quantitative analysis (numerical value of quantity) unless directed otherwise. When an analyte (substance being analyzed) is measured in multiple specimens from different sources or in specimens that are obtained at different times, the analyte is reported separately for each source and for each specimen.

Example

Chemistry Codes

82127 Amino acids; single, qualitative, each specimen

82128 multiple, qualitative, each specimen

82131 single, quantitative, each specimen

Please keep in mind, if the clinical information compiled from the results of laboratory data is calculated mathematically, it is considered part of the test and is not expected to be reported separately.

 Indexing Tip:

When indexing codes for drug testing, drug assays, and chemistry, look under the name of the substance (analyte) being analyzed.

Example:

Aminolevulinic acid, delta (ALA)

Index: Aminolevulinic acid

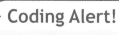 Coding Alert!

Consultations

A clinical pathology consultation is a service, including a written report, rendered by the pathologist in response to a request from an attending physician in relation to a test result requiring additional medical interpretive judgment.

 Think Like A Coder 9.1

Choose the correct codes for the following problems.

1. A physician ordered an ACTH stimulation panel for 3 beta-hydroxydehydrogenase deficiency in a 21-year-old female.

   80418

   80400

   80406

   80402

2. A physician ordered the following test panel: general health panel including comprehensive metabolic panel, automated complete blood count, and automated differential white blood count for a 37-year-old male.

   80050

   80050, 80053, 85027, 85004

   80053, 85027, 85004

   80050, 80053, 85025

Hematology and Coagulation

Hematology is the study of the blood and blood diseases. Coagulation is the clumping together of blood cells to form a clot. Hematology and coagulation codes are used to report laboratory tests that involve analyzing the blood for clotting, **prothrombin** time, thrombin time, platelet counts, complete blood counts (CBC), white blood counts (WBC), bone marrow, and smear interpretation. Please remember to pay special attention to the different types of procedures that involve hematology and coagulation. There are two different types of testing: automated and manual. Automated testing is the use of laboratory instruments/equipment that assay (calculate, arrange, group) mechanically. Manual testing is performed by methods that involve less mechanical intervention, such as the use of a counting chamber (hemacytometer) to calculate manually WBCs or red blood counts by using a microscope (see Figure 9.2).

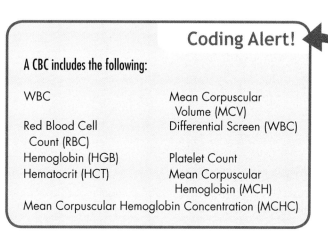

Coding Alert!

A CBC includes the following:

WBC	Mean Corpuscular Volume (MCV)
Red Blood Cell Count (RBC)	Differential Screen (WBC)
Hemoglobin (HGB)	Platelet Count
Hematocrit (HCT)	Mean Corpuscular Hemoglobin (MCH)

Mean Corpuscular Hemoglobin Concentration (MCHC)

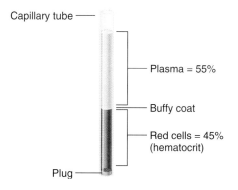

Figure 9.2

A blood-filled capillary tube after centrifuging shows the packed red blood cells at the bottom of the tube that is read at 45 percent by volume. The middle layer is the buffy coat and the top layer consists of 55 percent plasma. The packed red blood cells or the "Hematocrit" is read directly out of the centrifuge by the technician.

From D. Shier et al., Hole's Human Anatomy & Physiology, 11e. Copyright © 2007 The McGraw-Hill Companies. Reprinted with permission.

Immunology

Immunology codes are used to report tests performed on components of the immune system and their functions. The following definitions provide a better understanding of immunology:

- An *adjuvant* is a variety of substances that increase the antigenic response.
- *Antibodies* are immunoglobulins that combine with specific antigens to control or destroy them to provide protection against most common infections.
- *Antigens* are proteins on the surface of a cell that identify the cell and aid in the formation of antibodies.
- An **immunoglobulin** is a protein capable of acting as an antibody to help fight infection.

Think Like A Coder 9.2

Choose the correct code(s) for the following problem.
A physician ordered allergen-specific immunoglobulin G semiquantitative testing of four allergens for a 15-year-old male.

    86003
    86003 × 4
    86001
    86001 × 4

Microbiology

Microbiology is the study of microorganisms (bacteria or protozoan). The codes in the Microbiology subsection aid in the identification of different types of bacteria. Microbiology codes include:

- Bacteriology—the scientific study of bacteria; type and function
- Mycology—the scientific study of fungi; type and function
- Parasitology—the scientific study of parasites; type and function
- Virology—the scientific study of viruses; type and function

Microbiology subsection notes define the following types of identification for microorganisms:

- Presumptive identification—identification of microorganisms by colony **morphology,** growth on selective media, Gram stains, or up to three tests.
- Definitive identification—identification to the genus or species level that requires additional tests. If additional tests involve molecular probes, chromatography, or immunological techniques, these should be reported separately. For multiple specimens/sites, use modifier -59. For repeat laboratory tests performed on the same day, use modifier -91.

Coding Alert!

Remember to report multiple procedures when various microbiology testing procedures are performed.

Example: A physician ordered a bacterial urine culture with quantitative count and a fungi isolation culture on the patient's hair with presumptive identification.

Coding Assignment: 87086, 87101

Indexing Tip:

For quick and accurate coding assignment in the Microbiology subsection, index terms such as "culture," "smear/stain," "cytopathology," and the infectious agent itself, such as candida, hepatitis, and neisseria.

Cytopathology

Cytopathology is the study of the cellular changes in disease. Subsection notes indicate the various cytopathology procedures:

- Fluids, washings, or brushings
- Vaginal or cervical cytopathology; physician and interpretation
- Sex chromatin identification
- Cytohistological study with fine needle aspiration
- Flow cytometry

Please note that Papanicolaou smear screening is reported by the use of the Bethesda or non-Bethesda System. The Bethesda System is a system for reporting cervical or vaginal cytologic diagnosis. The Bethesda System replaces the numerical designations, class 1-5 of the Papanicolaou smear, with descriptive diagnoses of cellular changes.

Example

Code: 88164 Cytopathology, slides, cervical or vaginal (the Bethesda System); manual screening under physician supervision

Surgical Pathology

Surgical pathology is the study of the nature and cause of disease, which involves changes in structure and function. The unit of service in surgical pathology is referred to as a specimen. A specimen is tissue or tissues that are submitted for individual and separate attention, requiring examination and pathologic diagnosis. Keep in mind the basis of reporting is determined by the number of labeled specimens. Two or more such specimens from the same patient are each appropriately assigned an individual code that reflects the proper level of service. Services 88300-88309 include accession (number assigned to indicate the order of tissue acquisition), examination, and reporting. Levels I-VI are outlined in Table 9.2.

Think Like A Coder 9.3

Choose the correct code for the following problem. A pathologist performed the gross and microscopic examination of an 81-year-old female's left lower leg after a nontraumatic amputation.

27598

27598, 88305

88307

88309

Coding Alert!

When a physician has examined two or more specimens, separate codes should be used to identify the appropriate levels for each.

Table 9.2 Surgical Pathology Levels

Level	Physician Work	Example
Level I	Surgical pathology, gross examination only	Gross examination of renal calculi
Level II	Surgical pathology, gross and microscopic examination	Gross and microscopic examination of vaginal mucosa
Level III-VI	Surgical pathology, gross and microscopic examination	All other specimens that require gross and microscopic examination with ascending levels of physician work
	Level III Surgical pathology, gross and microscopic examination	Ganglion cyst
	Level IV Surgical pathology, gross and microscopic examination	Lung, transbronchial biopsy
	Level V Surgical pathology, gross and microscopic examination	Eye, **enucleation**
	Level VI Surgical pathology, gross and microscopic examination	Fetus, with dissection

APPLYING CODING THEORY TO PRACTICE

Choose the correct pathology and laboratory coding assignment. (Please see Appendix A for answers and rationale)

1. A physician ordered a urinalysis, automated with microscopy, for a 23-year-old female for bilirubin, glucose, hemoglobin, ketones, leukocytes, nitrite, pH, protein, specific gravity, and urobilinogen.
   A. ❑ 81099
   B. ❑ 81003
   C. ❑ 81001
   D. ❑ 81001, 83020, 82247

2. A physician conducted a pathology consultation during surgery with frozen section of three specimens.
   A. ❑ 88332 × 3
   B. ❑ 88329, 88332
   C. ❑ 88240
   D. ❑ 89352

3. PATHOLOGY REPORT:
   TISSUE: Appendix
   HISTORY: Right shoulder pain, lower quadrant stomach pain
   PATHOLOGICAL REPORT: The specimen was labeled "appendix" and was received in formalin. The specimen measures 4 × 1 × 0.5 cm. After gross and microscopic examination some purulent fibrinous material is noted. The serosa surface has fibrinoid material attached to it.
   DIAGNOSIS: Acute appendicitis with periappendicitis
   A. ❑ 44950
   B. ❑ 88302
   C. ❑ 88304
   D. ❑ 88319

4. A physician ordered blood gases pH, pC02, p02, C02, and HC03 including 02 saturation only, by direct measurement except pulse oximetry, for a 63-year-old male suspected of chronic obstructive pulmonary disease.
   A. ❑ 82820
   B. ❑ 82805
   C. ❑ 82803
   D. ❑ 82800

5. OBGYN, obstetrics and gynecology, a physician ordered a chemistry test for gonadotropin, luteinizing hormone (LH) and luteinizing release factor (LRF). Later that day the physician ordered the LH test again to ensure proper dates and calculations.
   A. ❑ 83002 × 2, 83727
   B. ❑ 83002-91, 83727
   C. ❑ 83001-91, 83727
   D. ❑ 83002-90, 86277

6. A physician ordered molecular diagnostics for a 41-year-old female for four nuclei acid sequences.
   A. ❑ 83890, 83901 × 4
   B. ❑ 83901 × 4
   C. ❑ 83890, 83901
   D. ❑ 83890, 83901-59

7. During evocative or suppressive agents testing, physician attendance and monitoring is reported with codes from the:
   A. ❑ Chemistry subsection of Pathology and Laboratory section
   B. ❑ Medicine section
   C. ❑ Evaluation and Management section
   D. ❑ Evocative/Suppression Testing subsection of the Pathology and Laboratory section

8. A physician ordered a Chlamydia culture on a 16-year-old male.
   A. ❑ 87270
   B. ❑ 87320
   C. ❑ 87110
   D. ❑ 87491

9. An outside laboratory performed a gross and microscopic autopsy on a 78-year-old female, including the brain.
   A. ❑ 88037-90
   B. ❑ 88036-59
   C. ❑ 88099-52
   D. ❑ 88025-90

10. A physician collected a cervical specimen in preservative fluid with automated thin layer fluid and preparation. Screening was automated and under the supervision of a physician.
    A. ❑ 88148-77
    B. ❑ 88166-90
    C. ❑ 88174
    D. ❑ 88161

11. Fresh sperm identification from testis tissue and semen analysis for motility and count was performed.
    A. ❑ 89257, 89310
    B. ❑ 89264, 89310
    C. ❑ 89260
    D. ❑ 89335

12. PATHOLOGY REPORT:
    TISSUE: LEFT BREAST MASS
    PATHOLOGICAL REPORT: The specimen was received in fresh state and labeled with the patient's name. No radiographs or skin was received. The sample consists of fibro-adipose breast tissue, 3.5 × 1.8 × 0.8 cm. Noted, through gross examination, is a sharply circumscribed rubbery mass measuring 1.5 × 0.3 × 1 cm with a gray-tan, bulging cut surface. One third of the margin is inked in black.
    DIAGNOSIS: Fibroadenoma of the left breast.
    A. ❑ 88307
    B. ❑ 88305
    C. ❑ 19101
    D. ❑ 88309

13. A physician ordered a chromosome analysis, count 18 cells, 2 karotypes with banding for a 3-year-old male.
    A. ❑ 88273
    B. ❑ 88285
    C. ❑ 88248
    D. ❑ 88262

14. A physician ordered testing of blood for levels of T3 uptake and thyroid-stimulating hormone for a 28-year-old female of 22 weeks' gestation.
    A. ❒ 84443, 84479
    B. ❒ 80438
    C. ❒ 80438, 84479
    D. ❒ 84479

15. A physician ordered a quantitative chemistry for one specimen analysis of seven amino acids for a 32-year-old male.
    A. ❒ 82139
    B. ❒ 82131 × 7
    C. ❒ 82139 × 7
    D. ❒ 82136

16. A 27-year-old female underwent a clotting test for factor XIII with fibrin stabilizing.
    A. ❒ 85291, 85335
    B. ❒ 85246
    C. ❒ 85290
    D. ❒ 85244, 85384

17. A CA 19-9 immunoassay for quantitative tumor antigen was performed for a 56-year-old male's bladder.
    A. ❒ 51530
    B. ❒ 86301
    C. ❒ 86294
    D. ❒ 86316

18. A physician ordered an outside lab to perform a semiquantitative infectious agent antigen detection by enzyme immunoassay technique, multiple step method for HIV-1 for a 22-year-old female presenting with multiple organ system failure.
    A. ❒ 87300, 87390-90
    B. ❒ 87301, 87390
    C. ❒ 87391-90
    D. ❒ 87390-90

19. A physician performed an extended culture of three embryos for 5 days.
    A. ❒ 89251
    B. ❒ 89272
    C. ❒ 89280
    D. ❒ 89272 × 3

20. A physician ordered a CCP cyclic citrullinated peptide antibody test for a 63-year-old female who presented with symptoms of rheumatoid arthritis.
    A. ❒ 86147
    B. ❒ 86185
    C. ❒ 86200
    D. ❒ 82030

21. PATHOLOGY REPORT:
    NAME: XXXX XXXXX
    DOB: xx xx xxxx
    HISTORY OF CASE: Multiple TURB, transurethral resection of the bladder, for grade II TCC, transitional cell carcinoma, with microinvasion; multiple tumors

    CLINICAL DIAGNOSIS: Carcinoma of bladder
    POSTOPERATIVE DIAGNOSIS: Carcinoma of the bladder
    DESCRIPTION: The specimen was received in one part. Cassette was labeled #1, "biopsy bladder tumor." Cassette #1 consists of multiple fragments of gray-brown tissue that appear slightly hemorrhagic. They are submitted in their entirety for processing.
    MICROSCOPIC: Section of bladder contains areas of transitional cell carcinom No area of invasion can be identified. A marked acute and chronic inflammatory reaction with eosinophils is noted, together with some necrosis. Sections are examined at six levels.
    DIAGNOSIS

    1. Papillary transitional cell carcinoma, grade II, bladder, biopsy.

    2. Acute and chronic inflammation, most consistent with recent biopsy procedure.
    A. ❒ 88184, 88307
    B. ❒ 88305
    C. ❒ 88307
    D. ❒ 88309, 88329

22. PATHOLOGY REPORT:
    NAME: XXXX XXXXX
    DOB: xx xx xxxx
    HISTORY OF CASE: Ten-year history of gastric ulcer
    CLINICAL DIAGNOSIS: Carcinoma of the stomach
    POSTOPERATIVE DIAGNOSIS: Carcinoma of the stomach
    GROSS DESCRIPTION: Two specimens were received. The first specimen consisted of a portion of the stomach measuring 12 × 8 × 3.5 cm. There was a portion of the mesentery attached to the lesser curvature, and there was a firm indurated area in the wall of the lesser curvature. The ulcer was 4 cm from the proximal portion of the specimen and 6 cm from the distal portion. The edges of the ulcer were firm, and no involvement was noted surrounding the mucosa.The rugae radiated toward the left of the ulcer from the anterior side. The entire specimen was admitted for examination.
    The second specimen consisted of a portion of the left anterior vagus. Specimen consisted of a piece of tan-white, soft tissue measuring 1.3 cm in length. The entire specimen was submitted for examination.
    MICROSCOPIC: Microscopically there is a ragged ulcer penetrating to within 7 mm of the serosal surface. The ulcer is surrounded by connective tissue and chronic inflammatory infiltrate. Several of the sections of the ulcer reveal malignant changes. The cells are pleomorphic with small amounts of eosinophilic cytoplasm. The tumor proper does not extend below the mucosa, but a single group of malignant cells is seen in a submucosal lymphatic space.
    DIAGNOSIS: Superficial spreading carcinoma in the margin of a chronic gastric ulcer.
    A. ❒ 88307
    B. ❒ 88307, 88309
    C. ❒ 88309 × 2
    D. ❒ 88309, 88302

23. A physician ordered HLA, human leukocyte antigen, typing for the donor of a 42-year-old male lung transplant patient with "A" multiple antigens, mixed lymphocyte culture, and DR/DQ single antigen, for tissue typing of a possible donor match.

A. ❏ 86812, 86813, 86817, 86821

B. ❏ 86813, 86816, 86822

C. ❏ 86813, 86816, 86821

D. ❏ 86920, 86813, 86816, 86821

24. A physician ordered a total ceratine kinase for a 13-year-old girl with isoenzymes and MB fraction only.

A. ❏ 82550, 82552, 82553

B. ❏ 82540, 82552, 82553

C. ❏ 82565, 82657, 83570

D. ❏ 82565, 82552, 83570

25. A physician ordered quantitative blood levels drawn on a 33-year-old female psychiatric patient who was suspected of having overdosed on haloperidol.

A. ❏ 80100, 80173

B. ❏ 80173

C. ❏ 81001, 80173

D. ❏ 85004, 80173

CHAPTER 10

Medicine Section Review

Learning Objectives

- The student will review all of the standards and guidelines organization, format, and content of the Medicine section.

- The student will review and interpret Medicine notes and assign codes accordingly.

- The student will review and assign all modifiers that are pertinent in the Medicine section.

- The student will review the difference between noninvasive and minimally invasive procedures.

- The student will review and apply the guidelines of reporting Evaluation and Management codes with immunization administration.

- The student will review areas of medical specialties.

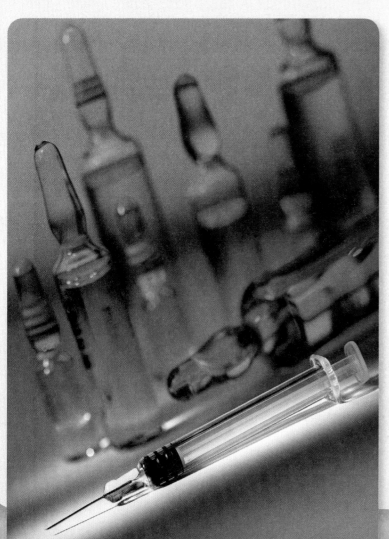

Key terms

Dialysis	Otorhinolaryngologic
Disseminated	Polysomnography
Hydration	Prophylactic
Maladaptive	Psychotherapy
Normocephalic	Spirometry
Opacification	Toxoid

From the Author...

"The Medicine section of the CPT manual is the last section of the CPT manual. It is unique, in that it is broken down into medical specialties and contains some very exclusive procedures and services. This is another section that contains a large variety of 'notes' that follow subsections and categories. Study these notes and become very familiar with the exclusive procedures and services offered in this section. Indexing will play an important role in this section as many of the codes seemingly fit into other sections of the CPT manual, such as Evaluation and Management (E&M) or Surgery. Don't be tricked and make sure that all appropriate modifiers are selected for final assignment."

The Medicine section of the CPT Manual includes the following subsections:

- Immune Globulins
- Immunization Administration for Vaccines/**Toxoids**
- Vaccines and Toxoids
- **Hydration,** Therapeutic, **Prophylactic,** and Diagnostic Injections and Infusions
- Psychiatry
- Biofeedback
- Dialysis
- Gastroenterology
- Ophthalmology
- Special **Otorhinolaryngologic** Services
- Cardiovascular
- Non-Invasive Vascular Diagnostic Studies
- Pulmonary
- Allergy and Clinical Immunology
- Endocrinology
- Neurology and Neuromuscular Procedures
- Medical Genetics and Genetic Counseling Services
- Central Nervous System Assessments/Tests
- Health and Behavior Assessment/Intervention
- Chemotherapy Administration
- Photodynamic Therapy
- Special Dermatological Procedures
- Physical Medicine and Rehabilitation
- Medical Nutrition Therapy
- Acupuncture
- Osteopathic Manipulative Therapy
- Chiropractic Manipulative Treatment
- Education and Training for Patient Self-Management
- Non–Face-to-Face Nonphysician Services
- Special Services, Procedures, and Reports
- Qualifying Circumstances for Anesthesia
- Moderate (Conscious) Sedation
- Other Services and Procedures
- Home Health Procedures/Services
- Medication Therapy Management Services

The Medicine section contains codes for evaluation, therapeutic, and diagnostic procedures and services that are generally not invasive. Noninvasive procedures require no surgical excision or incision and are considered closed procedures. Minimally invasive procedures such as injections and infusions include percutaneous access. The Medicine section has multiple subsections, and you must read the subsection information and instructions that pertain to the group codes that follow. The codes in this section may be used in conjunction with codes in all other CPT sections. If E&M services are performed and indicate the necessity of other procedures, it is appropriate to code both. Codes in this section do not include supplies used in testing, therapy, or diagnostic treatments unless specifically stated in the code description. Code supplies, including drugs, separately unless otherwise instructed in the code information.

Coding Alert!

Reporting E&M Codes with Immunization Administration

When a separate E&M service is provided in addition to the immunization administration of a vaccine/toxoid, the E&M code should be reported in addition to the immunization code. To identify that a significant, separately identifiable E&M service was indicated by the same physician in the same day, modifier -25 must be added to the E&M code reported.

Example

A physician administered immunization injections for a 2-year-old female established patient that included measles, mumps, rubella, and varicella vaccine. The mother of the child indicated that the toddler was suffering from an ache in the left ear. The physician performed an expanded-problem focused history and exam on the patient and indicated, without further testing, that the child suffered from otitis media and prescribed an antibiotic.

Coding Assignment: 90471, 90710, 99213-25

Modifiers

The most commonly used modifiers used in the Medicine section have been reviewed extensively in previous chapters, such as Chapter 7. Table 10.1 outlines the modifiers most common to the Medicine section as previously reviewed.

Special Report

You must always attach a "special report" to aid in the determination of medical appropriateness when a procedure or service is rarely provided, unusual, or new. Important information should include a detailed description of the nature, extent, and the need for the procedure or service and the time, effort, and equipment necessary to provide the service to the patient. Additional items that may be included for special reports are:

- Complexity of symptoms presented
- Final diagnosis
- Pertinent physical findings, such as size, locations, and number of lesions
- Diagnostic and therapeutic procedures including major and supplementary surgical procedures
- Concurrent problems
- Follow-up care

Table 10.1 Commonly Used Modifiers in the Medicine Section

Modifier	Modifier Description
-22	Increased Procedural Services
-32	Mandated Services
-50	Bilateral Services
-51	Multiple Procedures
-53	Discontinued Procedure
-58	Staged or Related Procedure or Service by the Same Physician during the Postoperative Period
-59	Distinct Procedural Service
-63	Procedure Performed on Infants Less Than 4 kg
-76	Repeat Procedure by the Same Physician
-77	Repeat Procedure by Another Physician
-99	Multiple Modifiers

Separate Procedures

Separate procedures are commonly performed as an integral component of a total service or procedure. When you encounter "separate procedure" listed in parenthesis () beside the procedure, you should bill only for the major procedure. The procedure identified as separate procedure should *not* be billed. When this phrase appears before the semicolon, all intended descriptions that follow are covered by it. Separate procedures are often improperly reported as related procedures. Remember, related procedures are performed for the same diagnosis and within the same operative area. A separate procedure can be a component of, or incidental to, a larger, related procedure.

Add-On Codes

Please remember that add-on codes are reported for procedures and services performed in addition to a primary procedure performed. All add-on codes found in the CPT manual are exempt from the use of modifier -51 (multiple procedures), as these procedures are not reported as stand-alone codes. Remember, these additional or supplemental procedures are identified in the CPT manual with a "+" in front of the code number.

Example

Code 92627 appears as:

+92627 Evaluation of auditory rehabilitation status; each additional 15 minutes (List separately in addition to code for primary procedure).

Unlisted Service or Procedure

An unlisted procedure and service code is assigned when there is no specific code that accurately describes the procedure or service performed. The service is identified by the appropriate "Unlisted Procedure" code, and a special report is submitted to indicate the service.

Unlisted procedures are typically found at the end of every section or subsection.

Medicine Coding Notes

Immunization Administration for Vaccines/Toxoids

As you review the Medicine section of the CPT manual, please remember that separate codes exist for the administration of immunization procedures of vaccines and toxoids and for the toxoid products themselves. Codes 90465-90474 must be reported in addition to the vaccine and toxoid codes 90476-90749. Codes 90465-90474 indicate the administration of the immunization itself. Codes 90476-90749 indicate the vaccine or toxoid being administered.

Report codes 90465-90468 only when the physician provides face-to-face counseling to the patient and family during the administration of a vaccine. These same code ranges are for patients eight years of age or younger when physician counsels the patient regarding immunizations. For the administration of any vaccine that is not accompanied by face-to-face physician counseling to the patient/family, report codes 90471-90474.

If a significant separately identifiable E&M service is performed, the appropriate E&M service code should be reported in addition to the vaccine and toxoid administration.

Example

1. A physician subcutaneously administered measles, mumps and rubella virus vaccine to a 5-year-old male.
   Codes: 90465, 90707
2. Nurse administered a live oral typhoid vaccine to a 25-year-old male.
   Codes: 90473, 90690

Immunization codes can appear similar and contain the same descriptions of toxoids or vaccines with the exception of a few words or phrases that determine the code. Make sure you carefully read the descriptor of each immunization code before assignment. Figure 10.1 is an example of codes for typical toxoids and vaccines.

Indexing Tip:

Remember to not confuse Medicine section code numbers with E&M code numbers. Medicine code numbers begin with 90281 and end with 99607.

Think Like A Coder 10.1

Choose the correct code for the following problem.

A physician administered, by intramuscular injection, a diphtheria and tetanus toxoids to a 6-year-old male patient and provided counseling with the parents before administering the vaccines.

- ▢ 90847, 90714
- ▢ 90847, 90702
- ▢ 90465, 90702
- ▢ 90471, 90702

Hydration, Therapeutic, Prophylactic, and Diagnostic Injections and Infusions (Excludes Chemotherapy)

The hydration, therapeutic, prophylactic, and diagnostic injections and infusions (excluding chemotherapy) services typically involve the endorsement of treatment plans and direct supervision of staff. These codes report the physician's work related to the infusion, hydration, or injection. The following services are included if performed to facilitate injections or infusions:

- Use of local anesthesia
- Intravenous (IV) start
- Access to indwelling IV or subcutaneous catheter or port
- Flush at conclusion of infusion
- Standard tubing, syringes, and supplies

Coding Alert!

When reporting codes for which infusion time is a factor, use the actual time over which the infusion is administered.

CPT 2007	Medicine / Hydration, Therapeutic, Prophylactic, Diagnostic Injections, Infusions	**90675—90749**

⊘ **90675** Rabies vaccine, for intramuscular use

⊘ **90676** Rabies vaccine, for intradermal use

⊘ **90680** Rotavirus vaccine, pentavalent, 3 dose schedule, live, for oral use

⊘ **90690** Typhoid vaccine, live, oral

⊘ **90691** Typhoid vaccine, Vi capsular polysaccharide (ViCPs), for intramuscular use

⊘ **90692** Typhoid vaccine, heat- and phenol-inactivated (H-P), for subcutaneous or intradermal use

⊘ **90693** Typhoid vaccine, acetone-killed, dried (AKD), for subcutaneous use (U.S. military)

⊬⊘ **90698** Diphtheria, tetanus toxoids, acellular pertussis vaccine, haemophilus influenza Type B, and poliovirus vaccine, inactivated (DTaP - Hib - IPV) for intramuscular use

⊘▲ **90700** Diphtheria, tetanus toxoids, and acellular pertussis vaccine (DTaP), when administered to younger than 7 years, for intramuscular use

⊘ **90701** Diphtheria, tetanus toxoids, and whole cell pertussis vaccine (DTP), for intramuscular use

⊘▲ **90702** Diphtheria and tetanus toxoids (DT) adsorbed when administered to younger than 7 years, for intramuscular use

⊘ **90703** Tetanus toxoid adsorbed, for intramuscular use

⊘ **90721** Diphtheria, tetanus toxoids, and acellular pertussis vaccine and Hemophilus influenza B vaccine (DtaP-Hib), for intramuscular use

⊘ **90723** Diphtheria tetanus toxoids, acellular pertussis vaccine, Hepatitis B, and pollovirus vaccine, inactivated (DtaP-HepB-IPV), for intramuscular use

⊘ **90725** Cholera vaccine for injectable use

⊘ **90727** Plague vaccine, for intramuscular use

⊘▲ **90732** Pnemococcal polysaccharide vaccine, 23-valent, adult or immunosuppressed patient dosage, when administered to 2 years or older, for subcutaneous or intramuscular use

⊘ **90733** Meningococcal polysaccharide vaccine (any group(s)), for subcutaneous use

⊘ **90734** Meningococcal conjugate vaccine, serogroups A, C, Y and W-135 (tetravalent), for intramuscular use

⊘ **90735** Japanese encephalitis virus vaccine, for subcutaneous use

⊘ **90736** Zoster (shingles) vaccine, live, for subcutaneous injection

⊘ **90740** Hepatitis B vaccine, dialysis or immunosuppressed patient dosage (3 dose schedule), for intramuscular use

⊘ **90743** Hepatitis B vaccine, adolescent (2 dose schedule), for intramuscular use

⊘ **90744** Hepatitis B vaccine, pediatric/adolescent dosage (3 dose schedule), for intramuscular use

Figure 10.1

Example of Codes for Vaccines and Toxoids from the CPT Manual

Source: *Current Procedural Terminology,* American Medical Association, 2008.

Hydration

Codes 90760 and 90761 are used for hydration IV infusion. Code 90706 is indicated for the initial (up to 1 hour) infusion. Code 90761 is indicated for each additional hour, up to 8 hours. Hydration codes are to be assigned when reporting hydration IV infusion that consists of a prepackaged fluid and/or electrolyte solutions.

Psychiatry

Psychiatry is the branch of medicine that deals with the diagnosis, treatment and prevention of mental illness. Codes 99221-99233 involve hospital care by the attending physician that is partial, initial, or subsequent. Some patients may receive hospital E&M services only, whereas others receive E&M services along with other procedures. Psychiatric treatment is at the same time as Evaluation and Management Service. Report one code for psychotherapy with E&M. Time is a major billing factor, and the record must indicate session time, or time spent with patient. Codes are divided based on interactive or insight-oriented psychotherapy, inpatient or outpatient, with or without E&M service, or individual or group. If other procedures such as behavior modification or **psychotherapy** are provided in addition to hospital E&M services, these should be assigned separate codes.

The E&M services should not be reported separately when the following codes are reported:

- 90805
- 90807
- 90809
- 90811
- 90813
- 90815
- 90817
- 90819

- 90822
- 90824
- 90827
- 90827

General Diagnostic and Evaluative Interview Procedures

Codes 90801 and 90802 typically include a psychiatric diagnostic interview evaluation that includes history, mental status, and disposition and may include communication with family or other outside sources. An interactive psychiatric diagnostic interview examination is usually provided to children (code 90802). It involves the use of physical aids and nonverbal communication to overcome barriers to therapeutic interaction between the clinician and the child patient. Table 10.2 breaks down the procedures included in these interview services.

> ### Indexing Tip:
>
> *When looking for codes in the Psychiatry subsection, index terms such as "psychiatric diagnosis," "psychiatric treatment," and "psychotherapy" for quick and accurate assignment.*

Psychiatric Therapeutic Procedures

Psychotherapy is used for the treatment of mental illness and behavioral disturbances. Psychotherapy involves a level of trust that is initiated between the clinician and the patient in order for the patient to express his or her thoughts, feelings, and disturbances. The clinician listens intently and encourages personality growth and development, alleviates emotional disturbances, and tries to reverse or change **maladaptive** behavior expressed by the patient. The two broad categories for reporting psychotherapy are (1) Interactive

Table 10.2 Interview Service Procedures

Psychiatric Diagnostic/Evaluative Interview Procedures	Interactive Psychiatric Diagnostic Interview Procedures
History/disposition	Orientation to person, place, and time
Mental status examination	Memory assessment
Patient disposition	Concentration ability
Communication with family/other sources	Language/communication; expressive
Ordering and medical interpretation of laboratory/diagnostic studies	Language/communication; responsive

Psychotherapy and (2) Insight Oriented, Behavior Modifying and/or Supportive Psychotherapy. As noted before, interactive therapy is typically rendered to children whereas insight-oriented behavior modification is rendered to all patients.

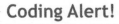

Coding Alert!

Please note that some psychotherapy codes factor in the amount of "time" spent with the patient. If the amount of time in the descriptor is less than or more than the time described, remember to use modifiers -22 (increased procedural services) or -52 (reduced services).

Think Like A Coder 10.2

Choose the correct codes for the following problems.

1. A psychiatrist provided individual interactive psychotherapy for a 10-year-old female inpatient with mechanisms used for nonverbal communication. The psychiatrist spent about 50 minutes face to face with the patient while rendering an E&M service.

   ❑ 90812, 99253

   ❑ 90827

   ❑ 90812

   ❑ 90819

2. A psychiatrist administered sodium amobarbital (Amytal) to a 27-year-old male patient for psychiatric diagnosis and therapeutic treatment.

   ❑ 90801

   ❑ 90880

   ❑ 90862

   ❑ 90865

Dialysis

Dialysis is described as the process of diffusing blood to remove toxic materials from the body to maintain fluid, electrolyte, and acid-based balance. The three subheadings in the Dialysis subsection include:

- End-stage renal disease services
- Hemodialysis
- Miscellaneous dialysis procedures

End Stage Renal Disease Services

Codes 90918-90921 are only reported once per month to distinguish age-specific services related to the patient's end-stage renal disease (ESRD) performed in an outpatient setting. Month is defined as 30 days, if less than a full month of service use codes (90922-90925) per day. Codes are used to report outpatient dialysis services for ESRD patient. Do not use these codes if the physician also submits hospitalization codes during the month. For ESRD and non-ESRD dialysis services performed in an inpatient setting and for non-ESRD

dialysis services performed in and outpatient setting, use codes 90935-90937 and 90945-90947. Codes 90922-90925 are reported when outpatient ESRD related services are not performed consecutively during an entire full month. The appropriate age-related code from this series (90922-90925) is reported daily less the days of hospitalization. For reporting purposes, each month is considered 30 days.

Example

End-Stage Renal Disease Services

Full month of ESRD for a 12-year-old female that includes monitoring for the adequacy of nutrition, assessment of growth and development, and counseling of parents.

Code: 90919 End-stage renal disease (ESRD) related services per month; For patients between two and eleven years of age to include adequacy of nutrition, assessment of growth and development, and counseling of parents.

Hemodialysis

Hemodialysis is the process of removing metabolic waste products, toxins, and excess fluids from the blood (see Figure 10.2). Codes 90935 and 90937 are reported to describe the hemodialysis procedure with all E&M services related to the patient's renal disease on the day of the hemodialysis Fprocedure. Use modifier -25 with E&M codes for separately identifiable services unrelated to the dialysis procedure or renal failure that cannot be rendered during the dialysis session.

Miscellaneous Dialysis Procedures/Peritoneal Dialysis

Peritoneal dialysis provides infusion of a fluid into the peritoneum that allows for diffusion between the dialyzing fluid and the body fluids containing waste products, which are then removed through a catheter. Codes 90945, 90947 describe dialysis procedures other than hemodialysis and all E&M services related to the patient's renal disease on the day of the procedure. Code 90945 is reported if only one evaluation of the patient is required related to that procedure. Code 90947 is reported when patient reevaluation(s) is (are) required during a procedure. Use modifier -25 with E&M codes for separately identifiable services unrelated to the dialysis procedure or renal failure that cannot be rendered during the dialysis session.

Ophthalmology

Ophthalmology is the study of the diseases and disorders of the eye by a physician who specializes in this area. The ophthalmology subsection is broken down into new and established patients, defined as:

Established Patient—An individual who has received professional services within the past 3 years from the opthamologist or group of physicians.

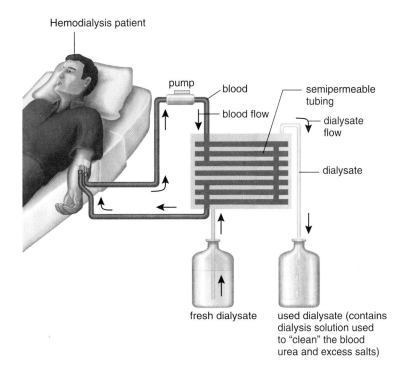

Figure 10.2

Hemodialysis – The patient's blood is pumped through dialysis tubing and is exposed to a dialysis solution. Wastes exit from blood in the solution, the blood is cleansed, and acid balances can be adjusted.

New Patient—An individual who has not received any professional services within the past 3 years from a physician or group of physicians. Opthalmology code descriptors are written to describe bilateral services. Use modifier -52 for reduced services if only a procedure on one eye is performed.

Opthalmology code descriptors are written to describe bilateral services. Use modifier -52 for reduced services if only a procedure on one eye is performed.

Indexing Tip:

When searching for ophthalmology procedures, for quick and accurate assignment, index "Ophthalmology, Diagnostic."

Table 10.3 provides the levels for ophthalmological services demonstrated in the code descriptors for this subsection.

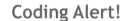

Coding Alert!

Contact lenses are not a part of the general ophthalmological services. However, the follow-up of successfully fitted extended wear lenses is reported as part of the general ophthalmological service.

Special Otorhinolaryngological Services

Otorhinolaryngology is the study of the disease and disorders of the ears, nose, and throat by a physician who specializes in this area. Services in this area include:

- Vestibular function tests, with observation and evaluation by the physician without electrical recording

Table 10.3 Levels of Ophthalmological Services

Intermediate ophthal-mological services	Evaluation of a new or existing condition complicated with a new diagnostic or management problem not necessarily relating to the primary diagnosis.
Comprehensive ophthalmological services	Evaluation of the complete visual system. The comprehensive services constitute a single service entity but need not be performed at one session. The evaluation always includes initiation of diagnostic and treatment programs.
Special ophthamological services	Services in which (1) a special evaluation of part of the visual system is made, which goes beyond the services included under general opthalmological services or (2) special treatment is given.

- Vestibular function tests, with recording and medical diagnostic evaluation
- Audiological function tests with medical diagnostic evaluation
- Evaluative and therapeutic services
- Special diagnostic procedures

Special otorhinolaryngological services are those diagnostic and treatment services not usually included in a comprehensive otorhinolaryngological evaluation or office visit. These services are reported separately, using codes 92502–92700. All services include medical diagnostic evaluation. Technical procedures are often part of the service but should not be mistaken as the service itself.

Think Like A Coder 10.3

Choose the correct code for the following problem. A physician performed a diagnostic analysis of a cochlear implant on the right ear for a 4-year-old male; subsequent programming. The physician then spent an hour, face to face, evaluating the child's auditory rehabilitation status.

- ☐ 92601-22
- ☐ 92601, 92627 × 4
- ☐ 92602, 92626
- ☐ 92602-22

Cardiovascular

In the Medicine section, *cardiovascular* refers to all procedures and treatments that relate to the heart and the vessels that network in the cardiovascular system. Echocardiography, one of the frequently used diagnostic tests in medicine, includes obtaining ultrasonic signals from the heart and great arteries, with two-dimensional image and/or Dopler ultrasonic signal documentation and interpretation report. Remember to use modifier -26 if the interpretation is performed separately.

Cardiac catheterization is another frequently used diagnostic test in medicine and includes introduction, positioning and repositioning of catheters, recording of intracardiac and intravascular pressure, and obtaining blood samples for tests. If an injection procedure is performed without a prior cardiac catheterization, the injection procedures should be reported using codes in the Vascular Injection Procedures subsection of the Surgery section.

Injection Procedures

When injection procedures are performed in conjunction with cardiac catheterization, these services do not include introduction of catheters but do include repositioning of catheters when necessary and use of automatic power injectors. Injection procedures 93539-93545 represent separate identifiable services and may be coded in conjunction with one another when appropriate. The technical details of angiography supervision of filming and processing, interpretation, and report are not included. To report radiological supervision, interpretation, and report for 93542 or 93453, use 93555. To report radiological supervision and interpretation, and report for 93539, 93540, 93541, 93544, or 93545, use code 93556. Modifier -51 should not be appended to 93539-93556.

Example

Injection procedure for a cardiac catheterization

Code: 93540 Injection procedure during cardiac catheterization; For selective **opacification** of aortocoronary venous bypass grafts, one or more coronary arteries.

Intracardiac Electrophysiological Procedures/Studies

Electrophysiology is the study that involves the analysis of the relationships of body functions to electrical phenomenon. Electrophysiological testing is performed on patients with cardiac arrhythmias that result in physical symptoms such as syncope and/or cardiac arrest. Patients who experience these physical symptoms are typically evaluated by the methods described in Table 10.4.

Indexing Tip:

When searching for Intracardiac Electrophysiological Procedures/Studies, the quickest and most accurate way is to index "Electrophysiology Procedures." You will find codes 93600-93660 listed.

Table 10.4 Electrophysiological Studies Methods

Arrhythmia induction	Induction of arrhythmias from single or multiple sites within the heart. Arrhythmia induction is achieved by performing pacing at different rates.
Mapping	Mapping is a distinct procedure performed in addition to a diagnostic electrophysiological procedure and should be reported separately. Do not report standard mapping in addition to three-dimensional mapping.
Ablation	Once the part of the heart involved in the tachycardia is localized, the tachycardia may be treated by ablation (the destruction of cardiac tissue by radio frequency energy).

Think Like A Coder 10.4

Choose the correct codes for the following problems.

1. An emergency physician provided allergen immunotherapy services for the supervision, preparation, and provision of antigens for wasps stings suffered by a 15-year-old female during a summer camp activity.

   ❏ 95010
   ❏ 95165
   ❏ 95145
   ❏ 95147

2. ABSTRACT:

PATIENT: xxxx xxxxx

DATE: xx xx xxxx

CHART NUMBER: xxx-xxxx

SEX: Male

CHIEF COMPLAINT: Sleeping difficulties

HISTORY: A 50-year-old male was admitted for a sleep study because of difficulty when falling asleep and staying asleep. The patient states that, when he feels tired, he lies down and cannot go to sleep or will eventually fall asleep and awake suddenly and cannot fall back asleep. The patient states that he will fall asleep at inappropriate times during the day. The patient denies any medication and is otherwise healthy. The patient acknowledges a mild amount of stress at his job.

PAST MEDICAL HISTORY: The patient denies drug abuse and drinks alcoholic beverages on the weekend. Denies smoking and drinks only mild amounts of caffeine. Patient states he had a cholecystectomy 4 years ago. He has had sleeping disturbances for over 1 month.

EXAMINATION: Vital Signs: Temp: 98.4, Respirations: 16, Pulse: 76, BP: 114/66. Heart: Normal sinus rhythm. HEENT: **Normocephalic.** Full extraocular movements. PERRLA. Throat: Clear. Chest: Clear to PA.

PROCEDURE: The unattended sleep study lasted over 6 hours, and during that time the patient's heart rate was normal and oxygen saturation was 90%; however, absence of breathing was noted at intermittent times during his sleep. The patient seemed restless and at times wheezing occurred. The patient was referred to an otorhinolaryngologist for diagnostic intervention.

   ❏ 780.55, 95807
   ❏ 780.53, 95805
   ❏ 780.51, 95806
   ❏ 780.55, 95806

Indexing Tip:

When searching for codes in the cardiovascular subsection, index terms such as "cardiac," "cardiac catheterization," and "cardiology" to find most of the procedures outlined in this subsection.

Pulmonary

The Pulmonary subsection of the Medicine section deals with pulmonology, which is the study of the lungs and respiratory system in the human body. Pulmonary services in the Medicine section include ventilator management, allergy and clinical immunology, allergy testing, and allergy immunotherapy. Of those services, **spirometry,** the measurement of the air capacity in the lungs, and continuous positive airway pressure, assistance to increase airway pressure, are most commonly performed. Additional Evaluation and Management Service is reported separately.

Neurology and Neuromuscular Procedures

Neurology is the study of the nervous system in the human body and its diseases and disorders. In the Medicine section neurology codes are used for diagnostic and therapeutic services and do not include surgical procedures. Contains codes to report tests, such as sleep test, muscle tests (electromyography), range-of-motion measurements, EEG (electroencephalogram), analysis and programming of neurostimulators, many bundled services, and services usually provided in addition to E&M service. Table 10.5 outlines and defines the various tests, procedures and services covered in this subsection.

Think Like A Coder 10.5

Choose the correct code for the following problem.

A physician performed a needle electromyography with related paraspinal areas for the left and right arms and the left leg of a 43-year-old female with a history of suspected **disseminated** sclerosis.

   ❏ 95863
   ❏ 95861-50
   ❏ 95857-50
   ❏ 95874

Coding Alert!

Please keep in mind that Health and Behavior Assessment and Intervention subsection is not relating to mental health; rather it focuses on biophysical factors affecting physical health problems such as chronic illnesses. These codes can be used by mental health professionals with training in health and behavior assessment.

Table 10.5 Neuromuscular Procedures and Services

Sleep testing	Sleep studies and **polysomnography** refer to the continuous and simultaneous monitoring and recording of various physiological and pathological parameters of sleep for 6 or more hours with physician review, interpretation, and report.
Routine electoencephalography (EEG)	EEG codes include hyperventilation and/or phobic stimulation when appropriate. Routine EEGs include 20 to 40 minutes of recording. Extended codes include reporting more than 40 minutes.
Muscle range of motion testing	This procedure includes muscle testing, range-of-motion measurements, and reports (see Figure 10.3).
Electromyography and nerve conduction tests	Needle electromyographic procedures include the interpretation of electrical waveforms measured by equipment that produces both visible and audible components of electrical signals recorded from the muscle.
Intraoperative neurophysiology	An intraoperative neurophysiology testing code is reported when intraoperative neurophysiology is performed during a surgical procedure.
Autonomic function tests	These tests evaluate autonomic functions such as the lungs and heart.
Evoked potentials and reflex tests	The responsiveness of the body's skin and internal structures is evaluated by electrically stimulating the nerves.
Neurostimulators, analysis-programming	This test assesses battery status, pulse amplitude, pulse duration, etc., in a previously implanted neurostimulator pulse generator system.
Motion analysis	This analysis is part of a major therapeutic or diagnostic decision-making process performed in a dedicated motion analysis laboratory.
Functional brain mapping	Brain mapping includes selection and administration of testing of language, memory, cognition, movement, and sensation.
Medical genetics and genetic counseling services	These services are provided by trained genetic counselors may include obtaining a structured family genetic history, pedigree construction, and analysis for genetic risk assessment.
Central nervous system assessments	These tests assess the cognitive function of the central nervous system.

Chemotherapy Administration

Chemotherapy is a treatment for disease by the application or administration of chemicals that have a specific and toxic effect on disease-causing microorganisms. Codes used to report chemotherapy treatments are 96401-96549. Chemotherapy services are typically highly complex in nature and require direct physician supervision for patient assessment, consent, and safety oversight. If a separate E&M service is provided, report E&M code with a -25 modifier. Report all drugs/substances separately. Keep in mind that codes are not limited to patients with diagnosis of cancer and codes also include infusion of anti-neoplastic agents, monoclonal antibody agents, and biological response modifiers for treatment of non-cancer diagnoses. If these services are used to facilitate the injection or infusion, the following are included and not reported separately:

- Use of local anesthesia
- IV start
- Access to indwelling IV subcutaneous catheter or port
- Flush at conclusion of infusion
- Standard tubing, syringes, and supplies
- Preparation of chemotherapy agents

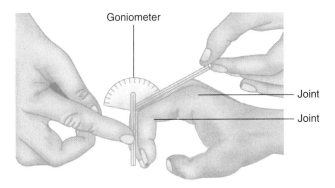

Goniometer

Joint

Joint

Figure 10.3
Range of Motion Test—A goniometer is used to measure the range of motion of a joint.

When reporting codes for a service in which infusion time is a factor, remember to use the actual "time" over which the infusion is administered as your guide for correct assignment. Report separate codes for each parenteral method of administration employed when chemotherapy is administered by different techniques. Report both the specific service as well as code(s) for the specific substance(s) or drug(s) provided. The fluid used to administer the drug(s) is considered incidental hydration and is not separately reportable.

Injection and Intravenous Infusion Chemotherapy

Intravenous or intra-arterial push is defined as (1) an injection in which the health care professional who administers the substance/drug is continuously present to administer the injection and observe the patient or (2) an infusion of 15 minutes or less.

Acupuncture

Acupuncture is reported based on 15-minute increments of personal, face-to-face contact with the patient, not the duration of acupuncture needle(s) placement. If no electrical stimulation is used during a 15-minute increment, use codes 97810, 97811. If electrical stimulation of any needle is used during the 15-minute increment, use codes 97813, 97814. Only one code may be reported for a 15-minute increment. Use either 97810 or 97813 for the initial 15-minute increment. Only one initial code is reported per day.

Osteopathic and Chiropractic Manipulative Treatment

Osteopathic manipulative treatment is a form of manual treatment applied by a physician to eliminate or alleviate somatic dysfunction and related disorders. Codes 98925-98929 are used to report these services.

Chiropractic manipulative treatment (CMT) is a form of manual adjustment treatment to influence joint and neurophysiological function. This treatment may be accomplished by using a variety of techniques. The CMT codes 98940-98943 include a premanipulative patient assessment.

Additional E&M services may be reported separately by using modifier -25, if the patient's condition requires a significant separately identifiable E&M service above and beyond the usual preservice and postservice work associated with the procedure.

The five spinal regions referred to in CMT are:

- Cervical region
- Thoracic region
- Lumbar region
- Sacral region
- Pelvic region

The five extraspinal regions referred to are:

- Head
- Temporomandibular joint
- Lower extremities
- Upper extremities
- Rib cage
- Abdomen

On-Line Medical Evaluation

An on-line electronic medical evaluation is a non–face-to-face assessment and management service by a qualified health care professional in response to an on-line inquiry by a patient using Internet resources. Reportable services involve the qualified health care professional's personal timely response to the patient's inquiry and must include permanent storage of the encounter. This service is reported only once for the same episode of care during a 7-day period, although multiple qualified health care professionals can report their exchange with the same patient. A reportable service encompasses the sum of communication, such as a related telephone call, prescription provision, and laboratory orders, pertaining to the on-line patient encounter.

Example

On-line Medical Evaluation
Code: 98969

On-line assessment and management service provided by a qualified nonphysician health care professional to an established patient, guardian, or health care provider not originating from a related assessment and management service provided within the previous 7 days, using the Internet or similar electronic communications network.

Moderate Conscious Sedation

Moderate conscious sedation is a technique used during various procedures in which the patient is in a state of depression of consciousness but can respond to verbal commands and maintain his or her own airway. Please refer to Appendix G, which contains codes that include moderate (conscious) sedation. The codes that include moderate (conscious) sedation are identified in the CPT manual with a "bulls-eye" symbol. When reporting moderate sedation, the following services are included and cannot be reported separately:

- Assessment of the patient (not included in intraservice time)

- Establishment of IV access and fluids to maintain patency, when performed

- Administration of agent

- Maintenance of sedation

- Monitoring of oxygen saturation, heart rate, and blood pressure

- Recovery (not included in intraservice time)

Coding Alert!

Intraservice Time; Moderate Sedation

Intraservice time starts with the administration of the sedation agent, requires face-to-face attendance, and ends at the conclusion of personal contact by the physician.

Category II Codes

Category II codes are found immediately following the Medicine section in the CPT manual. Category II codes are optional codes used as tracking codes and are represented by an alphanumerical character with a letter at the end of the numerical character, for example, **2001F Weight recorded (HF)**[1]. This category II code helps describe the aspects of a physical examination or clinical assessment.

Category II codes are intended to decrease administrative burden by facilitating data collection about the quality of care patients are receiving. Performance measures can be gauged when services or test results are assigned these codes and contribute to higher quality patient care. The following box describes how the American Medical Association defines and acknowledges Category II Codes.

CPT category II codes are arranged according to the following categories derived from standard clinical documentation format:

- Composite Measures   0001F-0012F
- Patient Management   0500F-0509F
- Patient History   1000F-1111F
- Physical Examination   2000F-2031F
- Diagnostic/Screening Processes or Results   3006F-3210F
- Therapeutic, Preventive, or Other Interventions   4000F-4124F
- Follow-up or Other Outcomes   5005F-5015F
- Patient Safety   6005F-6020F

Category II Codes Standards

Category II CPT codes are supplemental tracking codes used to measure performance. It is anticipated that the use of these codes will decrease the need for record abstraction and chart review and thereby minimize the administrative burden on providers and any other entity interested in measuring the quality of patient care. They are intended to facilitate data collection about the quality of care rendered by coding certain services and test results that support nationally established performance measures and that have an evidence base as contributing to quality patient care.

The use of these codes is optional. The codes are not required for correct coding and may not be used as a substitute for category I codes. These codes describe clinical components that may be typically included in evaluation and management services or clinical services and, therefore, do not have a relative value associated with them. Category II codes may also describe results from clinical laboratory or radiology tests and other procedures, identified processes intended to address patient safety practices, or services reflecting compliance with state or federal law.

The category II codes described in this section make use of alphabetical characters as the fifth character in the string (i.e., four digits followed by the letter F). These digits are not intended to reflect the placement of the code in the regular (category I) part of CPT. When you determine the need to implement the use of these codes and their associated measures, please reference appropriate information about performance measurement exclusion modifiers, measures, and the measurer's source. Use the letter "F"; for example, the Physical Examination (number 2000) is written 2000F.

Category II codes are reviewed by the Performance Measures Advisory Group (PMAG), an advisory body to the CPT Editorial Panel and the CPT/HCPAC (Health Care Provided Advisory Committee). The PMAG is comprised of performance measurement experts representing the Agency for Healthcare Research and Quality (AHRQ), the American Medical Association (AMA), the Centers for Medicare and Medicaid Services (CMS), the Joint Commission on Accreditation of Healthcare Organizations (JCAHO), the National Committee for Quality Assurance (NCQA), and the Physician Consortium for Performance Improvement. The PMAG may seek additional expertise and/or input from other national health care organizations, as necessary, for the development of tracking codes. These may include national medical specialty societies, other national health care professional associations, accrediting bodies, and federal regulatory agencies.

Category II codes are published biannually: January 1 and July 1. The most current listing, along with guidelines and forms for submitting code change proposals for category II codes, may be accessed on the Internet at www.ama-assn.org/go/cpt.

Table 10.6 Category II Code Modifiers

Modifier	Description
1P—Performance measure exclusion modifier due to medical reasons	• Not indicated (absence of organ or limb, already received/performed, other)
	• Contraindicated (patient allergy history, potential adverse drug interaction, other)
	• Other medical reasons
2P—Performance measure exclusion modifier due to patient reasons	• Patient declined
	• Economic, social, or religious reasons
	• Other patient reasons
3P—Performance measure exclusion modifier due to system reasons	• Resources to perform the services not available
	• Insurance coverage/payor-related limitations
	• Other reasons attributable to health care delivery system
8P—Performance measure reporting modifier: action not performed, reason not otherwise specified	Action described in a measure's numerator is not performed and the reason is not otherwise specified

To promote understanding of these codes and their associated measures, users are referred to Appendix H, which contains information about performance measurement exclusion modifiers, measures, and each measure's source.

 Think Like A Coder 10.6

Choose the correct answer and fill in the blank for the following problems.

1. Code 0500F of the category II codes is assigned for an initial prenatal care visit. What information is included with this service?

   ☐ Obstetrical care only

   ☐ Special report

   ☐ Obstetrical care, date of visit, and LMP (last menstrual period).

   ☐ Special report, obstetrical care, date of visit and LMP

2. Current smokeless tobacco user.

Category II code _____

Modifiers Used With Category II Codes

Category II modifiers are used to indicate that a service specified in the associated measure(s) was considered, but because of either medical, patient, or system circumstance(s) documented in the medical record, the service was not provided. These modifiers serve as denominator exclusions from the performance measure. The user should note that not all listed measures provide for exclusions (Refer to Appendix H). Category II modifiers should be reported only with Category II codes; they should not be reported with category I or category III codes. Table 10.6 outlines the category II code modifiers.

Category III Codes

Category III codes are found immediately after the category II codes included after the Medicine section. Category III codes contain "emerging technology" temporary codes assigned for data collection purposes and like category II codes are assigned an alphanumerical character. Category III codes are intended for the data collection of emerging technology services that are part of ongoing research. The following box describes how the American Medical Association defines and acknowledges category III codes.

Category III Codes Standards

Category III codes are a set of temporary codes for emerging technology, services, and procedures. Category III codes allow data collection for these services/procedures. Use of unlisted codes does not offer the opportunity for the collection of specific data. If a Category III code is available, this code must be reported instead of a Category I unlisted code. This is an activity that is critically important in the evaluation of health care delivery and the formation of public and private policy. The use of the codes in this section allows physicians and other qualified health care professionals, insurers, health services researchers, and health policy experts to identify emerging technology, services, and procedures for clinical efficacy, utilization, and outcomes.

The inclusion of a service or procedure in this section neither implies nor endorses clinical efficacy, safety, or applicability to clinical practice. The codes in this section may not conform to the usual requirements for CPT category I codes established by the Editorial Panel. For category I codes, the Panel requires that the service/procedure be performed by many health care professionals in clinical practice in multiple locations and that Federal Drug Administration approval, as appropriate, already be received. The nature of emerging technology, services, and procedures is such that these requirements may not be met. For these reasons, temporary codes for emerging technology, services, and procedures have been placed in a separate section of the CPT codebook, and the codes are differentiated from category I codes by the use of alphanumerical characters.

 Think Like A Coder 10.7

Choose the correct answer and fill in the blank for the following problems.

1. What category III code would be assigned for placement of visceral extension prosthesis for endovascular repair of abdominal aortic aneurysm involving visceral vessels and each visceral branch, with radiological supervision and interpretation?

   ❑ 0075T

   ❑ 00079T

   ❑ 00081T

   ❑ 0027T

2. What category III code would be assigned to an ECG, 64 leads or greater with graphic presentation and analysis, with interpretation and report?

   Code _____

APPLYING CODING THEORY TO PRACTICE

Choose the correct Medicine coding assignment. (Please see Appendix A for answers and rationale).

1. A physician administered a hemophilus influenza b vaccine (Hib) and a four-dose PRP-T protein-rich polypeptide conjugate to a 53-year-old male.
   A. ☐ 90474, 90648
   B. ☐ 90471, 90648
   C. ☐ 90471, 90648 × 4
   D. ☐ 90471, 90647

2. A physician provided face-to-face education and training for 60 minutes to a mother and daughter for health assessment and training for daily diabetic testing.
   A. ☐ 96040-22
   B. ☐ 90806
   C. ☐ 98961 × 2
   D. ☐ 96152 × 4

3. A 46-year-old male received CMT for five regions.
   A. ☐ 98942
   B. ☐ 98943
   C. ☐ 98925-22
   D. ☐ 98940 × 5

4. Dialysis is reported _____ time(s) per month to distinguish age-specific services related to the patient's ESRD performed in an outpatient setting.
   A. ☐ Twice
   B. ☐ As often as needed
   C. ☐ Three
   D. ☐ Once

5. A psychiatrist provided pharmacological management for the prescription of 100 mg of Zoloft for a 17-year-old male with obsessive-compulsive disorder. The physician also provided review of medication and minimal psychotherapy.
   A. ☐ 92605
   B. ☐ 90862
   C. ☐ 90862, 90804
   D. ☐ 90816, 90862

6. A physician provided individual psychotherapy in the office for an established 7-year-old patient suspected of autism. The therapy was interactive and included physical devices and mechanisms of nonverbal communication. The entire session lasted a little over 70 minutes face to face with the child along with medical E&M services.
   A. ☐ 99213, 90828
   B. ☐ 90826-22
   C. ☐ 90815
   D. ☐ 99214, 90814

7. An audiologist performed an electrocoustic evaluation for a 91-year-old female patient's left ear for hearing aids.
   A. ☐ 92587
   B. ☐ 92591-52
   C. ☐ 92595-52
   D. ☐ 92594

8. A physician provided review and interpretation of comprehensive computer-based motion analysis, dynamic plantar pressure measurements, dynamic surface electromyography during walking, dynamic fine wire electromyography, and two other functional activities with written report for a 32-year-old male.
   A. ☐ 96001, 96002, 96003
   B. ☐ 96001, 96002
   C. ☐ 96004-22
   D. ☐ 96004

9. A physician measured the gastric electrical activity of a 49-year-old female by placing electrodes on the skin of the patient's stomach, which indicated increased activity in the large intestine. Provocative testing was also performed.
   A. ☐ 91020
   B. ☐ 91133
   C. ☐ 91052
   D. ☐ 91299

10. A 65-year-old male was administered IV infusion chemotherapy drugs over the span of 2 hours.
    A. ☐ 96415-2
    B. ☐ 96413, 96417
    C. ☐ 96413, 96415
    D. ☐ 96420, 96423

11. A 51-year-old male underwent a cardiovascular stress test using maximal bicycle exercise with continuous electrocardiographic monitoring and pharmacological stress with physician supervision only.
    A. ☐ 93016
    B. ☐ 93017
    C. ☐ 93015-2
    D. ☐ 93005

12. A 71-year-old female underwent 45 minutes of water exercises for therapy of arthritis of the arms and physical rehabilitation after surgery on a broken knee.
    A. ☐ 98925
    B. ☐ 97530
    C. ☐ 97113 × 3
    D. ☐ 97022

13. A 42-year-old male with alcoholic psychosis met face to face with a health care professional for initial assessment and intervention for nutrition therapy for approximately 1 hour.
    A. ☐ 99404
    B. ☐ 97802 × 4
    C. ☐ 99412
    D. ☐ 98960 × 2

14. A physician performed a percutaneous transluminal coronary thrombectomy and angioplasty of right coronary artery for a 37-year-old male. Also, the placement of a percutaneous

intracoronary stent of the right circumflex without therapeutic intervention was performed.

A. ❏ 92984, 92973

B. ❏ 92995, 92997

C. ❏ 92982, 92973, 92980

D. ❏ 92995, 92998, 92973

15. Attended by a technologist, a 13-year-old female underwent a sleep study for 5 hours including an ECG, recordings of ventilation, respiratory effort, breathing, and O₂ saturation.

A. ❏ 93303, 95808

B. ❏ 93303, 95808, 95807-26

C. ❏ 93318, 95806-52

D. ❏ 95806-52

16. Qualifying circumstances in the Medicine section are for _____ codes.

A. ❏ Moderate Sedation

B. ❏ Home Infusion Procedures

C. ❏ Anesthesia

D. ❏ Special Services, Procedures and Reports

17. A physician performed a laser treatment for psoriasis on a 52-year-old male for a total area of 390 sq cm on the left leg.

A. ❏ 96921

B. ❏ 17108

C. ❏ 17266

D. ❏ 96921, 17226

18. What code would be assigned for the home visit for a 97-year-old home-bound female for respiratory therapy and apnea evaluation?

A. ❏ 99190

B. ❏ 99510

C. ❏ 99503

D. ❏ 97535

19. An emergency physician administered ipecac to a 21-year-old male who ingested over 1 L of alcohol and was continued on observation until his stomach was emptied. Also performed was a diagnostic gastric lavage to rule out vessel bleeding. He was subsequently transferred to an inpatient treatment facility.

A. ❏ 91105

B. ❏ 99175, 91105

C. ❏ 99282, 99175, 91105

D. ❏ 99282, 99175

20. Before having a total abdominal hysterectomy, a 48-year-old female underwent collection processing of her blood for storage in the event that hemorrhaging might occur postoperatively. During the procedure, the patient's vital signs began to fall to critical status, and the procedure was terminated.

A. ❏ 99195-52

B. ❏ 86890-52

C. ❏ 36415-52

D. ❏ 36450-52

CHAPTER 11

HCPCS Level II Coding Review

Learning Objectives

- The student will review the history and usage of HCPCS Level II codes.

- The student will review the breakdown of code groupings from the HCPCS Level II Manual.

- The student will review how to locate HCPCS Level II codes.

- The student will review and practice the indexing and assignment of HCPCS Level II codes.

- The student will review the modifiers for HCPCS Level II codes and their application to CPT codes.

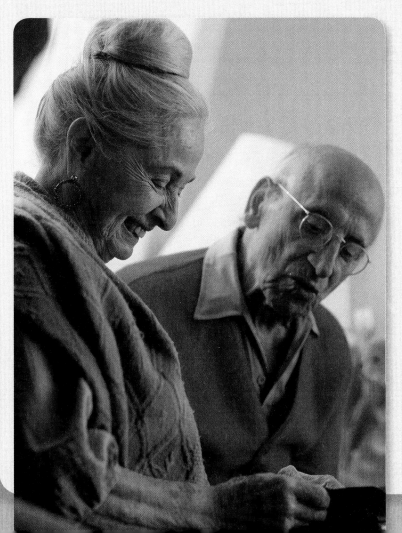

Key terms

Decubitus Ulcer
Intravenous
Mastectomy
Medicaid
Orthotic
Tracheostomy

From the Author...

"HCPCS Level II codes are very similar to CPT Level I codes and at the same time are very different. While CPT Level I codes contain five numerical digits, HCPCS Level II codes contain five characters with the first being an alpha character and the last four being numerical digits. The same coding principles apply when finding the correct HCPCS Level II codes. Look up the durable medical equipment, drugs, treatment services, and other services by indexing first and then verifying the code before assignment. Understand when to assign a HCPCS Level II code, and you will find yourself flying through this section."

HCPCS Level II Code Set is a standard set of codes used for Medicare and other health insurance programs in the United States to ensure that medical claims are processed in an orderly and consistent manner. The HCPCS is divided into two principal subsystems, referred to as Level I and Level II of the HCPCS. Level I of the HCPCS constitutes *Current Procedural Terminology,* a numerical coding system maintained by the American Medical Association (AMA). The CPT is a uniform coding system consisting of descriptive terms and identifying codes that are used primarily to identify medical services and procedures furnished by physicians and other health care professionals. These health care professionals use the CPT to identify services and procedures for which they bill public or private health insurance programs. Decisions regarding the addition, deletion, or revision of CPT codes are made by the AMA. The CPT codes are republished and updated annually by the AMA. Level I of the HCPCS, the CPT codes, does not include codes needed to separately report medical items or services that are regularly billed by suppliers other than physicians.

Level II of the HCPCS is a standardized coding system that is used primarily to identify products, supplies, and services not included in the CPT codes, such as ambulance services and durable medical equipment, prosthetics, orthotics, and supplies used outside a physician's office. Because Medicare and other insurers cover a variety of services, supplies, and equipment that are not identified by CPT codes, the HCPCS Level II codes were established for submitting claims for these items. The development and use of Level II of the HCPCS began in the 1980s. Level II codes are also referred to as alphanumerical codes because they consist of a single alphabetical letter followed by four numerical digits (J9165), whereas CPT codes consist of five numerical digits (33250).

Coding Alert!

HCPCS Level II Codes

HCPCS Level II codes consists of five digit alphanumerical codes beginning with an alpha character (A-V, excluding X) followed by four numbers.

Example

E1620 Blood pump for hemodialysis replacement

J9000 Doxorubicin HCl, 10 mg

M0301 Fabric wrapping of abdominal aneurysm

S2325 Hip core decompression

HCPCS Level II Codes Section Breakdowns

HCPCS Level II codes are divided into the following sections:

A Codes	Transportation Services, Including Ambulance
B Codes	Enteral and Parenteral Therapy
C Codes	Outpatient Prospective Payment System (OPPS)
D Codes	Dental Procedures
E Codes	Durable Medical Equipment (DME)
G Codes	Temporary (Procedures/Professional Services)
H Codes	Alcohol and Drug Abuse Treatment Services
J Codes	Drugs Administered Other Than by Oral Method
K Codes	Temporary (Durable Medical Equipment Regional Carriers)
L Codes	**Orthotic** Procedures, Prosthetic Procedures
M Codes	Medical Services
P Codes	Pathology and Laboratory Services
Q Codes	Temporary (Miscellaneous Services)
R Codes	Diagnostic Radiology Services
S Codes	Temporary National Codes
T Codes	National T Codes
V Codes	Vision Services, Hearing Services

 Indexing Tip:

The index to HCPCS code manual is in alphabetical order in the back of the book. You may have to think of alternative names for equipment that is assigned by the physician. Sometimes physicians use different names for durable-medical equipment and supplies.

General Guidelines for HCPCS Coding Assignments

The same set of rules apply to HCPCS Level II coding assignment as to any coding assignment:

1. Choose the name of the procedure or service that accurately describes the service performed.

Coding Alert!

Codes with Measurements

When assigning codes for anything with measurements, such as drugs, you may have to code twice or three times to cover the entire bill.

Example: The physician prescribed vincristine sulfate, 10 mg. The HCPCS code J9380 is presented in the HCPCS manual as:

J9380 vincristine sulfate, 5 mg

The coding assignment would be: J9380 × 2

2. Search for main terms in the alpha index that identifies the service that was performed.

3. Never assign a code directly from the index; it is only a reference to find the correct code and its descriptor.

4. Always verify the code to make sure the description is accurate and complete. Proper use of the index is vital for accurate code assignment.

HCPCS Table of Drugs

HCPCS Level II codes contain a Table of Drugs that begin with the alpha character "J." J codes describe drug names that sometimes are generic, or a physician may use another name. This can make finding the correct drug code very challenging. You should always have a pocket-size PDR (Physician's Drug Reference) or NDR (Nurse's Drug Reference) on hand to reference while assigning drugs from the HCPCS Level II Table of Drugs. Table 11.1 outlines the abbreviations used to designate the route of administration for all drugs.

Think Like A Coder 11.1

Table of Drugs

The following excerpt from the Table of Drugs demonstrates routes of administration:

Leuprolide acetate	per 1 mg	IM	J9218
Levofloxacin	250 mg	IV	J1956
Levonorgestrel	52 mg	OTH	J7302
Levorphanol tartrate	up to 2 mg	SC, IV	J1960

A 69-year-old female with breast cancer is 1 week post-op of a radical **mastectomy** of the left breast. Her physician ordered Paciltaxel 30 mg IV in combination of other chemotherapy drugs. Using the Table of Drugs in your HCPCS reference manual, choose the correct code.

❑ J9264
❑ J9265
❑ J2501
❑ J9305

Medical and Surgical Supplies A4000–A8999

The Medical and Surgical Supplies section covers a wide variety of medical, surgical, and some durable medical equipment (DME)–related supplies and accessories, maintenance, and repair required to ensure the proper functioning of this equipment is generally covered by Medicare under the prosthetic devices provision.

Example

HCPCS Medical and Surgical Supplies

The following are examples of HCPCS codes found in the Medical and Surgical Supplies section:

A4281:
Adhesive skin support attachment for use with external breast prosthesis, each

A4339:
Ostomy irrigation supply; cone/catheter, including brush

A8001:
Helmet, protective, soft, prefabricated, includes all components and accessories

Think Like A Coder 11.2

Medical and Surgical Supplies

1. Please code for the 23-square-inch foam dressing acting as a wound covering without adhesive border for a **decubitus ulcer** on the buttocks of a 81-year-old female inpatient at a nursing facility.

Code(s) _____

2. Please code for the **tracheostomy** care kit for a 90-year-old male patient who has just undergone a tracheostomy for the first time.

Code(s) _____

Table 11.1 Abbreviations for Routes of Administration

Route of Administration	Abbreviation
Intra-arterial	IA
Intrathecal	IT
Intravenous	IV
Intramuscular	IM
Subcutaneous	SC
Inhalant solution	INH
Various routes	VAR
Oral	ORAL
Other routes	OTH

Dental Procedures

The "D," or dental, codes are a separate category of national codes. The Current Dental Terminology (CDT-2007–2008) code set is copyrighted by the American Dental Association (ADA). CDT-2007/2008 codes are included in the HCPCS Level II. Decisions regarding modification, deletion, or addition of DCT-2007–2008 codes are made by the ADA and not the national panel responsible for the administration of HCPCS. The Department of Health and Human Services has an agreement with the AMA pertaining to the use of CPT codes for physician services; it also has an agreement with the ADA to include CDT-2007/2008 as a set of HCPCS Level II codes for use in billing for dental services.

 Think Like A Coder 11.3

Dental Procedures

1. Please assign the HCPCS code for a root canal anterior excluding final restoration.

Code _____

2. Please assign the HCPCS code for a repair of four broken teeth for a complete denture.

Code _____

Durable Medical Equipment

"E" codes include durable medical equipment such as canes; crutches; walkers; commodes; decubitus care, bath, and toilet aids; hospital beds; oxygen and related respiratory equipment; monitoring equipment; pacemakers; patient lifts; safety equipment; restraints; traction equipment; fracture frames; wheelchairs; and artificial kidney machines.

 Think Like A Coder 11.4

Durable Medical Equipment

1. Please assign the HCPCS code for a heavy-duty folding walker without wheels for a 74-year-old female patient at an assisted living facility.

Code _____

2. Please assign the HCPCS code for a TENS transcutaneous electrical nerve stimulation unit with six leads for a 68-year-old male patient in chronic pain as a result of advanced colon cancer.

Code _____

Alcohol and Drug Abuse Treatment Services

The "H" codes are used by state **Medicaid** agencies mandated by state law to establish separate codes for indentifying mental health services that include alcohol and drug treatment services.

 Think Like A Coder 11.5

Alcohol and Drug Abuse Treatment Services

1. Please assign the HCPCS code for acute detoxification for alcohol dependence in an outpatient program.

Code _____

2. Please assign the HCPCS code for 1 hour and 15 minutes of therapeutic behavioral services for an 11-year-old boy with severe attention deficit.

Code _____

Orthotic and Prosthetic Procedures

The "L" codes are used for orthotic and prosthetic procedures and devices, as well as scoliosis equipment, orthopedic shoes, and prosthetic limbs.

 Think Like A Coder 11.6

Orthotic and Prosthetic Procedures and Devices

1. Please assign the HCPCS code for the procedure of a hip orthosis with abduction control of hip joints, static, plastic, that includes fitting and adjustment.

Code _____

2. Please assign the HCPCS code for a Seattle Carbon Copy II foot prosthesis for a 67-year-old male who lost his left foot because of gangrene.

Code _____

HCPCS Level II Modifiers

HCPCS Level II modifiers function in the same way that CPT code modifiers function. In some instances, insurers instruct providers that a HCPCS code must be accompanied by a code modifier to provide additional information regarding the service or item identified by the HCPCS code. Modifiers are used when the information provided by a HCPCS code descriptor needs to be supplemented to identify specific circumstances that may apply to an item of service. Table 11.2 presents a sample listing of modifiers used for HCPCS Level II codes. A complete listing of HCPCS modifiers can be found in Appendix 2 of your HCPCS Level II reference code book.

Table 11.2 Sample Listing of HCPCS Modifiers

HCPCS Modifiers	Descriptor	HCPCS Modifiers	Descriptor
E1	Upper left, eyelid	LD	Left anterior descending coronary artery
E2	Lower left, eyelid	LT	Left side
E3	Upper right, eyelid	QM	Ambulance service provided under arrangement by a provider service
E4	Lower right, eyelid	QN	Ambulance service furnished directly by a provider of services
F1	Left hand, second digit	RC	Right coronary artery
F2	Left hand, third digit	RT	Right side
F3	Left hand, fourth digit	T1	Left foot, second digit
F4	Left hand, fifth digit	T2	Left foot, third digit
F5	Right hand, thumb	T3	Left foot, fourth digit
F6	Right hand, second digit	T4	Left foot, fifth digit
F7	Right hand, third digit	T5	Right foot, great toe
F8	Right hand, fourth digit	T6	Right foot, second toe
F9	Right hand, fifth digit	T7	Right foot, third digit
FA	Left hand, thumb	T8	Right foot, fourth digit
GG	Performance and payment of a screening mammogram and diagnostic mammogram on the same patient, same day	T9	Right foot, fifth digit
GH	Diagnostic mammogram converted from screening mammogram on same day	TA	Left foot, great toe
LC	Left circumflex coronary artery		

APPLYING CODING THEORY TO PRACTICE

Choose the correct coding assignment. (Please see Appendix A for answers and rationale).

1. What is the HCPCS code for a power wheelchair, group 2 heavy duty, multiple power option, sling, solid seat with solid back, and a weight capacity of up to 450 pounds?
   - A. ❏ K0850
   - B. ❏ K0853
   - C. ❏ K0838
   - D. ❏ K0843

2. A physician fitted a diaphragm contraceptive device for 16-year-old female and provided instructions for its use.
   - A. ❏ 11975, A4260
   - B. ❏ 11975, A4266
   - C. ❏ 57160, A4266
   - D. ❏ 57170, A4266

3. What HCPCS code would be used to bill for small-size disposable underpads for a patient in a nursing home setting?
   - A. ❏ A4520
   - B. ❏ A4554
   - C. ❏ A4520
   - D. ❏ A4465

4. A physician prescribed an injection of furosemide 40 mg for a 47-year-old female.
   - A. ❏ J1940 × 2
   - B. ❏ J1441 × 2
   - C. ❏ J1451 × 3
   - D. ❏ J1455

5. What code would you assign for the extension line with easy lock connectors used with dialysis?
   - A. ❏ A4672
   - B. ❏ A4653
   - C. ❏ A4673
   - D. ❏ A4680

6. What HCPCS code would you assign for the transportation of portable electrocardiogram (EKG) equipment to a nursing home?

   Code(s) _____

7. What HCPCS code(s) would you assign if three patients underwent an EKG at the same facility on the same portable EKG equipment as described in question # 6?

   _____

8. Please assign the HCPCS code for screening mammography that produces a digital image, bilateral, all views. Included is the performance of a screening mammogram and diagnostic mammogram on and payment by the same patient, same day.

   Code _____

9. Please assign the HCPCS code for a splint applied to the left hand, fourth digit of a patient.

   Code _____

10. Please assign the HCPCS code for a gradient compression full-length stocking, chap style with 30-40mm Hg, for both legs.

    Code _____

Diagnoses Review

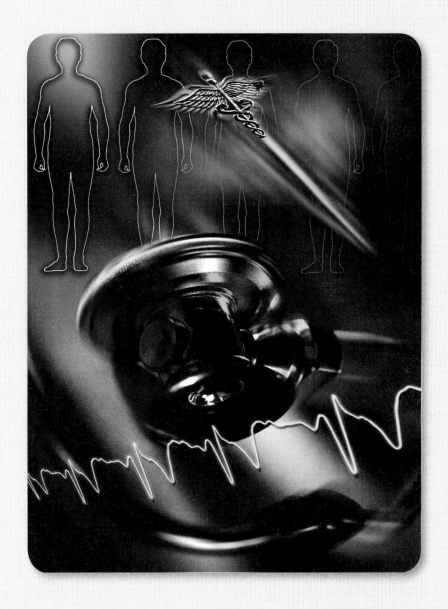

Chapter 12: ICD-9-CM Guidelines and Coding Conventions Review, Part I

Chapter 13: ICD-9-CM Guidelines and Coding Conventions Review, Part II

CHAPTER 12

ICD-9 CM Guidelines and Coding Conventions Review, Part I

Learning Objectives

- The student will review the organization of the ICD-9-CM Tabular List of Diseases, Index to Diseases, Index to Procedures, and Tabular List of Procedures.

- The student will review the official guidelines for coding and reporting of ICD-9-CM codes.

- The student will review all official coding conventions for ICD-9-CM codes and apply them when choosing the correct coding assignment.

- The student will review and apply all instructional notes as they appear in the Tabular List of Diseases.

- The student will review and apply all coding conventions and guidelines to E Codes and V Codes and codes for Infectious and Parasitic Diseases, Neoplasms, Endocrine System Diseases, Diseases of the Blood, Mental Disorders, Diseases of the Nervous System, Diseases of the Circulatory System, and Diseases of the Respiratory System.

- The student will review the Health Insurance Portability and Accountability Act.

- The student will review Coding from Abstracts.

- The student will review the Uniform Hospital Data Discharge Set.

Key terms

Carcinoma	Misadventure
Etiology	Myringotomy
Exanthema	Papilloma
Idiopathic	Psychogenic
Late Effect	Puerperium
Manifestation	Sarcoma

From the Author...

"Working knowledge of ICD-9 coding is vital to your success as a professional coder and is a central theme throughout both national coding

examinations. The CCS-P examination (AHIMA) has more emphasis on diagnosis coding than the CPC examination (AAPC). Please keep this in mind when choosing which credential to pursue. As you review the following chapter, remember that the same basic coding principles apply. Always index the diagnosis and verify the codes in the Tabular List.

It will really benefit you to memorize Table 12.1. If you have this information to call upon when choosing the correct ICD-9 code, it will help you rule out answers more quickly. Please read all coding instructions carefully, as the fourth and fifth digit assignments can sometimes become confusing or easy to miss. When you encounter a problem that includes both ICD-9 and CPT codes, make sure that the diagnosis code corresponds with the CPT code. You can very easily overlook this when choosing a group of codes for an answer on a national examination. Study hard and consistently and soon you will be a professional coder!"

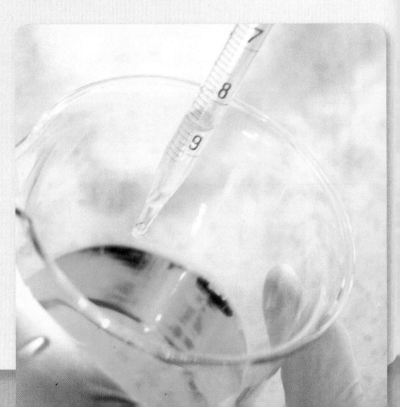

ICD-9-CM Coding Conventions and Guidelines

Review of the ICD-9-CM Coding Manual

The ICD-9-CM coding manual is composed of two indexes and two tabular lists. The Alphabetic Index to Diseases is separated by tabs labeled with the letters of the alphabet and contains diagnostic terms for illnesses, injuries, conditions, and reasons for encounters with health care professionals. The Table of Drugs and Chemicals is located within this section.

Following the Alphabetic Index to Diseases is the Tabular List of Diseases. The Tabular List of Diseases arranges the ICD-9-CM codes and their descriptors numerically (000–999). Table 12.1 lists the chapters in the Tabular List of Diseases and their corresponding disease categories.

The Tabular List of Diseases includes two official supplementary classifications:

- E Codes, Supplementary Classification of External Causes of Injury and Poisoning
- V Codes, Supplementary Classification of Factors Influencing Health Status and Contact with Health Services

There are four official appendices of the ICD-9-CM manual:

- Appendix A   Morphology of **Neoplasms**
- Appendix B   Deleted
- Appendix C   Classification of Drugs by AHFS List (American Hospital Formulary Services)
- Appendix D   Classification of Industrial Accidents According to Agency
- Appendix E   List of Three-Digit Categories

Table 12.1 Tabular List of Diseases

Chapter	Category of Disease
1	Infectious and Parasitic Disease
2	Neoplasms
3	Endocrine, Nutritional and Metabolic Disorders, and Immunity Disorders
4	Diseases of the Blood and Blood-Forming Organs
5	Mental Disorders
6	Diseases of the Nervous System and Sense Organs
7	Diseases of the Circulatory System
8	Diseases of the Respiratory System
9	Diseases of the Digestive System
10	Diseases of the Genitourinary System
11	Complications of Pregnancy, Childbirth, and the **Puerperium**
12	Disease of the Skin and Subcutaneous Tissue
13	Diseases of the Musculoskeletal System and Connective Tissue
14	Congenital Anomalies
15	Newborn (Perinatal) Guidelines
16	Symptoms, Signs, and Ill-defined Conditions
17	Injury and Poisoning

Next, is the procedure classification, the Alphabetic Index to Procedures. This index to procedures lists common surgical and procedural terminology and descriptions along with conventions to direct the coder to the correct area in the Tabular List of Procedures. Finally, the Tabular List of Procedures numerically lists the procedures codes and their descriptors. Procedures codes begin with 00.0, procedures and interventions, not elsewhere classified and end with 99.9, other miscellaneous procedures. Table 12.2 lists the chapters in the Tabular List of Procedures and their corresponding procedure categories.

ICD-9-CM Official Coding Conventions

ICD-9 official coding conventions can typically be found in the beginning of any coding manual and need to be reviewed carefully to ensure accurate coding and success for your national coding examination! As you know, the ICD-9-CM manual's Tabular List of Diseases includes abbreviations, symbols, punctuations, and other conventions.

Abbreviations

Abbreviations include:

- NEC—Not elsewhere classifiable. More information is needed to assign a more specific code and is not listed in the ICD-9-CM manual. The coder is directed to "other specified" code in the Tabular List of Diseases and Tabular List of Procedures.
- NOS—Not otherwise specified. This abbreviation means "unspecified" because of the lack of information the coder has received to assign a more specific four-digit code necessary to properly describe the disease or condition.

Punctuation

Punctuations include:

- Brackets [ ]. Brackets are used in the Tabular List of Diseases and the Tabular List of Procedures to indicate synonyms, alternative wording or terminology, and explanatory phrases.

> **Example**
>
> 253.6 Other disorders of neurohypophysis
> Syndrome of inappropriate secretion of antidiuretic hormone [ADH]

- Slanted Brackets *[ ]*. Slanted brackets are used in the Alphabetic Indexes to indicate **manifestation** codes, which indicates "code underlying first." Manifestation codes are always reported as secondary codes and must be reported to fully describe the condition or disease.

Table 12.2 Tabular List of Procedures

Chapter	Category of Procedures
0	Procedures and Interventions, Not Elsewhere Classified
1	Operations on the Nervous System
2	Operations on the Endocrine System
3	Operations on the Eye
4	Operations on the Ear
5	Operations on the Nose, Mouth, and Pharynx
6	Operations on the Respiratory System
7	Operations on the Cardiovascular System
8	Operations on the Hemic and Lymphatic Systems
9	Operations on the Digestive System
10	Operations on the Urinary System
11	Operations on the Male Genital Organs
12	Operations on the Female Genital Organs
13	Obstetrical Procedures
14	Operations on the Musculoskeletal System
15	Operations on the Integumentary System
16	Miscellaneous Diagnostic and Therapeutic Procedures

> **Example**
>
> *Arthritis, arthritic*
> urethritica 099.3 *[711.1]*

- Parentheses ( ). Parentheses are used in both the tabular lists and indexes to indicate nonessential modifiers that may be present as supplementary words that describe the disease without changing the code assignment.

> ### Example
>
> 300.00 Anxiety state, unspecified
>
> Anxiety:
> state (neurotic)

> ### Example
>
> Code 006.1
>
> Chronic intestinal amebiasis without mention of abscess
>
> Chronic:
>   amebiasis
>   amebic dysentery

- Colons: Colons are used in the tabular lists after an incomplete term to show that a modifier must be used to assure the correct code assignment.

Notes and Inclusion Terms

Table 12.3 outlines and defines notes and inclusion terms found in the Official ICD-9 Coding Conventions.

Table 12.3 Coding Conventions: Notes and Inclusion Terms

Note/Term	Definition/Usage
Includes	This note appears immediately under a three-digit code title to define, provide examples, or clarify content of the category.
Excludes	This note under a code indicates that the terms excluded from the code are to be assigned elsewhere.
Inclusion terms	Inclusion terms are listed under certain four- and five-digit ICD-9-CM codes found in the Tabular List of Diseases and Tabular List of Procedures. These terms indicate the conditions for which a code number is to be used. The terms may be synonyms or may be various other conditions assigned to that code.
Other	Codes that have "other" after them usually have a code with a fourth digit of 8 or a fifth digit of 9. This note is used when the information in the medical record provides detail for which a specific code does not exist.
Unspecified	Codes that usually have a fourth digit of 9 or a fifth digit of 0 are for use when the information provided is insufficient to assign a more specific code.
Etiology, manifestation code	This note indicates that the underlying disease needs to be coded first and, if applicable, the condition. It also indicates that the coder should use an additional code and look for diseases classified elsewhere.
And	This note should be interpreted as "and" or "or" when appears in a phrase or title.
With	This note appears in the Alphabetic Index and is sequenced immediately following the main term.
See and See Also	"See" indicates that another term should be referenced. "See Also" indicates that there is another term that should be taken into consideration and may be useful when clarifying an assignment.
Use additional code	This note prompts the coder that an additional code will be useful for clarifying and providing a more complete picture of the diagnosis.
Omit code	This note instructs the coder that no code is to be assigned.

Indexing Tip:

Remember when you look in the Alphabetic Indexes to Diseases or Procedures that the main term is always in bold and subterms are indented to the right and below the main term.

   308.3   Other acute reactions to stress
                 Acute situational disturbance

ICD-9-CM Official Coding Guidelines

Please review all coding guidelines before your attempt to assign ICD-9-CM codes in this chapter. By reviewing the guidelines first, you are "setting the stage" for assigning diagnosis codes with a renewed sense of order. Once that "order" has been achieved, assigning diagnosis codes will become easier and more accurate than ever before. Intimate awareness of all coding guidelines will aid in the expeditious passing of any national examination. In general, Table 12.4 lists the general coding guidelines you will need to prepare properly.

Think Like A Coder 12.1

Choose the correct answers for the following problems.

1. "Excludes" notes are found in the:
   - ☐ Tabular List of Diseases only
   - ☐ Tabular List of Diseases and Tabular List of Procedures
   - ☐ Indexes to Diseases and Procedures
   - ☐ Index to Procedures

2. The note "Manifestation codes (etiology)":
   - ☐ is found enclosed in slanted brackets
   - ☐ means that the code is not elsewhere classified
   - ☐ identifies terms that are excluded from a code
   - ☐ contains a "use additional code" note for clarification

Table 12.4 General Coding Guidelines

Order of Guidelines (Mental Process)	Guidelines
1	Use both the Alphabetic index and tabular lists
2	Locate each term in the Alphabetic index
3	Code to the highest level/detail
4	Select disease codes from 001.0-999.9
5	Select procedure codes from 00.0-99.9
6	Interpret/indicate signs and symptoms
7	Keep in mind conditions that are an integral part of a disease process
8	Keep in mind conditions that are not part of an integral disease process
9	Use multiple coding for a single condition when necessary or instructed to
10	Designate and discriminate between the difference between "chronic" and "acute" conditions
11	Remember to use codes in combination when instructed to do so
12	Differentiate conditions that are late effects and not the condition/disease itself
13	Take into consideration impending or threatened conditions while assigning codes
14	Read all chapter-specific coding guidelines

V Codes and E Codes: Supplementary Classifications

Chapter 18: Classification of Factors Influencing Health Status and Contact with Health Service (V01-V86)

Note: Chapter 18 and 19 of the ICD-9-CM manual are presented first in this chapter. Coding problems throughout this chapter require the use of many V and E codes. It is best to review these chapters first to ensure you are prepared to assign the correct codes to maximize the most of your review for your national coding examination!

V codes (V01-V86) are a supplementary classification provided to deal with occasions when circumstances other than a disease or injury are recorded as a diagnosis or problem. V codes also further clarify the reason for a patient's encounter and are used to report additional factors that provide important information concerning the patient receiving care. V codes are used for four primary reasons:

1. To indicate when a healthy individual receives health services for some specific reason, such as prophylactic care, immunizations, health screenings, or organ donations.

> **Example**
>
> *V70.0 Routine general medical examination at a health care facility*

2. To indicate when an individual with a chronic or long-term condition requires continuous care or when an individual requires special aftercare or follow-up care, such as dialysis or chemotherapy, after disease or injury.

> **Example**
>
> *V58.77 Aftercare following surgery of the skin and subcutaneous tissue, NEC*

3. To indicate when an individual who is not currently ill or injured encounters circumstances or problems that influence his or her health status.

> **Example**
>
> *V16 Family history of malignant neoplasms*
>
> *V16.0 Gastrointestinal tract*

4. To indicate the status of birth of a newborn.

> **Example**
>
> *V21.32 Low birth weight status, 500-999 grams*

Coding Alert!

V Codes

V codes are always reported as diagnosis codes, not as procedure codes.

Indexing Tip:

V codes can be indexed in the Index to Diseases; however it can be difficult to locate main terms for V codes. Table 12.5 presents a list of terms that will help you locate terms for V codes in the index. Memorization of these "keywords" will aid in quick and accurate coding assignment.

For further review, Table 12.6 outlines the breakdown of V codes into categories found in the ICD-9-CM manual. Like memorization of Table 12.5, memorization of this table will aid in quick and accurate coding assignment. Remember to refer to the V Code Table in the Official Coding Guidelines in your ICD-9 manual for updates on all V codes. The table contains columns for first listed, first or additional, additional only, and non-specific V codes. Each code of category is listed in the left-hand column in this table and the allowable sequencing of the code or codes within the category is noted under the appropriate column.

Table 12.5 List of Keywords to Locate V Codes in the Index

Admission	Observation
Aftercare	Outcome of delivery
Body mass	Personal history
Complications	Pregnancy
Contraception	Problem
Counseling	Screening
Encounter	Status
Examination	Supervision
Exposure	Test
Fitting	Therapy
Follow up	Vaccination
History of	Delivery
Newborn	

Table 12.6 ICD-9 CM Categories of V Codes

V Codes	Categories
V01-V06	Persons with health hazards related to communicable diseases
V07-V09	Persons who need isolation or have other potential health hazards, and prophylactic measures
V10-V19	Persons with potential health hazards related to personal and family history
V20-V29	Persons receiving health services in circumstances related to reproduction and development
V30-V39	Liveborn infants according to type of birth
V40-V49	Persons with conditions that influence their health status
V50-V59	Persons receiving health services for specific procedures and aftercare
V60-V68	Persons receiving health services in other circumstances
V69	Problems related to lifestyle
V70-V82	Persons without reported diagnoses encountered during examination and investigation of individuals and populations
V83-V84	Genetics
V85	Body Mass Index (BMI)

V Codes Use in Any Health Care Setting

V codes are for use in any health care setting. V codes may be used as either a first-listed or secondary code, depending on the circumstances of the encounter.

Personal and Family History

There are two types of history V codes, personal and family. Personal history codes are used for medical conditions that no longer exist and for which patients are not receiving any treatment but that have the potential for recurrence and therefore may require continued monitoring. The exceptions to this general rule are category V14, personal history of allergy to medicinal agents, and subcategory V15.0, allergy, other than medicinal agents. A person who has had an allergic reaction to a substance or food in the past should always be considered allergic to the substance.

Family history codes are used when a patient has a family member(s) who has had a particular disease that causes the patient to be at higher risk of also contracting the disease.

Screening

Screening is the testing for disease or disease precursors in seemingly well individuals so that early detection and treatment can be provided for those who test positive for the disease. The testing of a person to rule out or confirm a suspected diagnosis because that patient has some sign or symptom is a diagnostic examination, not a screening. In these cases, the sign or symptom is used to explain the reason for the test.

Observation

There are two observation V code categories. They are for use in very limited circumstances when a person is being observed for a suspected condition that is ruled out. The observation codes are not for use if any injury or illness or any sign or symptom related to the suspected condition is present. In such cases the diagnosis/symptom code is used with the corresponding E code to identify any external cause.

The observation codes are to be used as principal diagnosis only. The only exception to this is when the principal diagnosis is required to be a code from the V30, liveborn infant, category. Then the V29 observation code is sequenced after the V30 code.

Aftercare

Aftercare visit codes cover situations in which the initial treatment of a disease or injury has been performed and the patient requires continued care during the healing or recovery phase or for the long-term consequences of the disease.

Follow-up

The follow-up codes are used to explain continuing surveillance following completed treatment of a disease, condition, or injury. They imply that the condition has been fully treated and no longer exists. They should not be confused with aftercare codes that explain current treatment of a healing condition for its sequelae.

Donor

Category V59 are the donor codes and are used for living individuals who are donating blood or other body tissue for others only.

Counseling

Counseling V codes are used when a patient or family member receives assistance in the aftermath of an illness or injury or when support is required in coping with family or social problems.

Obstetrical and Related Conditions

Please refer to sections on ICD-9-CM Chapters 11 and 15 in Chapter 13 of this textbook.

Routine and Administrative Examinations

The V codes allow for the description of encounters for routine examinations, such as general check-ups, or examinations for administrative purposes, such as pre-employment physicals. The codes are used as first-listed codes only and are not to be used if an examination is for diagnosis of a suspected condition or for treatment purposes.

Think Like A Coder 12.2

Choose the correct answers for the following problems.

1. A female patient had breast cancer three years ago and underwent a radical mastectomy and received radiation and chemotherapy. She has had no treatment in the last 20 months. How is the status of the cancer reported for the patient?

   ❑ V16.3

   ❑ V13.2

   ❑ V10.3

   ❑ V10.44

2. A 25-year-old female with a personal history of schizophrenia received counseling on the use of oral contraceptives.

   ❑ V25.03, 295.90

   ❑ V25.01, V11.0

   ❑ V25.41, 295.90

   ❑ V25.40, V11.0

Chapter 19: Supplemental Classification of External Causes of Injury and Poisoning (E800-E999)

E codes are located in the ICD-9-CM Tabular List of Diseases and describe the external causes of injury, poisoning, or other adverse reactions affecting an individual's health. These codes are intended to provide data for injury research and evaluation of injury prevention strategies. E codes help describe how the injury or poisoning occurred (cause), the intent of the injury or poisoning, and the place where the event occurred. For further review, Table 12.7 outlines the breakdown of E codes into categories found in the ICD-9-CM manual.

Coding Alert!

E Code Rules to Remember

- E codes can be used with any ICD-9-CM code in the range of 001-V86.1.
- Use the full range of E codes.
- Assign as many E codes as necessary.
- Select the appropriate E code to accurately describe the scenario.
- E codes can *never* be used as principal diagnosis.

Indexing Tip:

E codes are indexed in the Alphabetic Index to External Causes of Injury or Poisoning and can be found at the end of the Index to Diseases.

If your ICD-9-CM manual does not have "tabs" for the E code index, apply self-made tabs to all pertinent sections for quick reference during your professional examination.

Range of E Codes

Use the full range of E codes to completely describe the cause, the intent, and the place of occurrence, if applicable, for all injuries, poisonings, and adverse effect of drugs.

Assignment of E Codes

Assign as many E codes as necessary to fully explain each cause. If only one E code can be recorded, assign the E code most related to the principal diagnosis.

E Code as Principal Diagnosis

An E code can *never* be a principal diagnosis.

Table 12.7 ICD-9 CM Categories of E Codes

E Codes	Categories
E800-E807	Railway accidents
E810-E819	Motor vehicle traffic accidents
E820-E825	Motor vehicle nontraffic accidents
E826-E829	Other road vehicle accidents
E830-E838	Water transport accidents
E840-E845	Air and space transport accidents
E846-E848	Vehicle accidents not elsewhere classifiable
E849	Place of occurrence
E850-E858	Accidental poisoning by drugs, medicinal substances, and biologicals
E860-E869	Accidental poisoning by other solid and liquid substances, gases, and vapors
E870-E876	Misadventures to patient during surgical and medical care
E878-E879	Surgical and medical procedures as the cause of abnormal reaction of patient or later complication, without mention of **misadventure** at the time of procedure
E880-E888	Accidental falls
E890-E899	Accidents caused by fire and flames
E900-E909	Accidents resulting from natural and environmental factors
E910-E915	Accidents caused by submersion, suffocation and foreign bodies
E916-E928	Other accidents
E929	Late effects of accidental injury
E930-E949	Drugs and medicinal and biological substances causing adverse effects in therapeutic use
E950-E959	Suicide and self-inflicted injury
E960-E969	Homicide and injury purposely inflicted by other persons
E970-E978	Legal intervention
E979	Terrorism
E980-E989	Injury undetermined whether accidentally or purposely inflicted
E990-E999	Injury resulting from operations of war

Place of Occurrence Guideline

Use an additional code from category E849 to indicate the place of occurrence for injuries and poisonings. The place of occurrence describes the place where the event occurred and not the patient's activity at the time of the event.

Adverse Effects of Drugs and Medicinal and Biological Substances Guidelines

- Do not code directly from the Table of Drugs and Chemicals; always refer back to the Tabular List of Diseases.
- Use as many codes necessary to describe.
- If the same E code describes the causative agent for more than one adverse reaction, assign the code only once.
- If two or more drugs are reported, code each individually unless the combination codes are listed in the Table of Drugs and Chemicals.
- When a reaction results from the interaction of a drug(s) and alcohol, use poisoning codes and E codes for both.

Intentional Injury

When the cause of an injury or neglect is intentional child or adult abuse, the first-listed E code should be assigned from categories E960-E968, homicide and injury purposely inflicted by other persons. An E code from code from category E967, child and adult battering and other maltreatment, should be added as an additional code to identify the perpetrator, if known.

Accidental Intent

In cases of neglect when the intent is determined to be accidental, E code E904.0, abandonment or neglect of infant and helpless person, should be the first-listed E code.

Use of Late Effect E Codes for Subsequent Visit

Use a **late effect** E code for subsequent visits when a late effect of the initial injury or poisoning is being treated. There is no late effect E code for adverse effects of drugs. Do not use a late effect E code for a subsequent visit for follow-up care of the injury or poisoning when no late effect of the injury has been documented.

Code Range E878-E879

Assign a code in the range of E878-E879 if the provider attributes an abnormal reaction or later complication to a surgical or medical procedure but does not mention misadventure at the time of the procedure as the cause of the reaction.

Cause of Injury Identified by the Federal Government as Terrorism

When the cause of an injury is identified by the federal government (Federal Bureau of Investigation) as terrorism, the first-listed E code should be a code from category E979, terrorism. Additional E codes from the assault categories should not be assigned.

Think Like A Coder 12.3

Choose the correct codes for the following problems.

1. A 26-year-old male suffered an open wound with tendon involvement of the great finger when broken glass from his windshield fell and cut his finger. The patient worked at a local factory where he drove a forklift.

   ☐ 882.2, E917, E849.3

   ☐ 886.0, E917.9, E849.9

   ☐ 883.2, E919.2, E849.3

   ☐ 883.1, E919.0, E849.6

2. What E code would be assigned to an accidental drowning of an individual while fishing?

   ☐ E910.1

   ☐ E910.2

   ☐ E849.4

   ☐ E910.8

Tables within the Index to Diseases

Table of Drugs and Chemicals

The Table of Drugs and Chemicals can be found at the end of the Index to Diseases. This table contains a classification of drugs and other chemical substances to identify poisoning and external causes of adverse effects, such as "accidental poisoning to." This table's extensive lists of drugs include industrial solvents, pesticides, toxic agents, corrosives, and gases. Specific drugs and chemical substances are listed alphabetically, and each of these substances is assigned a code to identify the drug or chemical. Table 12.8 outlines the seven-column table, in which the first column indicates the "drug or chemical" and the other five columns, titled "External Causes," list E codes for external causes depending on whether the circumstances involved in the use of the drug or chemical are accident, therapeutic use, suicide attempt, or assault or are considered undetermined.

Indexing Tip:

For identifying the place in which an accident or poisoning occurred, see the listing in the E Code index, "Accident, occurring."

Neoplasm Table

The Neoplasm Table can be found in the Index to Diseases under "neoplasm." Remember, a neoplasm is a "new" or abnormal tissue growth that exceeds in size and does not possess appearance of normal tissue growth. The Neoplasm

Table 12.8 Table of Drugs and Chemicals, External Causes (Sample)

Poisoning	Poisoning E-Code	Accident	Therapeutic Use	Suicide Attempt	Assault	Undetermined
Biligrafin	977.8	E858.8	E947.8	E950.4	E962.0	E908.4
Bilopaque	977.8	E858.8	E947.8	E950.4	E962.0	E908.4
Bioflavonoids	972.8	E858.8	E942.8	E950.4	E962.0	E908.4
Black (flag)	989.4	E863.4	_____	E950.6	E962.1	E980.7
Bleach	983.9	E864.3	_____	E950.7	E962.1	E980.6
Bleomycin	960.7	E856	E930.7	E950.4	E962.0	E908.4
Bone meal	989.89	E866.5	_____	E950.9	E962.1	E980.9
Borate	989.6	E861.3	_____	E950.9	E962.1	EE980.9

Table contains seven columns, of which three list malignant neoplasms, one describes the neoplasm itself, and the rest list neoplasms that are benign, exhibit uncertain behavior, or are unspecified. The code numbers for neoplasms are listed in alphabetical order by anatomical site. The description of the neoplasm often indicates which of the six columns fall under the appropriate type (see Table 12.9).

Major groups of neoplasms found in the Index to Diseases or in the Neoplasm Table are **sarcomas, carcinomas,** and mixed tissue tumors. The following steps are for review when using the Index to Diseases and the Neoplasm Table to code for neoplasms.

1. Locate the main neoplasm term in the alphabetical index.
2. Read subterms entries and notes and consider conventions.
3. If the site or neoplasm is not listed, refer to the Neoplasm Table.
4. Locate the anatomical site in the alphabetical table.
5. Select the behavior type for the neoplasm.
6. Select the appropriate neoplasm code and verify it in the Tabular List.

Table 12.9 Neoplasm Table, Malignancies (Sample)

Neoplasm Site	Primary	Secondary	Ca in situ	Benign	Uncertain Behavior	Unspecified
Thalamus	191.0	193.3	_____	225.0	237.5	239.6
Thigh NEC*	195.5	198.89	234.8	229.8	238.8	239.8
Thorax	195.1	198.89	234.8	229.8	238.8	239.8
Throat	149.0	198.89	230.0	210.9	235.1	239.0
Thumb	195.4	198.89	232.6	229.8	238.8	239.8
Tonsil	146.0	198.89	230.0	210.5	235.1	239.0
Tooth socket	143.9	198.89	230.0	210.4	235.1	239.0
Ureter/urethra	189.2	198.1	233.9	223.2	236.91	239.5

Indexing Tip:

Never index the term "mass" when referring to neoplasm. This will direct you to the site or organ-specific sections that are not referring to neoplasms.

Hypertension Table

The Hypertension Table can be found in the Index to Disease under "hypertension." Hypertension is the condition of abnormally elevated arterial blood pressure. The Hypertension Table can be difficult to read because of the various levels of indentations that are found in the table. Be careful when searching in the Hypertension Table and watch the difference between "terms" and "subterms." For instance, a *term* would be "cardiovascular disease" and the *subterm* would read, "with > heart failure."

Example

Cardiovascular disease (arteriosclerotic) (sclerotic)
..... 402.00
  with
    heart failure 402.01

Hypertension is classified in three ways: malignant, benign, and unspecified.

- Malignant hypertension: Malignant hypertension is the most severe hypertension, is difficult to treat than lower into normal ranges of hypertension. Malignant hypertension is usually diagnosed when the patient's systolic number (top number) is over 140.

- Benign hypertension: Benign hypertension is relatively mild, although sometimes chronic, but is normally treatable.

- Unspecified hypertension: Hypertension is unspecified when the treating physician does not classify the hypertension until further diagnostic tests are provided.

Table 12.10 provides a sample of the Hypertension Table.

Think Like A Coder 12.4

Choose the correct codes for the following problems.

1. An elderly prima gravida presented in the physician's office with a diagnosis of benign essential hypertension that was complicating her pregnancy. Upon further examination, the physician diagnosed the patient with preeclampsia and acute renal failure.

   - ☐ 646.23, 585.6
   - ☐ 642.73, 584.9
   - ☐ 642.43, 585.1
   - ☐ 642.43, 586

2. A patient presented in the office with lesions on the tongue and various areas of the mouth and complained of anorexia and difficulty when swallowing. After examinations and tests the physician diagnosed the patient with malignant cancer of the tongue on the anterior ventral surface and, secondary to the tongue, malignant mouth cancer located on the roof portion. The patient was referred to oncology.

   - ☐ 141.3, 145.5
   - ☐ 141.4, 141.9
   - ☐ 141.3, 198.89
   - ☐ 144.0, 198.89

ICD-9-CM Coding Notes for Review

Chapter-specific notes appear in all 17 chapters of the Tabular List of Diseases as outlined in Table 12.1. The notes reviewed in this chapter are the notes that should be of particular interest to you, as a coder who is seeking professional coding credentialing. The notes selected have been chosen for review because of the challenging nature of the disease, condition, or injury.

Chapter 1: Infectious and Parasitic Diseases (001-139)

In the Infectious and Parasitic Diseases section of the ICD-9-CM manual, infectious and parasitic diseases are classified into types of microorganisms that cause infections. These microorganisms are viruses, bacteria, parasites,

Table 12.10 Hypertension Table (Sample)

Hypertension/Hypertensive	Malignant	Benign	Unspecified
hypertension/hypertensive due to			
renal (artery)			
aneurysm	405.01	405.11	405.91
anomaly	405.01	405.11	405.91
kidney with lesser circulation	——	——	416.0
psychogenic	——	——	306.2
necrotizing	401.0	——	——
idiopathic	——	——	416.0

and fungi. Table 12.11 presents the subcategories of diseases and their corresponding code numbers for infectious and parasitic diseases.

Human Immunodeficiency Virus

The following are notes for coding human immunodeficiency virus (HIV) infections:

- Code only confirmed cases.
- If a patient is admitted for a HIV-related condition, the principal diagnosis should be 042.
- If a patient is admitted for an unrelated condition, the code for the unrelated condition should be the principal diagnosis. Other diagnoses are followed by 042.

- Code V08 should be applied when the patient, without any documentation of symptoms (asymptomatic), is listed as being "HIV positive," "known HIV," or "HIV test positive."
- Patients with inconclusive HIV serology may be assigned code 795.71.
- A patient admitted during pregnancy for an HIV-related illness should be assigned the principal diagnosis code of 647.6x.
- For a patient being seen to determine HIV status, code V73.89 should be used for unspecified viral disease. Code V69.8 should be used for problems relating to lifestyle.

Table 12.11 Infectious and Parasitic Diseases

Subcategory	Code Ranges
Intestinal Infectious Diseases	001-009
Tuberculosis	010-018
Zoonotic Bacterial Diseases	020-027
Other Bacterial Diseases	030-041
Human Immunodeficiency Diseases	042
Poliomyelitis and Other non-Arthropod-Borne Viral Diseases of Central Nervous System	045-049
Viral Diseases Accompanied by **Exanthem**	050-057
Other Human Herpesvirus	058

(Continued)

Table 12.11 Continued

Subcategory	Code Ranges
Arthropod-Borne Viral Diseases	060-066
Other Diseases Due to Virus and Chlamydiae	070-079
Rickettsioses and Other Arthropod-Borne Diseases	080-088
Syphilis and Other Venereal Diseases	090-099
Other Spirochetal Diseases	100-104
Mycoses	110-118
Helminthiases	120-129
Other Infectious and Parasitic Diseases	130-136
Late Effects of Infectious and Parasitic Diseases	137-139

Septicemia

The following are notes for coding septicemia and systemic inflammatory response syndrome (SIRS).

- If sepsis is present on admission and meets the definition of principal diagnosis, the underlying systemic infection code should be assigned as the principal diagnosis followed by the appropriate sepsis or SIRS code.
- Septicemia or sepsis (038) will include a code for streptococcal sepsis, from either streptococcal sepsis or streptococcal septicemia subcategories.
- The terms "sepsis" or "SIRS" must be documented to assign a code from subcategory 995.9.
- Categories 630-639 are used to code sepsis and septic shock associated with abortion, ectopic pregnancy, and molar pregnancies.
- Code 998.59 is used to report sepsis resulting from a postprocedural infection.

Coding Alert!

Patients who have been previously diagnosed with HIV illness (042) should never be assigned to nonspecific serologic evidence of HIV (795.71) or asymptomaticHIV (V08).

Chapter 2: Neoplasms (140-239)

Please refer to Table 12.9 to reference the Neoplasm Table. As stated earlier in this chapter, a neoplasm is a "new" or abnormal tissue growth that exceeds in size and does not possess appearance of normal tissue growth (see Figure 12.1). Table 12.12 presents the subcategories of neoplasms and their corresponding code numbers.

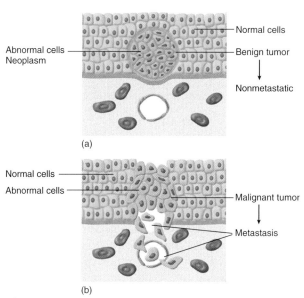

Figure 12.1

Neoplasms — a. Benign tumor; non-cancerous. b. Malignant tumor; cancerous with metastasis (spreading).

From N. Thierer and L. Breitbard, *Medial Terminology, Language for Health Care, 2e.* Copyright © 2006 The McGraw-Hill Companies, Inc. Reprinted with permission.

The following are notes for coding for neoplasms:

Treatment Directed at the Malignancy

If the treatment is directed at the malignancy, designate the malignancy as the principal diagnosis.

Treatment of Secondary Site

For patients who are admitted because of a primary neoplasm with metastasis but whose treatment is directed toward the secondary site only, the secondary neoplasm is

Table 12.12 Neoplasm Subcategories

Subcategory	Code Ranges
Malignant Neoplasm of Lip, Oral Cavity, and Pharynx	140-149
Malignant Neoplasm of Digestive Organs and Peritoneum	150-159
Malignant Neoplasm of Respiratory and Intrathoracic Organs	160-165
Malignant Neoplasm of Bone, Connective Tissue, Skin, and Breast	170-176
Malignant Neoplasm of Genitourinary Organs	179-189
Malignant Neoplasm of Other and Unspecified	190-199
Malignant Neoplasm of Lymphatic and Hematopoietic Tissue	200-208
Benign Neoplasms	210-229
Carcinoma In Situ	230-234
Neoplasms of Uncertain Behavior	235-238
Neoplasms of Unspecified Nature	239
Late Effects of Infectious and Parasitic Diseases	137-139

designated as the principal diagnosis despite the fact that the primary malignancy is still present.

Primary Malignancy Previously Excised

When a primary malignancy has been excised or eradicated and no further treatment such as chemotherapy or radiation is necessary, assign a V code to indicate a "personal history of malignant neoplasm." Any mention of extension, invasion, or metastasis (see Figure 12.1 for metastasis) to another site is coded as a secondary malignant neoplasm of that site.

Episode of Care Involving Surgical Removal of Neoplasm

When an episode of care involves the surgical removal of a neoplasm from a primary or secondary site, followed by adjunct chemotherapy or radiation treatment during the same episode of care, the neoplasm code should be assigned as principal or first-listed diagnosis, using codes in the 140-198 series.

Development of Complications by a Patient Admitted for Radiotherapy/Chemotherapy and Immunotherapy

When a patient is admitted for the purpose of radiotherapy, immunotherapy, or chemotherapy and develops complications such as uncontrolled nausea and vomiting or dehydration, the principal or first-listed diagnosis is V58.0 and so on.

Admission/Encounter to Determine Extent of Malignancy

When the reason for admission/encounter is to determine the extent of the malignancy or for a procedure such as paracentesis or thoracentesis, the primary malignancy or

> **Coding Alert!**
>
> Metastasis is the spread of malignant cells to another part of the body. When assigning codes for metastasis, read the problem carefully. Keep in mind that the phrases "metastatic to" and "metastatic from" can change the order of coding assignment.
>
> Example: Metastatic carcinoma from the breast to the lung. Breast is primary and lung is secondary.
>
> Example: Metastatic carcinoma to the liver from the prostate. Prostate is primary and liver is secondary.

appropriate metastatic site is designated as the principal or first-listed diagnosis, even though chemotherapy or radiotherapy is administered.

Think Like A Coder 12.5

Choose the correct codes for the following problems.

1. A 42-year-old male was diagnosed with a malignant neoplasm of the anterior wall of the urinary bladder, with a personal history of malignant neoplasm of the stomach.

   ❑ 188.2, V16.0

   ❑ 198.1, V10.04

   ❑ 188.3, V10.04

   ❑ 233.7, V16.0

12.B ABSTRACT:

Preoperative Diagnosis: Recurrent acute otitis media, intrinsic cartilaginous obstruction of the eustachian tube.

Postoperative Diagnosis: Same.

Operation: Unilateral **myringotomy** and tube.

Anesthesia: General endotracheal.

Complications: None

Blood Loss: 6 cc

Indications: The patient is a 45-year-old female who has recurrent otitis media and mild hearing loss in the left ear with cartilaginous obstruction of the eustachian tube.

Surgical Procedure: The patient was brought to the operating room and was prepped and draped in the usual fashion. Anesthesia was administered by an anesthesiologist without incident. The left ear was examined; finding no debris, the surgeon made an incision in the anterior inferior quadrant and placed a Teflon tube in the left ear. Xylocaine 1% containing epinephrine was administered to the left ear. The patient was extubated by the anesthesiologist and taken to the recovery room in good condition. The patient tolerated the procedure well and without complication.

   ❑ 381.60, 382.4, 20.01 69436-50

   ❑ 381.62, 382.9, 20.01, 69436

   ❑ 381.3, 382.1, 20.09, 20.01

   ❑ 381.62, 382.4, 20.09, 69436

Chapter 3: Endocrine, Nutritional, and Metabolic Diseases and Immunity Disorders (240-279)

Disorders of the endocrine system include various glandular disorders that can affect any of the body systems and cause hormonal disturbances that affect some of the body's most important physiological functions. Metabolic disorders include disturbances in the chemical processes that take place in the human body. Table 12.13 presents the subcategories of endocrine, nutritional, and metabolic diseases and immunity disorders and their corresponding code numbers.

Diabetes Mellitus

The category 250, diabetes mellitus, identifies complications and manifestations associated with this disease. A fifth digit is required for all category 250 codes in order to identify the type of diabetes mellitus and whether it is "controlled" or "uncontrolled."

Type of Diabetes Mellitus not Documented

"Type II" is the default diagnosis for diabetes if the type of diabetes is not noted in the medical record.

Diabetes Mellitus and the Use of Insulin

Type I diabetics must use insulin; however, the use of insulin does not necessarily mean that the patient is a type I diabetic. Some type II patients cannot control their blood sugar through diet alone and require the use of insulin. If the documentation in a medical record does not indicate the type of diabetes but does indicate that the patient uses insulin, the appropriate fifth digit for type II must be used. For type II patients who routinely use insulin, you should also assign code V58.67, long-term use of insulin, to indicate that the patient uses insulin. Code V58.67 should not be assigned if insulin is given temporarily to bring type II patient's blood sugar under control during an encounter.

Insulin Pump Malfunction

An "underdose" of insulin because of insulin pump failure should be assigned code 996.57, which is mechanical complication caused by the insulin pump. If the mechanical complication results in an overdose of insulin, assign code

Indexing Tip:

Remember to read all notes carefully when verifying diabetes codes in the Tabular List of Diseases. Many of the notes directly under the codes read, "Use additional code to identify manifestation . . ."

Table 12.13 Endocrine, Nutritional, and Metabolic Diseases and Immunity Disorders Subcategories

Subcategory	Code Ranges
Disorders of the Thyroid Gland	240-246
Diseases of Other Endocrine Glands	250-259
Nutritional Deficiencies	260-269
Other Metabolic Disorders	270-279

996.57 as the principal or first-listed code, followed by the appropriate diabetes mellitus code based on documentation (i.e., code 962.3 for poisoning by insulin).

Coding Alert!

Fifth Digits for Category 250

0: Type II or unspecified type, not stated as uncontrolled
1: Type I (juvenile type), not stated as uncontrolled
2: Type II or unspecified type, uncontrolled
3: Type I (juvenile type), uncontrolled

Chapter 4: Diseases of Blood and Blood-Forming Organs (280-289)

Anemia is one of the conditions in this category of diseases of blood and blood-forming organs. Anemia is a reduction of the number of red blood cells that make up the blood. Anemia exists when hemoglobin content is less than that required to provide the oxygen demands of the body. Although no real subcategories are outlined in the Disease of Blood and Blood-Forming Organs, Table 12.14 classifies diseases and disorders and their corresponding code numbers.

Anemia in Chronic Kidney Disease

- When assigning code 285.21, anemia in chronic kidney disease, it is necessary to assign a code from category 585, chronic kidney disease, to indicate the stage of chronic kidney disease.
- *Purpura* (287) is a condition with various manifestations and diverse causes, characterized by hemorrhages into the skin, mucous membranes, internal organs, and other tissues.

Think Like A Coder 12.6

Choose the correct codes for the following problems.

1. A physician diagnosed a 47-year-old male with diabetes mellitus, type 2 controlled, along with neutropenia and thrombocytopenia. The patient was referred to an endocrinologist.

   □ 250.23, 288.0, 287.4
   □ 250.21, 288.0, 287.3
   □ 250.00, 288.00, 287.5
   □ 250.02, 288.0, 287.3

2. A 67-year-old female with mild, chronic kidney disease had an encounter for kidney dialysis.

   □ 404.01, V56.8, 585.9
   □ 403.00, V56.0, 585.2
   □ 403.00, V56.0, 585.9
   □ V56.0, 585.2

Table 12.14 Diseases of Blood and Blood-Forming Organs

Diseases and Disorders	Code Ranges
Anemias	280-285
Coagulation Defects	286
Purpura and Other Hemorrhagic Conditions	287
Diseases of White Blood Cells	288
Other Diseases of Blood and Blood-Forming Organs	289

- *Thrombocytopenia* (287) is a condition in which there is an abnormal decrease in the number of the blood platelets in cells which can result in purpura. Secondary thrombocytopenia (287.4) is usually caused by underlying conditions such as tuberculosis and lupus erythematosus.
- *Agranulocytosis* is an acute disease characterized by a deficit or complete lack of white blood cells and is coded to category 288.0.
- *Polycythemia* is an excess of red blood cells in the body and is coded under the (289) category.

Chapter 5: Mental Disorders (290-319)

There are no official coding guidelines for ICD-9-CM for mental disorders; however, the World Health Organization offers the following guidelines for this category.

- Organically based illnesses are reported before functional illnesses.
- Within the functional group, the order is psychoses, neuroses, personality disorders, and others.
- When coding mental disorders associated with physical conditions, assign as many codes as necessary to fully describe the condition.

The American Psychiatric Association has developed a classification system to record diagnostic and statistical data on psychiatric patients. The clinical definitions of the diagnostic codes in ICD-9-CM and DSM-IV-TR are nearly identical. The *Diagnostic and Statistical Manual* (DSM-IV-TR) is based on a multiaxial system that evaluates patients on five different axes. These axes are outlined in Table 12.15.

Table 12.16 presents the subcategories of mental disorders and their corresponding code numbers.

Mental Retardation

The ICD-9-CM defines the levels of mental retardation as follows:

Mild mental retardation: IQ of 50 to 70

Moderate mental retardation: IQ of 35 to 49

Severe mental retardation: IQ of 20 to 34

Profound mental retardation: IQ under 20

Unspecified mental retardation: When medical documentation states the patient is mentally retarded but the level of functioning is not recorded.

Think Like A Coder 12.7

Choose the correct code for the following problem.

ABSTRACT:

PATIENT: 27-year-old male

DATE OF SERVICE: July 23, xxxx

BP: 142/80, Weight: 165 lbs, Height: 5'10", Pulse: 94, Temperature: 99.1

Patient was seen today in the office as the insistence of his friend who suspects chronic alcoholism and dependence.

The physical examination revealed:

HEENT: Normal

HEART: Increased heart rate, pulse 94

ABDOMEN: Hard, tender in the right lower quadrant.

PSYCHIATRIC: Not oriented to time and place. Patient speech is slurred, and patient admits to drinking heavily for the last four days. Admits to anorexia, heavy drinking since age 17, vomiting, diarrhea, hallucinations, and blood in the mouth.

DIAGNOSIS: Continuous chronic alcoholism, alcohol-induced psychotic disorder with hallucinations. Referral was made for inpatient treatment.

- ☐ 303.01, 291.1
- ☐ 303.92, 291.5
- ☐ 303.91, 291.3
- ☐ 303.90, 291.81

Chapter 6: Diseases of Nervous System and Sense Organs (320-389)

There are no official coding guidelines for ICD-9-CM for the Nervous System and Sense Organs; however, reviewed in this section will be some of the diseases with special coding instructions that are common to the nervous system and

Table 12.15 Five Axes of the DSM-IV-TR

Axis	Description
Axis I	Clinical Disorders, Other Conditions That May Be a Focus of Clinical Attention
Axis II	Personality Disorders, Mental Retardation
Axis III	General Medical Conditions
Axis IV	Psychosocial and Environmental Problems
Axis V	Global Assessment of Functioning

sense organs. Table 12.17 presents the subcategories of nervous system and sense organ diseases and their corresponding code numbers.

Category Organic Sleep Disorders (327) includes various conditions such as insomnia, hypersomnia, parasomnia, sleep apnea, and sleep-related hypoventilation and hypoxemia most of which include a note that reads, *"code first underlying disease."* This note prompts the coder as to where to look and lists "excludes" notes followed by codes that are excluded.

> **Example**
>
> *327.01 Insomnia due to medical condition classified elsewhere*
>
> *Code first underlying condition*
>
> *excludes insomnia due to mental disorder (327.02)*

Table 12.16 Mental Disorders

Disorders	Code Ranges
Organic Psychotic Conditions	290-294
Other Psychoses	295-299
Neurotic Disorders, Personality Disorders, and other Nonpsychotic Mental Disorders	300-316
Mental Retardation	317-319

Table 12.17 Nervous System and Sense Organs Diseases

Diseases	Code Ranges
Inflammatory Diseases of the Central Nervous System	320-326
Organic Sleep Disorders	327
Hereditary and Degenerative Diseases of the Central Nervous System	330-337
Pain	338
Other Disorders of the Central Nervous System	340-349
Disorders of the Peripheral Nervous System	350-359
Disorders of the Eye and Adnexa	360-379
Diseases of the Ear and Mastoid Process	380-389

- *Bacterial meningitis* (320) is the inflammation of the covering of the meninges on the brain or spinal cord. Meningitis (see Figure 12.2) can be caused by a variety of bacterial organisms, and you must be careful to assign the correct code and, if necessary, code first the underlying disease.
- *Alzheimer's Disease* (331.0) is a chronic, progressive disorder that accounts for half of all the dementias. The coder is instructed to assign an additional code to identify any mental condition, such as 290.3, senile dementia with delirium.
- *Parkinson's Disease* (332) is a chronic nervous disease characterized by a fine, slowly spreading tremor, muscular weakness, and rigidity. Parkinson's disease can be caused by the effects of drugs or chemicals and should be coded by assigning the appropriate poisoning agent and code 332.1.
- *Glaucoma* (365) is a group of eye diseases characterized by increased intraocular pressure, resulting in atrophy of the optic nerve and the possibility of blindness. Open-angle glaucoma (365.1) is marked by increased intraocular pressure despite free access of the aqueous humor. Primary angle-closure glaucoma (365.2) is marked by increase intraocular pressure caused by the iris occluding the anterior chamber structure of the eye.
- *Epilepsy* (345) is a recurrent disorder marked by sudden brief attacks of altered consciousness, motor activity, or sensory phenomena. Epilepsy can be intractable (fifth digit 0), without mention of intractable (fifth digit 1), or unspecified (345.9). Seizures can be classified as petit mal (345.2), grand mal (345.3), or localized.

Indexing Tip:

When indexing for seizures or related conditions, index the word "seizure" which will prompt you to look under "epilepsy" and "see also disease."

Coding Alert!

Hemiplegia

When coding for hemiplegia (paralysis on one side of the body), assign the following fifth digits to describe what side is affected.

0: Affecting unspecified side

1: Affecting dominant side

2: Affecting nondominant side

Please pay close attention of the assignment of late effects codes. Usually, hemiplegia is caused by a condition such as infectious or parasitic disease, abscess of the brain, or a cerebral vascular attack.

Chapter 7: Diseases of the Circulatory System (390-459)

Diseases of the circulatory system in the ICD-9-CM manual contain very specific guidelines and sometimes very complex instructions. When reviewing this category, it is very important to capture the correct coding assignments for your success on your national examination. Many of

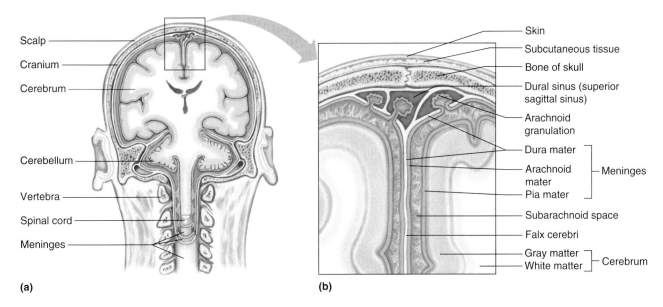

Scalp

Cranium

Cerebrum

Cerebellum

Vertebra

Spinal cord

Meninges

Skin

Subcutaneous tissue

Bone of skull

Dural sinus (superior sagittal sinus)

Arachnoid granulation

Dura mater

Arachnoid mater — Meninges

Pia mater

Subarachnoid space

Falx cerebri

Gray matter

White matter — Cerebrum

(a)

(b)

Figure 12.2

Meningitis – a. Brain, spinal cord, and meninges. b. The meninges include 3 layers—dura mater, arachnoid mater, and pia mater. When the meninges become inflamed because of bacterial organisms, meningitis occurs.

From D. Shier et al., Hole's *Human Anatomy & Physiology,* 11e. Copyright © 2007 The McGraw-Hill Companies. Reprinted with permission.

the conditions and diseases in this category are intricate and interrelated. Read the notes in the ICD-9-CM manual carefully before proceeding to assign codes. Table 12.18 classifies diseases of the circulatory system and their corresponding code numbers.

- Hypertension conditions and diseases are commonly found throughout the subcategory Diseases of the Circulatory System. Many circulatory system disorders are interrelated, complicated, or a late effect of hypertension. See Figure 12.3 for an illustration of the sphygmomanometer, the instrument used to measure blood pressure that aids in diagnosis of hypertension. Please refer to Table 12.10 for a sample and explanation of the Hypertension Table that is found under "hypertension" in the alphabetic index of the ICD-9-CM manual.

- Assign hypertension arterial, essential, primary, systemic and NOS to category 401 with the appropriate fourth digit to indicate malignant (0), benign (1), or unspecified (9).

- Heart conditions 425.8, 429.0-429.3, 429.8, and 429.9 are assigned to a code from category 402 when a casual relationship is stated (due to hypertension) or implied (hypertensive).

- Hypertensive kidney disease with chronic renal failure should be assigned from category 402, hypertensive kidney disease, when conditions in categories 585-587—chronic kidney disease, renal failure (unspecified), and renal sclerosis (unspecified)—are present.

- Hypertensive heart and kidney disease are assigned codes from a combination category of 404, hypertensive

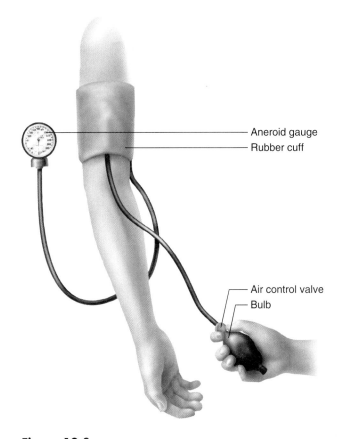

Aneroid gauge

Rubber cuff

Air control valve

Bulb

Figure 12.3

Measuring Blood Pressure – A sphygmomanometer is used to measure the force of blood exerted on the walls of the arteries, which can indicate hypertension.

Table 12.18 Diseases of the Circulatory System

Diseases	Code Ranges
Acute Rheumatic Fever	390-392
Chronic Rheumatic Heart Disease	393-398
Hypertensive Disease	401-405
Ischemic Heart Disease	410-414
Diseases of Pulmonary Circulation	415-417
Other Forms of Heart Disease	420-429
Cerebrovascular Disease	430-438
Diseases of Arteries, Arterioles, and Capillaries	440-449
Diseases of Veins and Lymphatics, and Other Diseases of Circulatory System	451-459

- Controlled hypertension is assigned codes from categories 401-405.
- Uncontrolled hypertension, not responding to therapy regimen, is assigned codes from categories 401-405.
- Cerebrovascular accident (CVA) and stroke are used interchangeably to designate a cerebral infarction. Both of these terms can be indexed to the default code of 434.91. Do not use code 436, acute, but ill-defined, cerebrovascular disease, when the documentation states "stroke" or "CVA."
- A cerebrovascular hemorrhage or infarction that occurs as a result of medical intervention is coded 997.02, iatrogenic cerebrovascular infarction or hemorrhage. This code should be assigned *only* when medical record documentation clearly specifies the cause-and-effect relationship between the medical intervention and the CVA. A secondary code from the code range 430-432 or from a code from subcategories 433 or 434 with a fifth digit of "1" should be used to identify the type of hemorrhage or infarct.

> ## Coding Alert!
>
> ### Category 413—Angina Pectoris
> When assigning a code from category 413, angina pectoris, never assign a code from category 410, AMI, in the same episode of care and site.

> ## Indexing Tip:
>
> *When you are indexing for cardiovascular diseases, some crucial key words include:*
>
> | | |
> |---|---|
> | arteriosclerosis | failure > renal |
> | arteritis | hypertension |
> | cardiomyopathy | ischemia |
> | disease > heart | myocardiopathy |
> | failure > heart | myocarditis |
> | late > effect(s) | |

heart and kidney disease, when both hypertensive heart and kidney disease are stated in the diagnosis. Remember to assume a relationship between the hypertension and the kidney disease even though the condition may not be stated. Assign an additional code from category 428, heart failure, to identify the type of heart failure.

- Code ranges 430-438 should be used to assign hypertensive cerebrovascular disease; then the appropriate hypertension code from code ranges 401405 should be assigned.
- Two codes are necessary to assign hypertensive retinopathy. First assign the code from subcategory 362.11, hypertensive retinopathy, then the appropriate code from categories 401-405 to indicate the type of hypertension.
- Two codes are necessary to identify hypertension, secondary. One code is used to identify the underlying condition/etiology and one from category 405 to identify the hypertension.
- Assign code 796.2, elevated blood pressure reading without diagnosis of hypertension, for transient hypertension.

- Category 438 is used to indicate conditions classifiable to categories 430-437 when the conditions are the causes of late effects (neurological deficits) classified elsewhere.
- Codes from category 438 may be assigned on a health care record along with codes from 430-437 if the patient has a current CVA and deficits from an old CVA.
- ICD-9-CM codes for acute myocardial infarction (AMI) identify the site, such as anterolateral wall or

Think Like A Coder 12.8

Choose the correct codes for the following problems.

1. A 71-year-old male with hemiplegia on left side (dominant), caused by an old spinal cord injury, was admitted to the hospital for isolation after coming in contact with infectious diseases.

   ❑ V01.9, 342.92, 907.1

   ❑ V07.0, 342.91, 907.2

   ❑ V01.8, 342.91, 952.9

   ❑ V01.89, 342.91, 952.9

2. ABSTRACT: The following is a pathology report for a 37-year-old male with a personal history of malignant neoplasm of the bladder.

PATHOLOGY REPORT:

DATE: March, xx, xxxx

CHART NUMBER: xxx-xxx

NAME: xxxx xxxxxx

DEPARTMENT: Medical-Surgical

TISSUE: Colonic polyp

HISTORY: Well-nourished 37-year-old male with history of malignant neoplasm of the lateral wall of the bladder. Colonic polyp 2 cm in diameter at 15 cm from anal verge.

PATHOLOGICAL REPORT: The specimen was received, placed in formalin, and labeled as colonic polyp consisting of a polypoid structure measuring 2 cm in diameter. Representation submitted.

MICROSCOPIC EXAMINATION: 1 slide

DIAGNOSIS: Tubular adenoma with mild superficial dysplasia

   ❑ 154.0, 88304

   ❑ 154.2, 211.3, 88305

   ❑ 211.4, 88307

   ❑ 211.3, 88305

true posterior wall. Subcategories 410.0, 410.6, and 410.8 are used for ST segment elevation myocardial infarction (STEMI). Subcategory 410.7 subendocardial infarction, is used for non-STEMI (NSTEMI) and nontransmural MIs.

Chapter 8: Disease of the Respiratory System (460-519)

The chapter on the respiratory system classifies disease and disorders that begin with the nose, sinuses, pharynx, larynx, trachea, bronchi, lungs, and alveoli. (See Chapter 2 for further review). Some conditions in the respiratory system can be complex to code because often they are classified under "Infectious and Parasitic Diseases." Be prepared to be prompted to code "underlying condition or disease" often when assigning codes for the respiratory system. Table 12.19 classifies diseases of the respiratory system and their corresponding code numbers.

COPD

Chronic obstructive pulmonary disease (COPD) is characterized by the difficult expiration of carbon dioxide from the lungs. The most common obstructive pulmonary diseases are asthma (see Figure 12.4), chronic bronchitis, and emphysema.

Conditions That Comprise COPD and Asthma

Conditions that comprise COPD are as follows: 491.2, obstructive chronic bronchitis; 492, emphysema. All asthma codes are under category 492, asthma. Code 496, chronic airway obstruction, NEC, is a nonspecific code that should be used only when the documentation in a medical record does not specify the type of COPD being treated.

Acute Exacerbation of Chronic Obstructive Bronchitis and Asthma

Codes for chronic obstructive bronchitis and asthma distinguish between uncomplicated cases and those in acute exacerbation (worsening of symptoms). An acute exacerbation is not equivalent to an infection superimposed on a chronic condition, though an exacerbation may be triggered by an infection.

Table 12.19 Diseases of the Respiratory System

Diseases	Code Ranges
Acute Respiratory Infections	460-466
Other Diseases of the Upper Respiratory Tract	470-478
Chronic Obstructive Pulmonary Disease and Allied Conditions	490-496
Pneumoconioses and other Lung Diseases Due to External Agents	500-508
Other Diseases of the Respiratory System	510-519

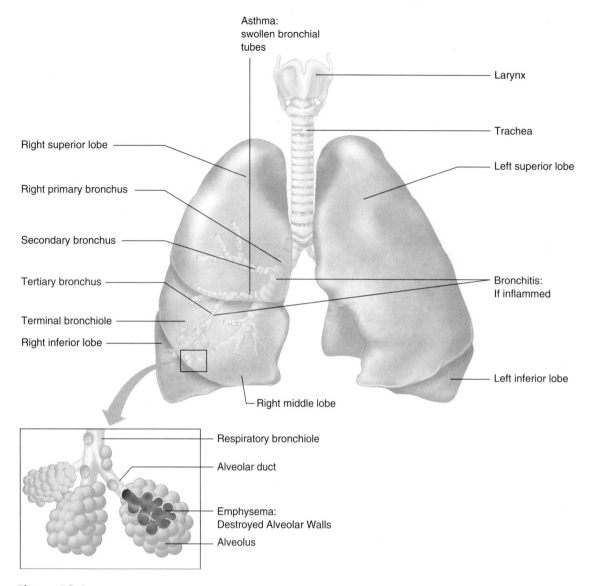

Asthma:
swollen bronchial
tubes

Larynx

Trachea

Right superior lobe

Left superior lobe

Right primary bronchus

Secondary bronchus

Tertiary bronchus

Bronchitis:
If inflammed

Terminal bronchiole

Right inferior lobe

Left inferior lobe

Right middle lobe

Respiratory bronchiole

Alveolar duct

Emphysema:
Destroyed Alveolar Walls

Alveolus

Figure 12.4

Emphysema – Damaged or destroyed alveolar walls no longer support and hold open the airways, and alveoli lose their property of passive elastic recoil. Both of the functions inhibit expiration of carbon dioxide.

From D. Shier et al., Hole's *Human Anatomy & Physiology*, 11e. Copyright © 2007 The McGraw-Hill Companies. Reprinted with permission.

Overlapping Nature of the Conditions That Comprise COPD and Asthma

Because of the interrelated and overlapping nature of the conditions that make up COPD and asthma, there are many variations in the way these conditions will be documented. Please remember that code selection *must* be based on the terms documented by the physician in the medical record. There are many instructional notes under the different COPD subcategories and codes. Please review *all* notes prior to choosing a coding assignment.

Acute Exacerbation of Asthma and Status Asthmaticus

Wheezing and shortness of breath are considered "acute exacerbation," an increase in the severity of symptoms with asthma. The term "status asthmaticus" refers to the patient's

failure to respond to treatment or therapy administered during an asthmatic episode and is life threatening. If status asthmaticus is documented by the physician with any type of COPD or with acute bronchitis, the status asthmaticus should be sequenced first.

Acute Bronchitis with COPD

Acute bronchitis, 466.0, is caused by an infectious organism. When acute bronchitis (see Figure 12.4) is documented with COPD, code 491.22, obstructive chronic bronchitis with acute bronchitis, should be assigned. It is not necessary to also assign code 466.0. If a physician documents in the medical record acute bronchitis with COPD with acute exacerbation, only code 491.22 should be assigned. The acute bronchitis included in code 491.22 supercedes the acute exacerbation. If the medical record documents COPD with acute exacerbation without mention of acute bronchitis, only code 491.21 should be assigned.

Emphysema

Emphysema (492) is an abnormal permanent enlargement of gas exchange airways accompanied by destruction of the alveolar walls (see Figure 12.4). Obstruction results from changes in lung tissue, rather than mucus production and inflammation as in chronic bronchitis.

Coding Alert!

Acute Exacerbation and Status Asthmaticus

It is inappropriate to assign an asthma code with the fifth digit of "2," with acute exacerbation, together with an asthma code with the fifth digit of "1," with status asthmaticus. ONLY the fifth digit "1" should be assigned.

Indexing Tip:

Pneumonia

Pneumonia is classified by infective organism such as aspergillosis, candidiasis, or streptococcusl. Always index "pneumonia" and peruse down the indentations to choose the correct infective organism.

Example: Pneumonia

> *due to*

> *Staphylococcus 482.40*

Think Like A Coder 12.9a

Choose the correct codes for the following problems.

1. A 56-year-old male with a social history of a two-pack-a-day cigarette habit was diagnosed with obstructive chronic bronchitis emphysematous with acute exacerbation. The patient was referred to a pulmonologist.

   ☐ 491.0, 491.8

   ☐ 491.0, 492.8

   ☐ 491.21

   ☐ 491.22

2. A 4-year-old female patient was diagnosed with acute bronchiolitis caused by respiratory syncytial virus along with chronic pharyngitis.

   ☐ 466.19, 079.6, 472.1

   ☐ 466.11, 472.1

   ☐ 466.11, 079.6, 472.1

   ☐ 466.0, 472.2

Review of Health Insurance Portability and Accountability Act Enforcement

Preventing Health Care Fraud and Abuse

Title II of the Health Insurance Portability and accountability Act (HIPAA) defines numerous offenses relating to health care and sets civil and criminal penalties for them. It also creates several programs to control fraud and abuse within the health care system. The most significant provisions of Title II are its Administrative Simplification rules. Title II requires the Department of Health and Human Services to draft rules aimed at increasing the efficiency of the health care system by creating standards for the use and dissemination of health care information. Included in the health care system are billing services, physicians/physician organizations that transmit health care data, and companies that cover health care plans. The five rules regarding Administrative Simplification are the Privacy Rule, the Transactions and Code Sets Rule, the Security Rule, the Unique Identifiers Rule, and the Enforcement Rule.

The Privacy Rule

The Privacy Rule establishes regulations for the use and disclosure of Protected Health Information (PHI). PHI (see Figure 12.5) is any information about health status, provision of health care, or payment for health care that can be linked to an individual, for example, any part of a patient's medical record or payment history. Covered entities must disclose PHI to the individual within 30 days upon request. They must also disclose PHI when required to do so by law, for example, child or elderly abuse.

A covered entity may disclose PHI to facilitate treatment, payment, or health care operations or if the covered entity has obtained authorization from the individual. When a covered entity discloses any PHI, it must take a reasonable effort to disclose only the minimum necessary information required to achieve its purpose. The Privacy Rule gives individuals the right to request that a covered entity correct any inaccurate PHI. It also requires covered entities to take reasonable steps to ensure the confidentiality of communications with individuals.

Transaction and Code Set Rules

Transactions are activities involving the transfer of health care information for specific purposes. Under the Health Insurance Portability and Accountability Act of 1996 (HIPAA), if a health care provider engages in one of the identified transaction, they must comply with the standard for that transaction. HIPAA requires every provider who does business electronically to use the same health care transactions, codes sets, and identifiers. HIPPA has identified ten standard transactions for Electronic Data

---

REPORT OF NEUROLOGICAL PHYSICAL SCREENING

Name: xxxx xxxxx

Med. Rec. #: xxxxxx xxxxxx

Admit #: xxxxxx xxxxx

Room #: Dxxxx

Age: 73

Hardness: Right/Left tendencies

Education: 12 years

Occupation: Retired secretary

Background Information:

XXXX XXXXX is 73-year-old, female, widowed who is currently an inpatient on the psychiatry service at XXX XXXXX. She was admitted on 2–15–XXXX with diagnosis of alcohol dependence and depressive disorder. Essentially, according to the chart, this patient has a long history of severe alcoholism who was found at her residence in a pool of blood on or about 2–11–XXXX. In the fall, Mrs. XXXX suffered a right scalp hematoma and closed head truma with left temporal cerebral contusion. The patient has been admitted three times in the last year for alcohol withdrawal and seizures....

Figure 12.5

Medical Record – Information that is Protected Health Information (PHI).

Interchange (EDI) for the transmission of health care data. Claims and encounter information, payment and remittance advice, and claims status and inquiry are several of the standard transactions. Code sets are the codes used to identify specific diagnosis and clinical procedures on claims and encounter forms. The HCPCS, CPT-4 and ICD-9 codes with which providers are familiar, are examples of codes sets for procedures and diagnoses.

The Security Rule

The Security Rule works in conjunction with the Privacy Rule. It lays out three types of security safeguards required for compliance. These security safeguards are administrative, physical, and technical. For each of these types, the Rule identifies various security standards and names both required and addressable implementation specifications. The standards and specifications are as follows:

Administrative Safeguards

Administrative safeguards are olicies and procedures designed to clearly show how the entity will comply with the act. Covered entities must adopt a written set of privacy procedures and designate a privacy officer. The policies and procedures must reference management oversight with the documented security controls. The procedures should clearly identify employees or classes of employees who will have access to PHI. Entities must show that an appropriate ongoing training program regarding the handling of PHI is provided to all employees. Covered entities that outsource some of their business processes to a third party (a clearinghouse) must ensure that their vendors also have a framework in place with which to comply with HIPAA requirements.

Physical Safeguards

Physical safeguards control physical access to protect against inappropriate access to PHI. Controls must govern the introduction and removal of hardware and software from the network. Access to equipment containing health information should be carefully controlled and monitored as well as access to hardware and software.

Technical Safeguards

Technical safeguards control access to computer systems and enabling covered entities to protect communications containing PHI transmitted electronically over open networks from being intercepted by anyone other than the intended recipient. Information systems housing PHI must be protected from intrusion, and the entity is responsible for ensuring that the data within its systems has not been changed or erased in an unauthorized manner.

The Unique Identifiers Rule and the Enforcement Rule

All covered entities using electronic communications, such as physicians, hospitals, health insurance companies, and third-party entities, must used a single new National Provider Identifier (NPI). The NPI replaces all other identifiers used by health plans, Medicare, Medicaid, and other government programs. The NPI does not replace a provider's Drug Enforcement Administration number, provider's state license number, or tax identification number. The NPI is 10 numerical digits that cannot contain any imbedded intelligence. The NPI is unique and national, it is never reused, and a provider will can usually have one NPI. The Enforcement Rule became effective on March 16, 2006. The Enforcement Rule sets civil money penalties for violating HIPAA rules and establishes procedures for investigations and hearings for HIPAA violations.

Review of Uniform Hospital Data Discharge Set

Procedures

The Uniform Hospital Data Discharge Set (UHDDS) requires all significant procedures to be reported. Medicare requires the reporting of any procedure that affects payment, whether or not it meets the definition of significant

Medical Record	Progress Notes
Date	
4–23–xxxx	Patient was admitted with symptoms of extreme dysuria, anuria, fever of 103.2 degrees F, and hematuria. Physician ordered automated urinalysis with microscopy. R/O UTI. **(Admitting Diagnosis)**
4–24–xxxx	Urinalysis revealed UTI with acute vaginitis. Physician ordered meds and patient was stabilized. **(Principal Diagnosis)**

Figure 12.6
Medical Record

procedure. Other procedures may be reported at the discretion of the hospital or medical facility. A significant procedure is defined by the following:

- Must be surgical in nature
- Carries a risk when administering anesthetics
- Carries a risk during the procedure
- Require specialized training

Surgical by nature includes all main keywords when indexing a procedure, such as destruction, amputation, introduction, insertion, repair, manipulation, endoscopy, laparoscopy, suturing, incision, and excision. All anesthetics carry risk except for topical anesthetics. Procedural risk can be defined as any procedure that has a recognized risk of physiological disturbance, function impairment, or trauma to the patient. Procedures that require specialized training include physicians with medical specialties, qualified technicians, and clinical or surgical teams specifically trained to perform procedures that are specific in nature. The Uniform Bill provides six spaces to report procedures. If more than six procedures are performed that relate to the principal diagnosis, they should be reported to the extent possible.

Diagnoses

Principal Diagnosis

The principal diagnosis is defined as the condition established after study to be chiefly responsible for admission to the patient to the hospital or short-term hospitals. The principal diagnosis is critical for reimbursement because many third-party payers, including Medicare, base reimbursement primarily on principal diagnosis. It is usually a first-listed diagnosis on the physician's notes and patient records; however, the coder must always review the record

carefully to determine the condition that should designate the principal diagnosis. Remember, it is not the admitting diagnosis on the medical record but the work-up or tests or even the outcome after surgery that define the principal diagnosis (see Figure 12.6).

 Think Like A Coder 12.9b

Choose the correct principal diagnoses for the following problems.

1. A 28-year-old female was admitted for work-up because of syncope and severe fatigue. The discharge diagnosis was recorded as severe fatigue caused by stress and hyperthyroidism.

   ❑ Fatigue

   ❑ Stress

   ❑ Hyperthyroidism

   ❑ Stress and hyperthyroidism

2. A 68-year-old male was admitted for encephalitis and encephalomyelitis caused by infectious mononucleosis.

   ❑ Encephalitis and encephalomyelitis

   ❑ Infectious mononucleosis

   ❑ Encephalitis

   ❑ Encephalomyelitis

APPLYING CODING THEORY TO PRACTICE

Choose the correct ICD-9 coding assignment. (Please see Appendix A for answers and rationale).

1. What codes are assigned for a patient admitted for chemotherapy for drug-induced aplastic anemia?

   A. ❏ 248.8, V58.11
   B. ❏ 284.8
   C. ❏ 284.8, V58.12
   D. ❏ 284.9

2. Health record of a newborn delivered in a birthing room: A male infant was born at XXXX XXXXX hospital at 1:19 a.m. on October 28, XXXX. He weighed 7 lbs, 4 oz and was 20 inches long with Apgars of 8 and 9. Dr. XXXX XXXXX performed a history and examination immediately following his vaginal delivery. There were no abnormal findings, and the male infant was discharged with his mother at 12:30 p.m. the same day.

   A. ❏ V30.0, 99435
   B. ❏ V30.2, 99431
   C. ❏ V30.2, 99435
   D. ❏ V30.00, 99435

3. A 24-year-old male presented to the hospital emergency room with symptoms of left and right upper quadrant pain, bloody diarrhea, severe stomach cramps, and extreme fatigue. An infectious consultation was obtained, and a diagnosis was made of infection by *Giardi lamblia* and *Clostridium difficile*.

   A. ❏ 008.46, 009.2, 008.45
   B. ❏ 009.2, 008.45, 007.1
   C. ❏ 007.1, 008.45
   D. ❏ 007.1, 008.5, 009.2

4. An 11-year-old female patient was admitted to the emergency room with severe chest pain and presented with pulmonary infiltrates. The patient has sickle-cell anemia Hb-SS. The treatment consisted of reducing the chest pain to improve breathing. A specialist was called in, and a diagnosis of sickle-cell crisis and acute chest syndrome with respiratory failure was made.

   A. ❏ 282.60, 518.81
   B. ❏ 282.61, 517.3, 518.81
   C. ❏ 282.64, 517.3, 289.52
   D. ❏ 282.62, 517.3, 518.81

5. A 52-year-old male patient with primary cancer of the lung was admitted to the hospital.However, the patient received treatment for his secondary cancer of the prostate. The principal diagnosis in this case would be:

   A. ❏ primary malignancy
   B. ❏ secondary malignancy

6. A 27-year-old male was admitted to the psychiatric ward with symptoms of insomnia, lethargy, disorientation and auditory hallucinations. The patient exhibited signs of difficulty maintaining wakefulness. A psychiatric evaluation was completed, and a diagnosis of heroin and diazepam addiction, transient disorder of insomnia, and drug-induced psychotic disorder with hallucinations was made. Arrangements for the patient to transfer to a detox unit were made.

   A. ❏ 304.70, 307.43, 292.12
   B. ❏ 307.42, 304.81, 292.0
   C. ❏ 305.50, 307.43, 292.12
   D. ❏ 305.50, 304,81, 290.9

7. A 37-year-old female was diagnosed with premature menopause that is symptomatic and ovarian failure. Please code for this diagnosis.

   A. ❏ 256.39
   B. ❏ 256.31, 627.2
   C. ❏ 256.2, 627.4
   D. ❏ 256.31, V49.81

8. Assign the appropriate E code for a self-inflicted injury by use of arsenic.

   Code _____

9. Assign the correct codes to the supervision of a normal first pregnancy and the outcome of delivery of twins who were stillborn.

   Codes _____

10. Health Record:
    Preoperative Diagnosis: Malignantneoplasm of the cervical esophagus, primary with metastasis to the epiglottis. PostoperativeDiagnosis: Cancer in situ of the epiglottis secondary to malignant neop lasm of the cervical esophagus. Indications: Bronchoscopy showed suspicious lesion in the cervical esophagus. Laser photoresection was planned for the excision of this lesion. Upon further inspection of the epiglottis, a darken nodule was visualized. A biopsy was performed on the anterior aspect of the epiglottis, and lab results indicated carcinoma in situ. Chemotherapy was recommended. Code for thediagnoses only.

    A. ❏ 150.4, 231.0
    B. ❏ 231.0, 150.0
    C. ❏ 150.0, 230.0
    D. ❏ 197.8, 197.3

11. An 81-year-old patient presents to the ER with symptoms of fatigue, confusion, left-sided hemiplegia, and dysphagia. The patient's past history includes congestive heart failure. A computed tomography scan was performed with contrast material. The patient suffered an allergic reaction to the latex gloves used by the technician. The emergency room physician diagnosed a CVA with evidence of embolism.

    A. ❏ 437.3, 434.9
    B. ❏ 434.11, 428.0, V15.07
    C. ❏ 437.3, 428.1
    D. ❏ 437.3, 428.1, V15.07

12. Please code for type I diabetes mellitus with an ophthalmic manifestation of blindness, profound impairment of both eyes.

    Code(s) _____

13. A patient diagnosed with AIDS (acquired immune deficiency syndrome) is admitted to the hospital for treatment of Kaposi's sarcoma of the lung. Assign the principle diagnosis.

    A. ❒ 176.4

    B. ❒ 042

    C. ❒ 176.1

    D. ❒ 176.1, 042

14. Many conditions and diseases have "late effects," such as a CVA. How much time must be present between the incident and the acute symptoms to be coded as a late effect?

    A. ❒ More than 48 hours

    B. ❒ No set time

    C. ❒ Six months

    D. ❒ None of the above

15. A 47-year-old female with diverticulitis of the colon and rectal bleeding underwent a colonoscopy. The colonoscopy identified as the cause of bleeding not the diverticulitis but angiodysplasia of the colon. What codes would be assigned?

    A. ❒ 569.85

    B. ❒ 569.85, 562.10

    C. ❒ 568.84

    D. ❒ 569.85, 562.11

ICD-9-CM Guidelines and Coding Conventions Review, Part II

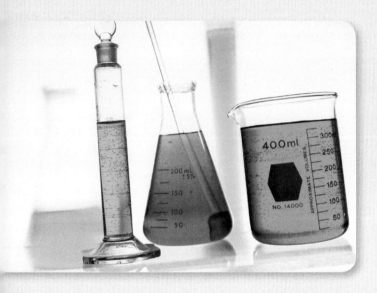

Key terms

Achalasia

Cellulitis

Cirrhosis

Copayment

Explanation of Benefits

Hypertrophy

Meconium

Osteomalacia

Sequela

Septicemia

Sialadenitis

Learning Objectives

- The student will review the organization of the ICD-9-CM Tabular List of Diseases, Index to Diseases, Index to Procedures, and Tabular List of Procedures.

- The student will review the official guidelines for coding and reporting of ICD-9-CM codes.

- The student will review and apply all instructional notes as they appear in the Tabular List of Diseases.

- The student will review and apply all coding conventions and guidelines to Diseases of the Digestive System, Diseases of the Genitourinary System, Complications of Pregnancy, Diseases of the Skin, Diseases of the Musculoskeletal System, Congenital Anomalies, Newborn Perinatal, Signs and Symptoms, and Injury and Poisoning.

- The student will review of Data Quality and Management.

From the Author...

"After working through Chapter 12, tackling all of the ICD-9 concepts presented may seem overwhelming. Do not let this dissuade you from your "bulls eye," which is to pass your national coding examination! As a medical coder, you are not going to know or recognize all diseases, conditions or injuries, however, you will be adept at finding them in the ICD-9 manual and verify if the code you have chosen is correct. Please keep in mind the concepts presented in Chapter One, Test Taking Skills, as you work through the remaining ICD-9 review. Those concepts include pre-reading strategies, knowing your strengths and weaknesses, how to attack difficult questions and problems, and comprehending medical records. I cannot emphasize enough how re-reading a problem for content and clarity is important. Early on as a medical coder, I would make many mistakes if I did not re-read the progress notes, operative notes or medical reports. Making sure you comprehend what you are reading is setting yourself up for success!"

ICD-9-CM Coding Notes for Review

Chapter 9: Diseases of the Digestive System (520-579)

The digestive system is made up of the digestive tract and other organs that aid in digestion. The digestive tract is a series of hollow organs joined in a long, twisting tube from the mouth to the anus, consisting of the following:

- Mouth
- Esophagus
- Stomach
- Small intestine
- Large intestine
- Rectum
- Anus

Organs that help with digestion, but are not part of the digestive tract, include the following:

- Tongue
- Glands in the mouth that make saliva
- Pancreas
- Liver
- Gallbladder

Table 13.1 presents the disorders of the digestive system found in Chapter 9 and their corresponding code numbers.

There are no official coding guidelines for ICD-9-CM for the digestive system disorders; however, the following are notes on specific subcategories outlined in the digestive system.

Diseases of the oral cavity, salivary glands, and jaws include diseases and disorders of the jaw, salivary and parotid glands, teeth, gingivae and periodontium, lips, oral mucosa, and tongue. When you are coding disorders of the oral cavity, understanding the structures of the oral cavity is helpful (see Figure 13.1). Some of these diseases include:

- Disorders of tooth development and eruption (520.0)
- Diseases of hard tissues of teeth (521)
- Diseases of pulp and periapical tissues (522)
- Gingival and periodontal diseases (523)

Diseases of the salivary glands include:

- Atrophy (527.0)
- **Hypertrophy** (527.1)
- **Sialadenitis** (527.2)
- Abscess (527.3)

Diseases of the jaw include:

- Developmental odontogenic cysts (526.0)
- Inflammatory conditions (526.4)
- Alveolitis of jaw (526.5)
- Exotosis of the jaw (526.81)

Table 13.1 Digestive System Diseases

Diseases	Code Ranges
Diseases of Oral Cavity, Salivary Glands, and Jaws	520-529
Diseases of Esophagus, Stomach, and Duodenum	530-538
Appendicitis	540-543
Hernia of Abdominal Cavity	550-553
Noninfectious Enteritis and Colitis	555-558
Other Diseases of Intestines and Peritoneum	560-569
Other Diseases of the Digestive System	570-579

Diseases and disorders of the esophagus, stomach, and duodenum include:

- **achalasia** and cardiospasm (530.0)
- esophagitis (530.1)
- gastric ulcer (531)
- duodenal ulcer (532)
- disorders of function of stomach (536), and
- other disorders of the stomach and duodenum (537).

> **Coding Alert!**
>
> ### Gastritis and Duodenitis (535)
> These illnesses are characterized by nausea, vomiting, stomach pain, and lack of appetite. The following fifth digit subclassifications are as follows:
> 0 without mention of obstruction
> 1 with obstruction

- *Appendicitis* (540-543) is the inflammation of the appendix and is frequently diagnosed in tandem with obstruction or generalized peritonitis.
- There are several types of hernias, such as inguinal, abdominal, femoral, umbilical, ventral, and hiatal.
  - *Inguinal hernias* (550) are protrusions of abdominal cavity contents through an area of the abdominal wall commonly referred to as the groin.

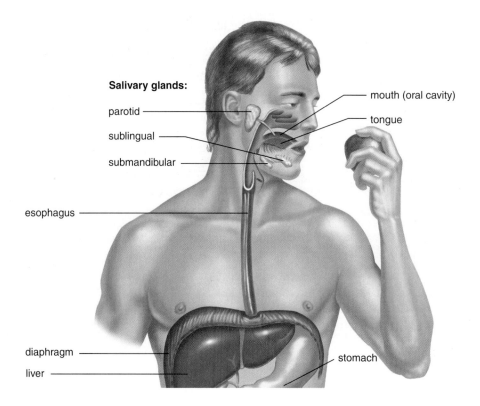

Salivary glands:

parotid

sublingual

submandibular

esophagus

diaphragm

liver

mouth (oral cavity)

tongue

stomach

Figure 13.1

Salivary Glands

From S. Mader, *Understanding Human Anatomy and Physiology,* 5e. Copyright © 2005 The McGraw-Hill Companies, Inc. Reprinted with permission.

- An *umbilical hernia* (553.1) is present at the site of the umbilicus (commonly called a navel or belly button) in the newborn.

- Important steps to remember when coding for hernia include (1) determining the site of the hernia, (2) determining if there is a complication, (3) determining if there is an obstruction, and (4) determining if a fifth digit is required for recurrent, non-recurrent, bilateral, or unilateral.

- *Crohn's disease* (also known as *regional enteritis* [555]) is a chronic, episodic, inflammatory condition of the gastrointestinal tract characterized by transmural inflammation (affecting the entire wall of the involved bowel) and skip lesions, which are areas of inflammation interspersed with areas of normal lining.

- *Ulcerative colitis* (556) is a form of colitis, a disease of the intestine, specifically the large intestine or colon, that includes characteristic ulcers or open sores in the colon.

- *Diverticulum* of the colon (562.1) is the formation of a pouch or sac in the colon. Congenital diverticula are herniations of the entire thickness of the intestinal wall. Conversely, acquired diverticula are herniations of the mucosa through the muscle.

- An *anal fissure* (565.0) is an unnatural crack or tear in the anus, usually extending from the anal opening

and located posteriorly in the midline. A fistula (565.1) is an abnormal connection or passageway between organs or vessels that normally do not connect.

- *Peritonitis* (567) is defined as inflammation of the peritoneum, which is the serous membrane that lines part of the abdominal cavity and some of the viscera the cavity contains.

- ***Cirrhosis*** of the liver (571) is a consequence of chronic liver disease characterized by replacement of liver tissue by fibrotic scar tissue as well as regenerative nodules, leading to progressive loss of liver function. Cirrhosis is most commonly caused by alcoholism and hepatitis C but has many other possible causes.

- *Hepatitis* (573) is an inflammation of the liver, with a variety of causes. Most cases of acute hepatitis are caused by viral infections. The following are a list of the various types of hepatitis:

  - hepatitis A
  - hepatitis B
  - hepatitis C
  - hepatitis B with D
  - hepatitis E
  - hepatitis F (discredited)
  - hepatitis G

Patients with CKD may also suffer from other serious conditions, most commonly diabetes mellitus and hypertension. The sequencing of the CDK code in relationship to codes for other contributing conditions is based on the conventions in the Tabular List of Diseases.

The following is a list of common diseases associated with the genitourinary system:

Chronic cystic mastitis (611), also called *fibrocystic disease,* a condition rather than a disease, is characterized by noncancerous lumps in the breast.

Pelvic inflammatory disease or *disorder* (PID, 614-616) is a generic term for infection of the female uterus, fallopian tubes, and/or ovaries as it progresses to scar formation with adhesions to nearby tissues and organs. Pay close attention to the coding note; it may instruct you to use additional codes to identify the infectious organism (see Figure 13.2).

Genital prolapse includes vaginal wall, uterus, and uterovaginal prolapse and vaginal enterocele. Prolapse may cause urinary incontinence, which should be identified by using an additional code as instructed (see Figure 13.2).

A *rectocele* (618.04) is an abnormal bulging of the rectovaginal septum, which is normally a semi-rigid divider between the rectum and vagina (see Figure 13.2).

- A *cystocele* (618.01-618.09) is a condition that occurs when the wall between a woman's bladder and her vagina weakens and allows the bladder to droop into the vagina (see Figure 13.2).
- *Amenorrhea* (626.0) is the absence of a menstrual period in a woman of reproductive age. All disorders of menstruation and other abnormal bleeding from female genital tract require a fourth digit.

Chapter 11: Complications of Pregnancy, Childbirth and Puerperium (630-677)

Chapter 11 of the ICD-9-CM manual classifies conditions that occur during pregnancy and childbirth and within 6 weeks after delivery. This chapter also includes codes for normal deliveries, obstetrical care, obstetrical complications, and medical care before and after delivery. It will be important for you to decide as a coder whether the condition specified in the diagnostic statement is a complication of pregnancy, labor, or delivery or whether it occurred after the delivery. This chapter can be confusing and at times complex, so make sure that you read all of the code descriptors carefully and assign the appropriate fourth and fifth digits to best describe the disease or condition. Table 13.3 presents the subcategories of the Complications of Pregnancy, Childbirth, and Puerperium chapter and their corresponding code numbers.

General Rules for Obstetrical Cases

The following notes consist of rules for obstetrical cases only.

Codes from Chapter 11 and Sequencing Priority

Codes from Chapter 11, Complications of Pregnancy, Childbirth and Puerperium, have sequencing priority over codes from other chapters. Additional codes from other chapters may be used in conjunction with Chapter 11 codes to further specify conditions. Should the provider document that the pregnancy is incidental to the encounter, then code V22.2 should be used in place of any Chapter 11 codes.

Chapter 11 Codes Used Only on the Maternal Record

Chapter 11 codes should be used only on the maternal record, never on the record of the newborn.

Chapter 11 Fifth Digits

Fifth digits used in categories 640-648 and 651-676 indicate whether the encounter is antepartum (before birth).

Selection of Obstetrical Principal or First-List Diagnosis

The following notes pertain to principal or first-listed obstetrical diagnosis codes.

Think Like A Coder 13.2

Choose the correct codes for the following problems.

1. A 62-year-old male presented in the office with symptoms of urinary difficulties and lower abdominal pain with sexual dysfunction. The physician's diagnosis was hyperplasia of prostate with urinary obstruction and urinary hesitancy. The patient was referred to urology for a comprehensive work-up and examination.

   - 600.20, 788.64
   - 600.91, 788.64
   - 600.21, 788.64
   - 600.91, 788.5

2. A 19-year-old female presented in the office complaining of severe feminine itching and discharge for over 3 days. After examination and tests, the gynecologist diagnosed the patient with unspecified vaginitis and vulvovaginitis caused by *Escherichia coli.* Also, upon examination, the physician noted a medium-sized fissure on the nipple of the left breast.

   - 616.10, 041.4, 611.2
   - 616.11, 611.9
   - 615.9, 611.9, 041.4
   - 616.10, 008.00, 611.2

Indexing Tip:

When coding for hepatitis categorized with viral diseases the coder is instructed to first code the underlying disease typically found in category, "Infectious and parasitic diseases" in the ICD-9-CM manual.

- *Choledocholithiasis* (574.3) is the presence of gallstones in the common bile duct, which causes jaundice and liver cell damage.
- *Acute pancreatitis* (577.0) is rapid-onset inflammation of the pancreas. It can have severe complications and high mortality despite treatment. Fourth digits "0" and "1" for category 577 are used to describe acute (0) or chronic (1).
- *Gastrointestinal bleeding* or *gastrointestinal hemorrhage* (578) describes every form of hemorrhage in the gastrointestinal tract, from the pharynx to the rectum.
- *Malabsorption* (579) is the state of impaired absorption of nutrients in the small intestine. It has many different potential causes, such as vitamin deficiencies, which lead to different patterns in malabsorption.

Think Like A Coder 13.1

Choose the correct codes for the following problems.

1. A 17-year-old female presented with anorexia, jaundice, malaise and fatigue, pain, nausea, and blood in the stool. The physician diagnosed the patient with acute duodenal ulcer with hemorrhage and obstruction caused by long-term use of doxycycline for acne therapy.

   - 534.01, E856
   - 532.41, 533.01
   - 533.01, E856
   - 532.01, E930.4

2. A 32-year-old female presented in the office with symptoms of severe upper gastric pain. After general examination and blood tests, the physician diagnosed hepatitis resulting from infectious mononucleosis.

   - 573.1, 070.12
   - 573.1, 075
   - 573.3, 070.30
   - 573.2, 070.51

Chapter 10: Diseases of the Genitourinary System (580-629)

The genitourinary system includes the urinary organs, the kidneys, the urinary bladder, and the organs of reproduction and their accessories. The ICD-9-CM category diseases of the genitourinary system classifies conditions nary system and the male and female genital t for separately identifiable genitourinary infec plasms, and conditions associated with compl pregnancy, childbirth, and the puerperium (Ch the ICD-9-CM).

Table 13.2 presents the genitourinary syster and their corresponding code numbers.

Chronic Kidney Disease

Chronic kidney disease (CKD) as classified b 9-CM is based on severity. The severity of CK nated by stages I-V. Stage II, code 585.2, equa CKD; and stage IV, code 585.4, equates to s Code 585.6 is assigned when the provider has end-stage renal disease (ESRD). If both a sta and ESRD are documented, you should assign only.

Patients who have undergone kidney tran still have some form of CKD because the kidne may not fully restore kidney function. Code V assigned with the appropriate CKD code for are status post-kidney transplant, based on post-transplant stage.

Use of code 585 (CKD) with V42.0 does no indicate transplant rejection or failure. Patients moderate CKD following a transplant should as having transplant failure unless it is docum medical record. For patients with severe CKD is appropriate to assign code 996.81, complicati planted organ, kidney transplant, when kidn failure is documented. If a post-kidney transpla CKD and the documentation is unclear about wh transplant failure or rejection, you must query t

Table 13.2 Genitourinary System Disorders

Disorder	Code R
Nephritis, Nephrotic Syndrome, and Nephrosis	580-5
Other Diseases of the Urinary System	590-5
Diseases of Male Genital Organs	600-6
Disorders of the Breast	610-6
Inflammatory Disease of Female Pelvic Organs	614-6
Other Disorders of Female Genital Tract	617-6

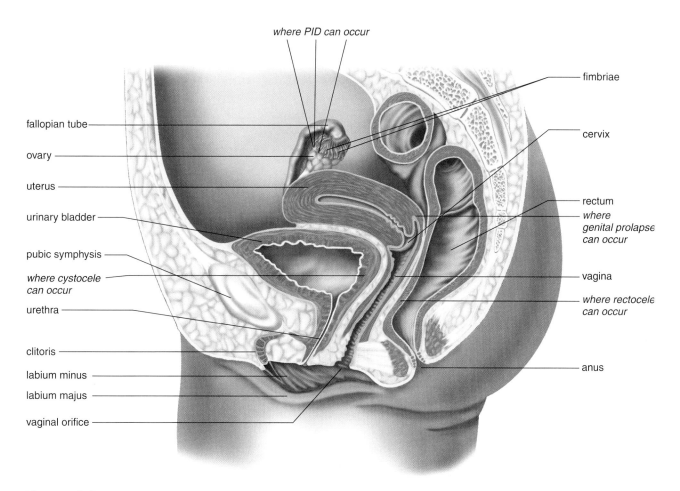

where PID can occur

fallopian tube

ovary

uterus

urinary bladder

pubic symphysis

where cystocele can occur

urethra

clitoris

labium minus

labium majus

vaginal orifice

fimbriae

cervix

rectum

where genital prolapse can occur

vagina

where rectocele can occur

anus

Figure 13.2

Female Reproductive System – Many diseases and disorders can occur in the different structures and organs in this system.

From S. Mader, *Understanding Human Anatomy and Physiology,* 5e. Copyright © 2005 The McGraw-Hill Companies, Inc. Reprinted with permission.

Routine Outpatient Visits for High-Risk Patients

Routine outpatient prenatal visits when no complications are present should be coded V22.2., supervision of normal first pregnancy, or V22.1, supervision of other normal pregnancy, and should be used as the first-listed diagnoses. Remember, these codes should not be used in conjunction with Chapter 11 codes.

Prenatal Outpatient Visits for High-Risk Patients

For prenatal outpatient visits for patient with high-risk pregnancies, use the code V23, supervision of high-risk pregnancy, as the principal or first-list diagnoses. These codes should not be used in conjunction with Chapter 11 codes.

Episodes When No Delivery Occurs

In episodes when no delivery occurs, the principal diagnosis should correspond to the principal complication of the pregnancy that necessitated the encounter. Should more than one complication exist, all of which are treated or monitored, any of the complication codes may be sequenced first.

When a Delivery Occurs

When a delivery occurs, the principal diagnosis should correspond to the main circumstances or complication of the delivery. In cases of cesarean delivery, the selection

Table 13.3 Complications of Pregnancy, Childbirth and Puerperium

Disorder	Code Ranges
Ectopic and Molar Pregnancy	630-633
Other Pregnancy With Abortive Outcome	634-639
Complications Mainly Related to Pregnancy	640-649
Normal Delivery, and Other Indications for Care in Pregnancy, Labor, and Delivery	650-659
Complications Occurring Mainly in the Course of Labor and Delivery	660-669
Complications of the Puerperium	670-677

of the principal diagnosis should correspond to the reason the cesarean delivery was performed unless the reason for admission/encounter was unrelated to the condition resulting in the cesarean delivery.

Outcome of Delivery

An outcome of delivery code, V27.0-V27.9, should be included on every maternal record when a delivery has occurred. These codes are not to be used on subsequent records or on the newborn record.

Fetal Conditions Affecting the Management of the Mother

The following notes concern fetal conditions that may or may not affect the management of the mother during pregnancy.

Fetal Condition Responsible for Modifying the Management of the Mother

Codes from category 655, known or suspected fetal abnormality affecting the management of the mother, and category 656, other fetal and placental problems affecting the management of the mother, are assigned only when the fetal condition is actually responsible for modifying the management of the mother. The fact that the fetal condition exists does not justify assigning a code from this series to the mother's record.

In Utero Surgery

In cases in which surgery is performed on the fetus, a diagnosis code from category 655, known or suspected fetal abnormalities affecting the management of the mother, should be assigned identifying the fetal condition. Procedure code 75.36, correction of fetal defect, should be assigned on the hospital inpatient record. No code from Chapter 15, Newborn (Perinatal), should be used on the mother's record to identify fetal conditions. Surgery performed in utero on a fetus should still be coded as an obstetric encounter.

Human Immunodeficiency Virus Infection in Pregnancy, Childbirth and Puerperium

During pregnancy, childbirth, or the puerperium, a patient admitted because of illness related to human immunodeficiency virus (HIV) should receive a principal diagnosis of 647.6x, other specified infectious and parasitic diseases in the mother classifiable elsewhere, but complicating the pregnancy, childbirth, or the puerperium, followed by 042 and the code(s) for the HIV-related illness(es). A patient with asymptomatic HIV infection status admitted during pregnancy, childbirth, or the puerperium should receive codes of 647.6x and V08.

Current Conditions Complicating Pregnancy

Assign a code from subcategory 648.x for patients who have current conditions when the condition affects the management of the pregnancy, childbirth, or puerperium. Use secondary codes from other chapters to identify the conditions, as appropriate.

Diabetes Mellitus in Pregnancy

Diabetes mellitus is a significant complicating factor in pregnancy. Pregnant women who are diabetic should be assigned code 648.0x, diabetes mellitus complicating pregnancy, and a secondary code from category 250, diabetes mellitus, to identify the type of diabetes. Code V58.67, long-term current use of insulin, should also be assigned if the diabetes mellitus is being treated with insulin.

Gestational Diabetes

Gestational diabetes can occur during the second and third trimester of pregnancy in women who were not diabetic before pregnancy. Gestational diabetes can cause complications in the pregnancy similar to those caused by pre-existing diabetes mellitus. It also puts the woman at greater risk of developing diabetes after pregnancy. Gestational diabetes is coded 648.8x, abnormal glucose tolerance. Code 648.0x and 648.8x should never be used together on the same record. Code V58.67, long-term current use of insulin, should also be assigned if the diabetes mellitus is being treated with insulin.

Normal Delivery

Code 650 is used in cases when a woman is admitted for a full-term normal delivery and delivers a single, healthy infant without any complications antepartum, during the delivery, or postpartum. Code 650 is always a principal diagnosis. It should not be used if any other code from Chapter 11 is needed to describe a current complication of the antenatal, delivery, or perinatal period. Additional codes from other chapters may be used with code 650 if they are not related in any way to complications of pregnancy.

> **Coding Alert!**
>
> ## Multiple Gestation (651)
> Category 651 is for multiple gestation, which indicates the patient is pregnant with twins, triplets, quadruplets, or other specified multiple fetus presence.

Normal Delivery with Resolved Antepartum Complication

Code 650 may be used if the patient had a complication at some point during her pregnancy but the complication is not present at the time of the admission for delivery.

V27.0 Single Liveborn, Outcome of Delivery

V27.0, Single liveborn, is the only outcome of delivery code appropriate for use with 650.

The Postpartum and Peripartum Periods

The following notes concern conditions, illnesses, and complications after birth and around the time of birth. The postpartum period begins immediately after delivery and continues for 6 weeks following delivery. The peripartum period is defined as the last month of pregnancy to 5 months postpartum.

Postpartum Complications

A postpartum complication is any complication occurring within the 6-week period.

> ## Coding Alert!
>
> ## Fifth Digits for Complications during Labor and Delivery and the Puerperium
>
> The following fifth digits are used to indicate the current episode of care:
>
> 0 – Unspecified as to episode of care or not applicable
> 1 – Delivered, with or without mention of antepartum condition
> 2 – Delivered, without mention of postpartum complication
> 3 – Antepartum condition or complication
> 4 – Postpartum condition or complication

Pregnancy-Related Complications after 6-Week Postpartum Period

Chapter 11 codes may also be used to describe pregnancy-related complications after the 6-week period should the provider document that a condition is pregnancy related.

Postpartum Complications Occurring during the Same Admission as Delivery

Postpartum complications that occur during the same admission as the delivery are identified with a fifth digit of "2." Subsequent admissions/encounters for postpartum complications should be identified with a fifth digit of "4."

Admission for Routine Postpartum Care after Delivery Outside Hospital

When the mother delivers outside the hospital before admission and is admitted for routine postpartum care with no noted complications, code V24.0, postpartum care and examination immediately after delivery, should be assigned as the principal diagnosis. A delivery diagnosis code should not be used for a woman who has delivered before admission to the hospital. Any postpartum conditions and/or postpartum procedures should be coded.

Late Effects of Complications of Pregnancy

The following notes concern "late effects" or a residual condition that develops after the end of pregnancy, childbirth, and puerperium.

Code 677

Code 677, late effect of complication of pregnancy, childbirth, and the puerperium, is for use in those cases when an initial complication of a pregnancy develops a **sequela** requiring care or treatment at a future date. Code 677 may be used at any time after the initial postpartum period.

Sequencing of Code 677

Code 677, like all late effects codes, must be sequenced following the code describing the sequela of the complication.

Abortions

The following notes concern the various types of abortions that take place as a result of a medical condition or a voluntary action.

Fifth Digits Required for Abortion Categories

Fifth digits are required for abortion categories 634-637. Fifth-digit "1," incomplete, indicates that all products of conception have not been expelled from the uterus. Fifth-digit "2," complete, indicates that all products of conception have been expelled from the uterus before the episode of care.

> ## Coding Alert!
>
> ## Legally Induced Abortion (635)
>
> Medical terms that apply to this category are (1) termination of pregnancy, (2) elective abortion, (3) legal abortion, and (4) therapeutic abortion.
> Remember – The fifth digits for this category are:
>
> 0 – unspecified
> 1 – incomplete
> 2 – complete

Code from Categories 640-648 and 651-659

A code from categories 640-648 or 651-659 may be used as an additional code with an abortion code to indicate the complication leading to the abortion.

Fifth-digit "3" is assigned with codes from these categories when used with an abortion code because the other fifth digits will not apply. Codes from the 660-669 series are not to be used for complications of abortion.

Code 639 for Complications

Code 639 is to be used for all complications following abortion. Code 639 cannot be assigned with codes from categories 634-638.

Abortion with Liveborn Fetus

When an attempted termination of a pregnancy results in a liveborn fetus, assign code 644.21, early onset of delivery, with an appropriate code from category V27, outcome of delivery. The procedure code for the attempted termination of pregnancy should also be assigned.

Retained Products of Conception Following an Abortion

Subsequent admissions for retained products of conception following a spontaneous or legally induced abortion are assigned the appropriate code from category 634, spontaneous abortion, or 635, legally induced abortion, with a fifth digit of "1" (incomplete). This advice is appropriate even when the patient was discharged previously with a discharge diagnosis of complete abortion.

Indexing Tip:

Many of the obstetrical codes can be found by using the following key words:

"Pregnancy," "Delivery," "Labor," "Puerperal," "Outcome of delivery," and "Abortion."

💡 Think Like A Coder 13.3

Choose the correct codes for the following problems.

1. A 28-year-old female, para 1, gravida 2, 15 weeks' gestation, suffered a complete spontaneous abortion complicated by renal failure. The patient was taken to the emergency room (ER) for a D&C (dilation and curettage.)

   - 636.32
   - 639.3
   - 634.32
   - 637.32

2. A 31-year-old female presented at the ER with an ectopic pregnancy complicated by salpingitis caused by group D streptococcus.

   - 633.80, 638.0, 041.04
   - 633.91, 639.0, 041.04
   - 633.10, 639.0, 041.04
   - 633.91, 638.0, 038.0

Chapter 12: Diseases of Skin and Subcutaneous Tissue (680-709)

Chapter 12 of the ICD-9-CM manual classifies diseases and disorders of the skin and subcutaneous tissue inclusive of the epidermis, dermis, subcutaneous tissue, sweat glands, hair, hair follicles, and nails. Table 13.4 presents the subcategories of the Skin and Subcutaneous Tissue disorders and their corresponding code numbers.

Although there are no official ICD-9-CM coding guidelines for the Skin and Subcutaneous Tissue chapter, the following are specific notes that can be used to gain a better understanding of this chapter.

- A *carbuncle* (680) is an abscess larger than a boil, usually with one or more openings draining pus onto the skin. It is usually caused by bacterial infection. A *furuncle* (680) is a skin disease caused by the

inflammation or hair follicles resulting in the localized accumulation of pus. The fourth digit will describe the anatomical site of the carbuncle or furuncle.

- **Cellulitis** and *abscess* (681-682) is an inflammation of the connective tissue that can be caused by a bacterial infection. Group A *Streptococcus* or *Staphylococcus aureus* are usually the cause; however, another organism can be involved as well. Category 681 includes lymphangitis and abcess, which is often associated with cellulitis of the skin. You may be directed to use an additional code to identify the infective organism.

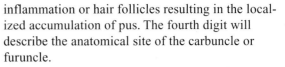

Coding Alert!

Category 681

- When cellulitis (681) occurs with chronic skin ulcer (707), remember to code both conditions.
- When cellulitis occurs secondary to an injury such as a burn, two codes are required, one for the cellulitis and one for the injury.

- *Pilonidal cyst* (685) is a term used for any type of skin infection near the tailbone that often drains through the opening at the postanal dimple. Fourth digits are "0," with abscess, and "1," without mention of abscess.
- Other inflammatory conditions of the skin and subcutaneous tissue (690-698) include *eczema, dermatitis* (seborrheic, atopic, and contact) *rosacea, lupus erythematosus, psoriasis,* and *lichen.*
- *Contact dermatitis* (692) is a skin reaction resulting from exposure to allergens or irritants. The fourth digit in this category will describe the type of irritant involved; fifth digits in this category involve solar radiation, sunburn, and metal agents.

Table 13.4 Skin and Subcutaneous Tissue Chapter Subcategories

Disorder	Code Ranges
Infections of Skin and Subcutaneous Tissue	680-686
Other Inflammatory Conditions of Skin and Subcutaneous Tissue	690-698
Other Diseases of Skin and Subcutaneous Tissue	700-709

- *Psoriasis* (696) is a disease that affects the skin and joints. It is commonly causes red, scaly patches to appear on the skin. The scaly patches are areas of excessive skin production and inflammation. The fourth digit describes similar forms of psoriasis.

- *Lichen* (697) is a pruritic (itching) skin disease marked by angular, flat-topped, violet-colored papules. Lichen may be acute and widespread over the body or chronic and localized.

- *Actinic keratosis* (702.0) is a premalignant condition of thick, scaly, or crusty patches of skin, most commonly found in fair-skinned people who are frequently exposed to the sun.

- *Hirsutism* (704.1) is excessive and increased hair growth in women in locations on the body where the occurrence of terminal hair (developed hair) normally is minimal or absent.

- A *sebaceous cyst* (706.2) is a closed sac or cyst below the surface of the skin that has a lining that resembles the uppermost part of a hair follicle and fills with fatty white material called keratin.

Indexing Tip:

Many of the Skin and Subcutaneous Tissue codes can be found by using the following key words:

"Carbuncle," "Furuncle," "Cellulitis," "Dermatitis," "Seborrhea," "Psoriasis," and "Ulcer."

Think Like A Coder 13.4

Choose the correct codes for the following problems.

1. A 17-year-old male presented in the office with complaint of painful burn by an open flame on his back along with a red, hot swollen patch that had become larger in the last 34 hours. After careful examination and tests, the physician diagnosed *Staphylococcus cellulitis* of a second-degree burn of the patient's back.

   - 681.10, 942.34, 041.11
   - 682.2, 942.34, 041.11
   - 681.10, 942.4, 041.10
   - 682.2, 942.4, 041.10

2. Upon examination of a 93-year-old female in a skilled nursing facility, the physician diagnosed pressure ulcers on the bedridden patient's hip, sacrum, and right elbow. The physician began an aggressive treatment plan immediately.

   - 707.11, 707.02, 707.01
   - 707.07, 707.03, 707.01
   - 682.5, 682.2, 682.3
   - 682.5, 707.03, 707.01

- *Decubitus ulcers* (707.0), or "bedsores," are lesions caused by unrelieved pressure to any anatomical site, especially over bony areas of the body. The fifth digit describes the anatomical part of the body that is the site of the decubitus ulcer.

- *Urticaria* (708), or "hives," is a common form of allergic reaction that caused raised red skin welts on the body. The fourth digit describes the type of urticaria involved in the diagnosis.

- *Vitiligo* (709.01) is a chronic skin condition that causes loss of pigment, resulting in irregular pale patches of skin.

Chapter 13: Diseases of Musculoskeletal System and Connective Tissue (710-739)

Chapter 13 of the ICD-9-CM manual classifies diseases and disorders of the musculoskeletal system and connective tissue. Injuries that affect the musculoskeletal system such as fractures are classified in Chapter 17, "Injury and Poisoning" of the ICD-9-CM manual. Table 13.5 presents the Musculoskeletal System and Connective Tissue disorders and their corresponding code numbers.

Although there are no official ICD-9-CM coding guidelines for the Musculoskeletal System and Connective Tissue chapter, the following are specific notes that can be used to gain a better understanding of this chapter. Table 13.6 illustrates the fifth-digit subclassifications for use with categories 711-712, 715-716, 718-719, and 730.

- *Systemic lupus erythematosus* (710.0) is a chronic autoimmune disease that is potentially debilitating and sometimes fatal as the immune system attacks the body's cells and tissue, resulting in tissue damage. The coder is directed to use an additional code to identify the manifestation.

- *Arthropathy* (710-719) is a disease of a joint. Arthropathies in category 711-713 use the fifth digit

Table 13.5 Musculoskeletal System and Connective Tissue Chapter Disorders

Disorder	Code Ranges
Arthropathies and Related Disorders	710-719
Dorsopathies	720-724
Rheumatism, Excluding the Back	725-729
Osteopathies, Chondropathies, and Acquired Musculoskeletal Deformities	730-739

Table 13.6 Fifth Digit Subclassifications for codes 711-712, 715-716, 718-719, and 730

Fifth Digit	Specified Site
0	Site unspecified
1	Shoulder region: acromioclavicular joint(s)
2	Upper arm: elbow joint, humerus
3	Forearm: radius, ulna, wrist joint
4	Hand: carpus, metacarpus, phalanges
5	Pelvic region and thigh: buttock, femur, hip
6	Lower leg: fibula, knee joint, patella, tibia
7	Ankle and foot: ankle joint, digits (toes), metatarsus, phalanges (foot), tarsus, other joints in foot
8	Other specified sites: head, neck, ribs, skull, trunk, vertebral column
9	Multiple sites

to describe the anatomical site. The coder is directed to use an additional code to code first the underlying disease.

- *Rheumatoid arthritis* (714.0) is considered a chronic, inflammatory autoimmune disorder that causes the immune system to attack the joints. The coder is directed to identify the manifestation as myopathy (359.6) or polyneuropathy (357.1).

- *Osteoarthritis* (715) is a condition in which low-grade inflammation results in pain in the joint because of wearing of the cartilage that covers and acts as a cushion inside the joints (see Figure 13.3). The fifth digits in this category describe the anatomical site.

- *Spondylosis* (721) is spinal degeneration and deformity of a joint(s) of two or more vertebrae that commonly occurs with the aging process.

- *Degeneration of the intervertebral disc* (722) is commonly referred to as "degenerative disc disease" of the spine that involves the lower part of the spine.

- *Torticollis* (723.5), or "wry neck," is a condition in which the head is tilted toward one side and the chin is elevated and turned toward the opposite side.

- *Adhesive capsulitis* (726.0) is a disorder in which the shoulder capsule, the connective tissue surrounding the glenohumeral joint of the shoulder, becomes inflamed and stiff.

- *Synovitis* (727.0) is inflammation of a synovial membrane that lines a synovial joint. The condition is usually painful when the joint is moves and normally swells because of fluid collection.

- A *ganglion cyst* (727.4) is a swelling that often appears on or around joints and tendons in the hand. Subcategories 727.1, 727.4, 727.5, 727.6, and 727.8 all require a fifth digit.

- *Osteomyelitis* (730) is an infection of bone or bone marrow, usually caused by pyogenic bacteria or mycobacteria. Please refer to Table 13.6 for the fifth digit subclassifications for this category.

- *Osteoporosis* (733.0) is a disease of the bone in which the bone mineral density is reduced, putting osteoporotic bones at risk for fractures.

- *Pathological fractures* (733.1) are due to bone structure weakening by the disease process. Code the underlying disease in addition to the appropriate codes from subcategory 733.1. Sequencing of the codes depends on whether the fracture only or the fracture and the underlying disease were treated.

- *Osteopenia* (744.9, unspecified disorder of the bone) is a decrease in bone mineral density that can be a precursor condition to osteoporosis.

- *Hallux valgus* (735.0) is a painful structural deformity of the bones and the joint between the foot and big toe. The fourth digit describes the type of condition in this category.

- *Kyphosis* (737.1) is curvature of the upper spine. Lordosis (737.2) is an inward curvature of a portion of the

Think Like A Coder 13.5

Choose the correct codes for the following problems.

1. Chapter 13, "Diseases of the Musculoskeletal System and Connective Tissue," contains the codes for all fractures in the ICD-9-CM manual.

   - True
   - False

2. A physician diagnosed an 11-year-old male with juvenile osteochondrosis of the left tibia along with a pathological fracture of the left fibula caused by **osteomalacia.**

   - 732.4, 733.16, 268.2
   - 732.3, 823.82, 269.0
   - 823.01, 823.00, 268.2
   - 732.4, 823.02, 268.2

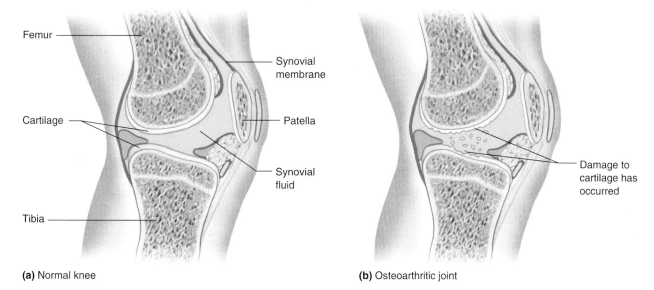

(a) Normal knee   **(b)** Osteoarthritic joint

Figure 13.3

Osteoarthritis – Illustration shows difference between a normal knee and an osteoarthritis knee.

From D. Shier et al., Hole's *Human Anatomy & Physiology*, 11e. Copyright © 2007 The McGraw-Hill Companies. Reprinted with permission.

vertebral column. Scoliosis (737.3) is a condition that involves complex lateral and rotational curvature and deformity of the spine.

- *Spondylolisthesis* (738.4) is an anteroposterior translatory movement of two spinal vertebrae in relationship to each other caused by instability between the two involved vertebrae.

Chapter 14: Congenital Anomalies (740-759)

Congenital anomalies are intrauterine developments of organs or structures that are abnormal in form, structure, or position. This chapter classifies conditions present at birth that include anomalies in most of the body's systems. The chapter is organized by organ system or anatomical site affected by the congenital anomaly. There are no subcategories in Chapter 14, Congenital Anomalies.

Codes in Categories 740-759, Congenital Anomalies

- Assign an appropriate code or codes from categories 740-759, Congenital Anomalies, when an anomaly is documented. A congenital anomaly may be the principal/first-listed diagnosis on a record or a secondary diagnosis. When a congenital anomaly does not have a unique code assignment, assign an additional code or codes for any manifestations that may be present.
- When the code assignment specifically identifies the congenital anomaly, manifestations that are an inherent component of the anomaly should not be coded separately. Additional codes should be assigned for manifestations that are not an inherent component.

- Codes from Chapter 14 may be used throughout the life of the patient. If a congenital anomaly has been corrected, a personal history code should be used to identify the history of the anomaly. Although present at birth, a congenital anomaly may not be identified until later in life. Whenever the condition is diagnosed by the physician, it is appropriate to assign a code from codes 740-759.
- For the birth admission, the appropriate code from category V30, liveborn infants, according to type of birth should be sequenced as the principal diagnosis, followed by any of the congenital anomaly codes 740-759.
- *Anencephaly* (740) is a cephalic disorder that results from a neural tube defect that occurs when the cephalic end of the neural tube fails to close, resulting in the absence of a major portion of the brain.
- *Ventricular septal defect* (745.4) is a defect in the ventricular septum, which is the wall dividing the left and right ventricles of the heart.
- *Atrial septal defect* (745.5) is a form of congenital heart disease that enables blood flow between the left and right atria via the interatrial septum.
- *Congenital hydrocephalus* (742.3) is fluid accumulation within the skull of the newborn that involves internal and external brain spaces (see Figure 13.4).
- *Pyloric stenosis* (750.5) is a condition that causes severe vomiting in the first few months of life as a result of the narrowing of the opening from the stomach to the intestines.
- *Hypospadias* (752.6) is a birth defect of the urethra in the male that involves an abnormally placed urethral meatus (opening).

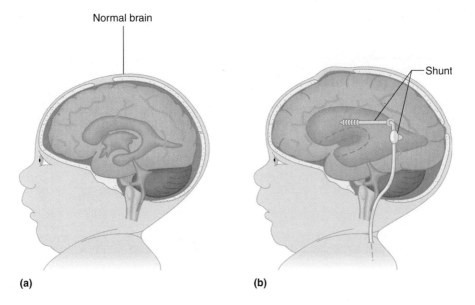

Normal brain

Shunt

(a)   (b)

Figure 13.4

Congenital Hydrocephalus – a. Normal brain of infant. b. Brain of infant with hydrocephalus where a shunt has been placed to relieve pressure.

From N. Thierer and L. Breitbard, *Medial Terminology, Language for Health Care,* 2e. Copyright © 2006 The McGraw-Hill Companies, Inc. Reprinted with permission.

 Indexing Tip:

Many of the diseases found in Congenital Anomalies are named after the physician who first discovered the disease. Example: Marfan Syndrome was discovered by Antoine Marfan in 1896 and can be indexed under "Marfan."

 Think Like A Coder 13.6

Choose the correct answers for the following problems.

1. If an individual's congenital anomaly has been corrected, the coder would:

   - Still code the congenital anomaly along with other diagnoses
   - Not code the congenital anomaly since it was corrected
   - Code the congenital anomaly and a V code (V10-V15) to describe a personal history of the congenital anomaly
   - Code only a V code (V10-V15) to indicate personal history of the individual

2. A pediatrician diagnosed a 2-day-old male infant with spina bifida along with Arnold-Chiari syndrome type II in the cervical region.

   - 742.3, 741.01
   - 741.01
   - 742.0, 742.3, 741.0
   - 742.3, 771.2

- *Pectus excavatum* (754.81) is a congenital deformity of the sternum, which is depressed into the chest, resulting in a sunken appearance.
- *Polydactyly* (755.0) is the abnormal condition consisting of more than the usual number of digits on the hands or the feet.
- *Down syndrome,* or *trisomy 21* (758.0), is a genetic disorder caused by the presence of all or part of an extra 21st chromosome.

Chapter 15: Conditions in the Perinatal Period (760-779)

The codes found in Chapter 15, Conditions in the Perinatal Period, are for the medical record of the fetus or newborn only and are never found or recorded in the medical record of the mother. The perinatal period, surrounding the birth of the newborn, is the time of birth up to 28 days after the birth. Table 13.7 presents the disorders found in the Conditions in the Perinatal Period chapter and their corresponding code numbers.

Table 13.7 Conditions in the Perinatal Period Chapter Disorders

Disorder	Code Ranges
Maternal Causes of Perinatal Morbidity and Mortality	760-763
Other Conditions Originating in the Perinatal Period	764-779

Sequencing of Perinatal Codes

Codes from Chapter 15 should be sequenced as the principal, or first-listed, diagnosis on the newborn record, with the exception of the appropriate V30 code for the birth episode, followed by codes from any other chapter that provide additional detail. The "use additional code" note at the beginning of the chapter supports this guideline. If the index does not provide a specific code for a perinatal condition, assign code 779.89, Other specified conditions originating in the perinatal period, followed by the code from another chapter that specifies the condition. Codes for signs and symptoms may be assigned when a definitive diagnosis has not been established.

Birth Process or Community Acquired Conditions

If a newborn has a condition that may be either due to the birth process or community acquired and the documentation does not indicate which it is, the default is "due to the birth process," and the code from Chapter 15 should be used. If the condition is community acquired, a code from Chapter 15 should not be assigned.

Clinically Significant Conditions

All clinically significant conditions noted on routine newborn examination should be coded. A condition is clinically significant if it has implications for future health care needs or requires:

- Clinical evaluation
- Therapeutic treatment
- Diagnostic procedures
- Extended length of hospital stay
- Increased nursing care and/or monitoring

Use of Codes V30-V39

When coding the birth of an infant, assign a code from categories V30-V39, according to the type of birth. A code from this series is assigned as a principal diagnosis and assigned only once to a newborn at the time of birth.

Newborn Transfers

If the newborn is transferred to another institution, the V30 series is not used at the receiving hospital.

Assigning a Code from Category V29

Assign a code from category V29, observation and evaluation of newborns and infants for suspected conditions not found, to identify those instances when a healthy newborn is evaluated for a suspected condition that is determined after study not to be present. Do not use a code from category V29 when the patient has identified signs or symptoms of a suspected problem; in such cases code the sign or symptom.

- A code from category V29 may also be assigned as a principal diagnosis for readmissions or encounters

when the V30 code no longer applies. Codes from category V29 are for use only for healthy newborns and infants for which no condition after study is found to be present.

- A V29 code should be used as a secondary code after the V30 outcome of delivery code.

Use of Other V Codes on Perinatal Records

V codes other than V309 and V29 may be assigned on a perinatal or newborn record. The codes may be used as a principal, or first-listed, diagnosis for specific types of encounters or for readmissions or encounters when the V30 code no longer applies.

Maternal Causes of Perinatal Morbidity

Codes from categories 760-763, maternal causes or perinatal morbidity and mortality, are assigned only when the maternal condition has actually affected the fetus or newborn. The fact that the mother has an associated medical condition or experiences some complication of pregnancy, labor, or delivery does not justify the routine assignment of codes from these categories to the newborn record.

> **Indexing Tip:**
>
> *Many of the conditions and complications found in this chapter can be index by the following keywords:*
>
> *"birth," "outcome of delivery," and "delivery."*

Congenital Anomalies in Newborns

For birth admission, the appropriate code from category V30, liveborn infants according to type of birth, should be used, followed by any congenital anomaly codes, categories 740-759. Use additional secondary codes from other chapters to specify conditions associated with the anomaly, if applicable.

Coding Additional Perinatal Diagnoses

Assigning Codes for Conditions That Require Treatment

Assign codes for conditions that require treatment or further investigation, prolong the length of stay, or require resource utilization.

Codes for Conditions Specified as Having Implications for Future Health Care Needs

Assign codes for conditions that have been specified by the provider as having implications for future health care needs.

Codes for Newborn Conditions Originating in the Perinatal Period

Assign codes for newborn conditions originating in the perinatal period (760-779) as well as for complications arising during the current episode of care classified in other chapters only if the diagnoses have been documented by the responsible provider at the time of transfer or discharge as having affected the fetus or newborn.

Prematurity and Fetal Growth Retardation

Providers use different criteria in determining prematurity. A code for prematurity should not be assigned unless it is documented. The fifth-digit assignment for codes from category 764 and subcategories 765.0 and 765.1 should be based on the recorded birth weight and estimated gestational age.

Newborn Sepsis

Codes 771.81, **septicemia** of newborn, should be assigned with a secondary code from category 041, bacterial infections in conditions classified elsewhere and of unspecified site, to identify the organism. It is not necessary to use a code from subcategory 995.9, systemic inflammatory response syndrome (SIRS), on a newborn record. Code 771.81 describes the sepsis.

Miscellaneous Notes

- *Fetal alcohol syndrome* (760.71) is a term used to describe the varied effects of alcohol consumption on the brain of the fetus during pregnancy.

Coding Alert!

Mother's Record versus Newborn's Record

Do not assign codes from Chapter 15 to the mother's record. Also, do not assign codes from Chapter 11, "Complications of Pregnancy, Childbirth and the Puerperium," to the newborn's record.

 Think Like A Coder 13.7

Choose the correct answers for the following problems.

1. The perinatal period is considered:

   - 28 days before the birth and the 28 days after the birth
   - Time of birth up to 28 days after the birth
   - Time of birth up to 6 weeks after the birth
   - 28 days before the birth and 6 weeks after the birth

2. In the ER a physician delivered a single, liveborn male infant with septicemia caused by hemophilus influenzae. The infant was taken to the critical care unit. The mother, who delivered vaginally, was taken to the recovery room and put under observation. (Code only for the newborn's chart.)

   - V27.0, 773.2, 038.4
   - V27.0, 771.81, 041.5
   - V30.00, 771.81, 041.5
   - V30.01, 771.81, 038.4

- **Meconium** *aspiration syndrome* (770.1) occurs when infants take meconium into their lungs during or before delivery.
- *Jaundice* (774.2), a yellowing of the skin, conjunctiva, and mucous membranes caused by increased levels of bilirubin in the human body, often affects newborns.

Chapter 16: Signs, Symptoms, and Ill-Defined Conditions (780-799)

This chapter includes signs, symptoms and abnormal results of laboratory or the investigative procedures, as well as ill-defined conditions for which there are no other specific diagnoses classified elsewhere in the ICD-9-CM manual. Codes from this chapter are used to report symptoms, signs, and ill-defined conditions that usually equate to two or more diagnoses or represent complications or problems that may affect the management of the patient.

Table 13.8 presents the disorders found in the Signs, Symptoms, and Ill-Defined Conditions chapter and their corresponding code numbers.

Although there are no official ICD-9-CM coding guidelines for the Signs, Symptoms, and Ill-Defined Conditions chapter, the following are specific notes that can be used to gain a better understanding of this chapter.

- Most all categories in this group could be designated as "not otherwise specified," or as "unknown etiology," or as "transient." The Alphabetic Index of Diseases should be consulted to determine which symptoms and signs are to be allocated here and which to more specific sections of the classification; the residual subcategories numbered .9 are provided for other relevant symptoms that cannot be allocated elsewhere in the classification.
- Burns are defined by degree of burn (first, second, and third degree) and location (site) of the burn on the body.
- *Seizures* (780.3) are temporary abnormal electrophysiological phenomena of the brain, resulting in abnormal synchronization of electrical neuronal activity manifested in the patient as alteration of mental state tonic or clonic movements and convulsions.

Table 13.8 Disorders Presented in the Signs, Symptoms, and Ill-Defined Conditions Chapter

Disorders	Code Ranges
Symptoms	780-789
Nonspecific Abnormal Finding	790-796
Ill-Defined and Unknown Causes of Morbidity and Mortality	797-799

- *Chronic fatigue syndrome* (780.71) is a syndrome of unknown and possibly multiple etiologies affecting the central nervous system and many other systems and organs.
- *Dysdiadochokinesia* (781.3) is the medical term for an inability to perform rapid, alternating movements.

Indexing Tip:

Many of the signs and symptoms found in this chapter can be indexed by the following keywords:

"Abnormal," "Decreased," "Elevation," and "Findings abnormal."

- A *petechia* is a small red or purple spot on the body caused by a minor hemorrhage.
- *Developmental milestones* (783.42) are tasks most children learn or physical developments that commonly appear in certain age ranges, e.g., the ability to lift the head and when crawling begins, speech begins, and puberty begins.
- *Epistaxis* (784.7) is a nosebleed that is a relatively common occurrence of hemorrhage from the nose.
- *Heart murmurs* (785.2) are generated by turbulent flow of blood that may occur inside or outside the heart.

Coding Alert!

Reporting Codes for This Chapter

Codes from this chapter are also used to report:

- Cases in which a more definitive diagnosis was not reached.
- Cases referred elsewhere for further diagnostic examination.
- Signs and symptoms present upon initial encounter but no longer existing.
- Provisional diagnosis for patients who failed to follow up as instructed.

Think Like A Coder 13.8

Choose the correct code for the following problem. Laboratory findings for a Pap smear of 57-year-old female included atypical squamous cells that cannot exclude a high-grade squamous intraepithelial lesion. Also indicated was a false positive serological test for syphilis.

- 795.04, 095.8
- 795.02, 095.8, 795.6
- 795.02, 795.6
- 795.03, 795.6, 097.1

Abnormal murmurs can be caused by stenosis restricting the opening of a heart valve, causing turbulence as blood flows through it.

- *Cheyne-Stokes respiration* (786.04) is an abnormal pattern of breathing characterized by periods of breathing with gradually increasing and decreasing tidal volume interspersed with periods of apnea.
- *Hemoptysis* (786.3) is the expectoration of blood or of blood-stained sputum from the bronchi, larynx, or lungs.
- *Viremia* (790.8) is a condition in which viruses enter the bloodstream; it is related to bacteremia, a condition in which bacteria enter the bloodstream, and septicemia.
- *Cachexia* (799.4) is loss of weight, muscle atrophy, fatigue, weakness, and anorexia in someone who is not actively trying to lose weight.

Chapter 17: Injury and Poisoning (800-999)

The Injury and Poisoning chapter is not confined to one particular anatomical site or body system but is rather a collection of injuries, burns, poisonings, adverse affects, and complications of surgical and medical care governed by specific coding guidelines. Table 13.9 presents the disorders found in the Injury and Poisoning chapter and their corresponding code numbers.

Coding of Injuries

When coding for injuries, assign separate codes for each injury unless a combination code is provided, in which case the combination code is assigned. Multiple injury codes are provided in ICD-9-CM but should not be assigned unless information for a more specific code is not available. These codes are not be used for normal, healing surgical wounds or to identify complications of surgical wounds.

Coding of Fractures

The principles of multiple coding of injuries should be followed in coding fractures. Fractures of specified sites are coded individually by site in accordance with both the provisions within categories 800-829 and the level of detail furnished by medical record content. Combination categories for multiple fractures are provided for use when there is insufficient detail in the medical record ,when the reporting form limits the number of codes that can be used in reporting pertinent clinical data, or when there is insufficient specificity at the fourth-digit or fifth-digit level.

Coding of Burns

Current burns, 940-948, are classified by depth, extent, and agent (E code). Burns are classified by depth as first degree, second degree, and third degree.

When coding burns, assign separate codes for each burn site. Category 946, burns of multiple specified sites, should be used only if the locations of the burns are not documented.

Table 13.9 Injury and Poisoning Chapter Disorders

Disorder	Code Ranges
Fractures	800-829
Fracture of Skull	800-804
Fracture of Neck and Trunk	805-809
Fracture of the Upper Limb	810-819
Fracture of the Lower Limb	820-829
Dislocation	830-839
Sprains and Strains of Joints and Adjacent Muscles	840-848
Intracranial Injury, Excluding Those With Skull Fracture	850-854
Internal Injury of Thorax, Abdomen, and Pelvis	860-869
Open Wound of Head, Neck, and Trunk	870-897
Open Wound of Upper Limb	880-887
Open Wound of Lower Limb	890-897
Injury to Blood Vessels	900-904
Late Effects of Injuries, Poisonings, Toxic Effects, and Other External Causes	905-909
Superficial Injury	910-919
Contusion with Intact Skin Surface	920-924
Effects of Foreign Body Entering through Orifice	930-939
Injury to Nerves and Spinal Cord	950-957
Certain Traumatic Complications and Unspecified Injuries	958-959
Poisoning by Drugs and Medicinal and Biological Substances	960-979
Toxic Effects of Substances Chiefly Nonmedical as to Source	980-989
Other and Unspecified Effects of External Causes	990-995
Complications of Surgical and Medical Care, not Elsewhere Classified	996-999

 Indexing Tip:

Many injuries and poisonings found in this chapter can be indexed by the following keywords:

"Injuries," "Fractures," "Burns," "Adverse Effects," "Poisonings," and "Toxic Effects."

Burns Classified According to Extent of Body Surface Involved

Assign codes from category 948, burns, when the site of the burn is not specified or when there is a need for additional data. It is advisable to use category 948 as additional coding when needed to provide data for evaluating burn mortality, such as that needed by burn units. It is also advisable to use category 948 as an additional code for reporting purposes when there is mention of a third-degree burn involving 20% or more of the body surface (see Figure 13.5).

Rule of Nines

Category 948 is based on the classic "rule of nines" in estimating body surface involved: head and neck are assigned 9%, each arm 9%, each leg 18%, and genitalia 1% (see Figure 13.5).

Coding of Debridement of Wound, Infection, or Burn

Excisional debridement involves an excisional debridement as opposed to mechanical (brushing, scrubbing) debridement.

Adverse Effects, Poisoning, and Toxic Effects

The properties of certain drugs, medicinal and biological substances, or combinations of such substances, may cause toxic reactions.

Poisoning

For errors made in drug prescription or in the administration of the drug by provider, nurse, patient, or other person, use the appropriate poisoning codes from the 960-979 series.

Overdose of a Drug Intentionally Taken

If an overdose of a drug was intentionally taken or administered and resulted in drug toxicity, code as a poisoning from the 960-979 series.

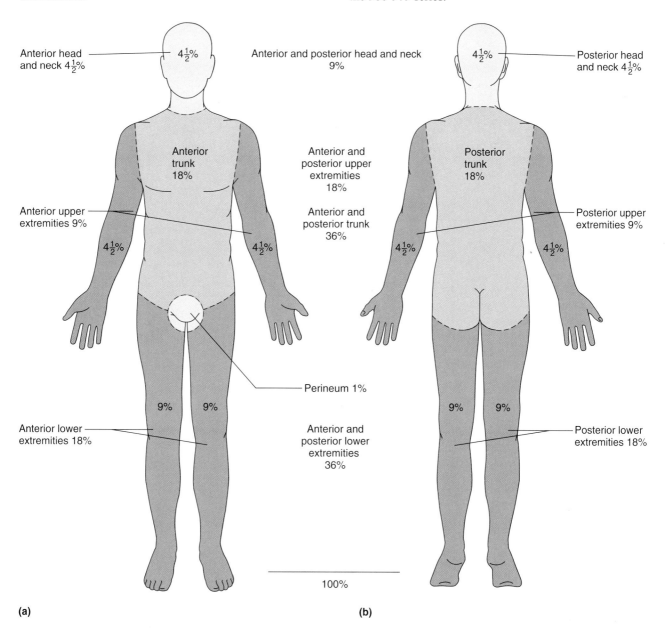

(a)   (b)

Figure 13.5

Burns: Rule of Nines — a. Anterior view of body regions. b. Posterior view of body regions.

From D. Shier et al., Hole's *Human Anatomy & Physiology*, 11e. Copyright © 2007 The McGraw-Hill Companies. Reprinted with permission.

Nonprescribed Drug Taken with Correctly Prescribed and Properly Administered Drug

If a nonprescribed drug or medicinal agent was taken in combination with a correctly prescribed and properly administered drug, any drug toxicity or other reaction resulting from the interaction of the two drugs would be classified as a poisoning.

Toxic Effect Codes

When a harmful substance is ingested or comes in contact with a person, this is classified as a toxic effect. A toxic effect code should be sequenced first, followed by the codes that identify the result of the toxic effect.

Coding Alert!

Burns (948)

When assigning a code from category 948:

- Fourth-digit codes are used to identify the percentage of total body surface involved in a burn (all degree).
- Fifth-digits are assigned to identify the percentage of body surface involved in third-degree burn.
- Fifth-digit zero (0) is assigned when less than 10% or when no body surface is involved in a third-degree burn.

💡 Think Like A Coder 13.9

Choose the correct answers for the following problems.

1. Burns are classified by two conditions, which are:

   - Degree, percentage(s) and site
   - Degree and site
   - Percentages, site
   - Degree, percentages

2. A 24-year-old male was the victim of an accidental overdose of ampicillin and suffered severe vomiting for the last 18 hours.

   - 960.3, 787.03
   - 960.03, 787.01
   - 960.0, 787.01, E856
   - 960.0, 787.03, E856

One of the following external cause codes should also be assigned to indicate intent: a code from categories E860-E869 for accidental exposure, either code E950.6 or E950.7 for intentional self-harm, category E962 for assault, or categories E980-E982 for undetermined.

Review of Data Quality and Management

The characteristics of managed health care are as follows:

- Patient health and preventive care education
- Treatment plan guides for high-cost disorders and diseases
- Patient and family collaboration with the health care providers to ensure patient compliance with treatment plans
- Utilization management performed by (1) prospective and retrospective review of treatment plans, (2) preauthorization, and (3) discharge planning
- Selective contracting with health care providers and institutions to achieve discount rates paid to these providers

Insurance Claims

The following is a review of terms used when following the life cycle of an insurance claim.

- A **copayment** is a provision in an insurance policy requiring the policyholder to pay a specific payment for each medical service or claim.
- An *encounter form* is used as a financial record to document diagnoses and services rendered to a patient during every visit.
- Allowed charges are the maximum amount the insurance company will pay for each procedure or service.
- An **explanation of benefits** (EOB) form is a statement from the insurance company that explains how the amount of reimbursement was disbursed to the company and the provider.

Processing Steps of an Insurance Claim Form

The following is a review outlining the processing steps performed on a claim form by an insurance company. The steps are documented in proper sequence (see Figure 13.6).

- The claim is examined for patient, policy, and group identification numbers.
- Procedure codes are correlated with diagnostic codes.
- Code numbers are matched with the benefits list.

Coding Alert!

Coding from Source Documents

When choosing the primary diagnosis, review the list of symptoms, complaints, and disorders in each source document and determine the primary diagnosis. After choosing the primary diagnosis, link the diagnosis with the procedure/service that was rendered.

NUCC

HEALTH INSURANCE CLAIM FORM

APPROVED BY NATIONAL UNIFORM CLAIM COMMITTEE XX/XX

PICA | PICA

CARRIER

1. MEDICARE (Medicare #) MEDICAID (Medicare #) CHAMPUS (Sponsor's SSN) CHAMPVA (VA File #) GROUP HEALTH PLAN (SSN or ID) FECA BLK LUNG (SSN) OTHER (ID)

1a. INSURED'S I.D. NUMBER (FOR PROGRAM IN ITEM 1)

2. PATIENT'S NAME (Last Name, First Name, Middle Initial)

3. PATIENT'S BIRTH DATE MM DD YY SEX M F

4. INSURED'S NAME (Last Name, First Name, Middle Initial)

5. PATIENT'S ADDRESS (No., Street)

6. PATIENT RELATIONSHIP TO INSURED Self Spouse Child Other

7. INSURED'S ADDRESS (No., Street)

CITY STATE

8. PATIENT STATUS Single Married Other

CITY STATE

ZIP CODE TELEPHONE (Include Area Code) ( )

Employed Full-Time Student Part-Time Student

ZIP CODE TELEPHONE (INCLUDE AREA CODE) ( )

9. OTHER INSURED'S NAME (Last Name, First Name, Middle Initial)

10. IS PATIENT'S CONDITION RELATED TO:

11. INSURED'S POLICY GROUP OR FECA NUMBER

a. OTHER INSURED'S POLICY OR GROUP NUMBER

a. EMPLOYMENT? (CURRENT OR PREVIOUS) YES NO

a. INSURED'S DATE OF BIRTH MM DD YY SEX M F

b. OTHER INSURED'S DATE OF BIRTH MM DD YY SEX M F

b. AUTO ACCIDENT? YES NO PLACE (State)

b. EMPLOYER'S NAME OR SCHOOL NAME

c. EMPLOYER'S NAME OR SCHOOL NAME

c. OTHER ACCIDENT? YES NO

c. INSURANCE PLAN NAME OR PROGRAM NAME

d. INSURANCE PLAN NAME OR PROGRAM NAME

10d. RESERVED FOR LOCAL USE

d. IS THERE ANOTHER HEALTH BENEFIT PLAN? YES NO ***If yes***, return to and complete item 9 a-d.

READ BACK OF FORM BEFORE COMPLETING & SIGNING THIS FORM.

12. PATIENT'S OR AUTHORIZED PERSON'S SIGNATURE I authorize the release of any medical or other information necessary to process this claim. I also request payment of government benefits either to myself or to the party who accepts assignment below.

SIGNED ______ DATE ______

13. INSURED'S OR AUTHORIZED PERSON'S SIGNATURE I authorize payment of medical benefits to the undersigned physician or supplier for services described below.

SIGNED ______

PATIENT AND INSURED INFORMATION

FOLD HERE / USE ENVELOPE NO. 1500E

14. DATE OF CURRENT: MM DD YY ILLNESS (First symptom) OR INJURY (Accident) OR PREGNANCY(LMP)

15. IF PATIENT HAS HAD SAME OR SIMILAR ILLNESS. GIVE FIRST DATE MM DD YY

16. DATES PATIENT UNABLE TO WORK IN CURRENT OCCUPATION FROM MM DD YY TO MM DD YY

17. NAME OF REFERRING PROVIDER OR OTHER SOURCE

17a.

17b. NPI#

18. HOSPITALIZATION DATES RELATED TO CURRENT SERVICES FROM MM DD YY TO MM DD YY

19. RESERVED FOR LOCAL USE

20. OUTSIDE LAB? YES NO $ CHARGES

21. DIAGNOSIS OR NATURE OF ILLNESS OR INJURY. (RELATE ITEMS 1,2,3 OR 4 TO ITEM 24E BY LINE)

1. ___ . __ 3. ___ . __

2. ___ . __ 4. ___ . __

22. MEDICAID RESUBMISSION CODE ORIGINAL REF. NO.

23. PRIOR AUTHORIZATION NUMBER

24. A. DATE(S) OF SERVICE From MM DD YY To MM DD YY	B. Place of Service	C. EMG	D. PROCEDURES, SERVICES, OR SUPPLIES (Explain Unusual Circumstances) CPT/HCPCS MODIFIER	E. DIAGNOSIS POINTER	F. $ CHARGES	G. DAYS OR UNITS	H. EPSDT Family Plan	I. ID. QUAL.	J. RENDERING PROVIDER ID. #
1								NPI #	
2								NPI #	
3								NPI #	
4								NPI #	
5								NPI #	
6								NPI #	

25. FEDERAL TAX I.D. NUMBER SSN EIN

26. PATIENT'S ACCOUNT NO.

27. ACCEPT ASSIGNMENT? (For govt. claims, see back) YES NO

28. TOTAL CHARGE $

29. AMOUNT PAID $

30. BALANCE DUE $

31. SIGNATURE OF PHYSICIAN OR SUPPLIER INCLUDING DEGREES OR CREDENTIALS (I certify that the statements on the reverse apply to this bill and are made a part thereof.)

SIGNED DATE

32. SERVICE FACILITY LOCATION INFORMATION

a. b.

33. BILLING PROVIDER INFORMATION & PHONE #

a. b.

PHYSICIAN OR SUPPLIER INFORMATION

www.nucc.org

Figure 13.6

Insurance Claim Form—CMS 1500

- The claim is checked against the patient file.
- Allowed charges are determined.
- The EOB form is completed.
- The EOB (explanation of benefits) and check are mailed or electronically sent.

Diagnostic Related Groups Review

The diagnostic-related group (DRG), a system to classify hospital cases into 1 of approximately 500 groups expected to have a similar hospital resource use, was developed for Medicare as part of the prospective payment system. DRGs are assigned by a "grouper" program based on ICD-9-CM diagnoses, procedures, age, sex, and the presence of complications or comorbidities. DRGs are used to determine how much Medicare pays the hospital, because patients within each category are similar clinically and are expected to use the same level of hospital resources. DRGs may be further grouped into Major Diagnostic Categories (MDCs).

Think Like A Coder 13.10

In the following coding scenario determine what, if any, errors have occurred.

A patient underwent laser surgery for destruction of four actinic keratoses lesions of the chest. The coder assigned the following codes: 17003 × 4,701.1.

- Coding assignment is accurate
- Procedure code is incorrect
- Diagnosis code is incorrect
- Diagnosis and procedure code are incorrect

Choose the correct ICD-9-CM coding assignment. (Please see Appendix A for answers and rationale).

1. A 53-year-old male construction worker was admitted through the emergency department following a fall from a ladder while framing a building under construction. He suffered an open intertrochanteric fracture of the femur and contusions on the face and scalp.

    A. ❑ 820.21, 873.50, 873.0, E849.3

    B. ❑ 820.31, 920, E881.0, E849.3

    C. ❑ 820.21, 873.50, E881.0

    D. ❑ 820.30, 920, 873.50, E881.0, E849.0

2. ABSTRACT:

    S: A 26-year-old female waitress presented with severe abdominal pain, nausea, and vomiting for the last 12 hours. The patient denied fever and acknowledged some diarrhea. The patient stated that she ate sushi on her 30-minute break.

    O: Pleasant, slightly confused woman who appears in great discomfort. Vital Signs: Temp: 101.4, Pulse: 82, Respirations: 18, BP: 132/76. HEENT (head eyes, ears, nose, throat): Unremarkable. Skin: Hot and sweaty. Neck: No JVD (jugular venous distension) or bruits. Lungs: Clear. Normal sinus.

    A: Food poisoning due to *Clostridium botulinum*

    P: Will order Phenergan for nausea; push fluids for 48 hours. Follow-up as needed.

    A. ❑ 005.1, 787.02

    B. ❑ 003.20, 787.02, 787.3

    C. ❑ 003.20, 787.02

    D. ❑ 005.1

3. A 72-year-old male presented in the office with chronic bleeding of the nose, lethargy, decreased appetite, and weight loss for over 1 month. After several diagnostic tests, the physician diagnosed acute promyelocytic leukemia.

    A. ❑ 204.00

    B. ❑ 205.00

    C. ❑ 203.0

    D. ❑ 204.20

4. The type of diabetes that is always considered insulin dependent is:

    A. ❑ Type I and Type II

    B. ❑ Type I

    C. ❑ Type II

    D. ❑ There is no specified type

5. A 24-year-old male who recently served in the Iraq war was diagnosed with anemia caused by blood loss from a chronic gastric ulcer of the stomach.

    A. ❑ 281.3, 532.40

    B. ❑ 280.1, 532.70

    C. ❑ 280.0, 531.40

    D. ❑ 281.9, 531.40

6. A 73-year-old female was recently admitted as an inpatient to the psychiatric ward at a local hospital with diagnoses of continuous alcohol dependence, Korsakoff's psychosis, alcoholic hallucinations, and delirium tremens. According to her chart, the patient, who has a long history of severe alcoholism, was found at her residence in a pool of blood during status epilepticus before her admission to the psychiatric ward.

    A. ❑ 303.01, 291.1, 291.0, 291.3

    B. ❑ 303.1, 291.1, 291.0

    C. ❑ 303.91, 291.1, 291.0, 291.3

    D. ❑ 303.1, 291.0, 291.3

7. A 31-year-old female presented with symptoms of sweating, chronic pain in the lower right leg, yellow-tan pallor, and severe edema. After examination by a neurologist, the patient was diagnosed with reflex sympathetic dystrophy of the lower right leg.

    A. ❑ 359.1, 337.21

    B. ❑ 337.22

    C. ❑ 359.1, 337.32, 338.1

    D. ❑ 337.22, 338.1

8. A 49-year-old male with a family history of ischemic heart disease was admitted to the local hospital for suffering an acute myocardial infarction. After a preliminary electrocardiogram was given, it was also noted that the patient demonstrated extrasystolic arrhythmia.

    A. ❑ 410.10, 427.60

    B. ❑ 410.31, 427.41

    C. ❑ V17.3, 410.90, 427.60

    D. ❑ V17.3, 410.31, 427.60

9. A 7-year-old male presented with multisystemic symptoms. Symptoms include rhinitis, watery eyes, sneezing, coughing, sore throat, swollen tonsils, and intermittent fever. The physician diagnosed allergic rhinitis with chronic tonsillitis and adenoiditis resulting from contact with the family's dog. The child was referred to an otorhinolaryngologist for examination of the tonsils and adenoids.

    A. ❑ 477.2, 474.02

    B. ❑ 477.0, 472.1, 474.02

    C. ❑ 473.8, 474.00, 474.01

    D. ❑ 477.2, 474.00, 474.01

10. A 45-year-old female presented in the office with symptoms of left neck and jaw pain and left back and arm pain accompanied with generalized pain in the teeth. These symptoms have persisted over the last year intermittently with recent exacerbation. The physician diagnosed the patient with temporomandibular joint arthralgia with odontogenesis imperfecta. The patient was referred to an endodontist for further evaluation.

    A. ❑ 520.0, 524.62

    B. ❑ 526.9, 524.62, 520.5

    C. ❑ 524.62, 520.5

    D. ❑ 520.0, 526.9, 524.62

11. A 66-year-old male with a personal history of malignant neoplasm of the bladder was diagnosed with acute renal failure with a lesion of the renal cortical. Later, biopsies showed malignant neoplasm of the renal parenchyma.

    A. ❏ 583.9, 233.0
    B. ❏ 583.9, V10.51, 233.9
    C. ❏ 584.6, V10.51, 189.0
    D. ❏ 233.9, V10.51, 584.8

12. The time before childbirth is called:

    A. ❏ Postpartum
    B. ❏ Periperium
    C. ❏ Perinatal
    D. ❏ Antepartum

13. An obstetrician delivered premature stillborn twins, for a 41-year-old elderly prima gravida.

    A. ❏ 644.12, 651.01, V32.00
    B. ❏ 644.12, 651.03, 656.79, V32.00
    C. ❏ 644.21, 656.41, 651.01, V27.4
    D. ❏ 644.00, 656.41, 656.79, V27.4

14. ABSTRACT:
    S: An 18-year-old female presented with complaints of increased acne on the face and back along with a "large sore" on the left cheek of her face.
    O: Examination revealed a well-nourished, slightly overweight female with lesions on the face and back and a large boil on the left cheek of her face. HEENT: Normal, no abnormalities noted. HEAD: Normocephalic. EYES: Clear and reactive to light. EARS: TMs (tympanic membrane) clear. SKIN: Unremarkable except for the acne on the face and back.
    A: Acne vulgaris, carbuncle on the left portion of the face.
    P: Patient referred to a dermatologist.

    A. ❏ 706.0, 708.3, 682.0
    B. ❏ 706.1, 680.0
    C. ❏ 686.00, 708.3
    D. ❏ 706.01, 682.0

15. A physician diagnosed an 86-year-old male with arthropathy with hyperparathyroidism and kyphosis resulting from radiation treatment. The patient has a history of bone cancer that currently is in remission.

    A. ❏ 252.1, 713.4, 737.11
    B. ❏ 252.08, 713.4, 737.22, V16.8
    C. ❏ 252.01, 713.7, 737.22, V10.81
    D. ❏ 252.00, 713.0, 737.11, V10.81

16. A 6-year-old female was seen in the ER for symptoms of medication overdose. The patient's mother stated that she read the dosage instructions incorrectly and administered too much antihistamine to the child. The physician noted on the patient's record that the medication overdose was accidental.

    A. ❏ 786.00, 786.50, 962.3, E857
    B. ❏ 963.0, E858.1
    C. ❏ 962.3, 786.00, E858.1
    D. ❏ 963.0, 786.50, E857

17. An infant was born in the hospital by cesarean section and was diagnosed with congenital lower left leg vessel anomaly and congenital absence of the external auditory canal resulting in conductive hearing loss of the external ear.

    A. ❏ V30.00, 747.63, 744.01, 389.01
    B. ❏ V27.1, 747.0, 389.01
    C. ❏ V27.0, 747.63, 744.02, 389.08
    D. ❏ V30.00, 747.63, 744.02, 389.08

18. Assign the appropriate E code for the following statements:
    A. Fracture of the tibia incurred during a suicide attempt by a patient who ran in front of a moving vehicle.
    B. Cerebral hematoma caused by a large rock that fell on a construction worker's head.

    A. ❏ A. E957.1 B. E919
    B. ❏ A. E958.0 B. E916
    C. ❏ A. E953 B. E913.3
    D. ❏ A. E958.0 B. E913.3

19. When an admission occurs for the treatment of renal dialysis, the coder should assign:

    A. ❏ E code
    B. ❏ V code and E code
    C. ❏ V code
    D. ❏ Only the code for the renal dialysis

20. ABSTRACT
    S: A 61-year-old female patient presented with pain in her right leg that has been intermittent for over a week and severe at times. The patient is currently ambulatory with an abnormal gait. The patient denies hypertension, diabetes and renal difficulties.
    O: HEENT: Reveals no adenopathy or thyromegaly. VITAL SIGNS: Temp: 99.0, Pulse: 66, Respiration: 14, BP: 150/82. LUNGS: Occasional rhonchi, no wheeze present. HEART: Regular rhythm. EXTREMITIES: Upon palpation of the right calf, pain is present; edema is present in the right leg.
    A: Endophlebitis of superficial vessels
    P: Immediately immobilize right leg and administer heparin; patient to return to office in 2 days.

    A. ❏ 451.11
    B. ❏ 451.0
    C. ❏ 451.19
    D. ❏ 451.2

21. A 51-year-old female was diagnosed with a malignant neoplasm of the lower-inner quadrant of the left breast. A modified radical mastectomy with axillary lymph nodes (Urban type) was performed. Gross and microscopic examination was performed to confirm the neoplasm. The coder assigned the following codes: 174.8, 19306, 88307-50 What codes were assigned incorrectly?

    A. ❏ No codes were assigned incorrectly
    B. ❏ 174.8 and 88307
    C. ❏ 174.8
    D. ❏ 88307 and 19306

22. What is the three-digit code for "other diseases and conditions of the teeth and supporting structures?"

    A. ❏ 250

    B. ❏ 525

    C. ❏ 520

    D. ❏ 523

23. Code the late effect: ataxia due to cerebrovascular accident.

    A. ❏ 438.84

    B. ❏ 438.21

    C. ❏ 432.0

    D. ❏ 438.81

24. A 44-year-old female with a history of breast cancer presented with a mass in her uterus after complaints of pain, bloating, and discharge. A biopsy was performed, and it was confirmed that the patient had carcinoma in situ of the uterus. The physician who diagnosed the patient and performed the surgery participated in a medical team conference and discussed the patient's prognosis for 65 minutes.

Please review the claim form and decide if there is incorrect information on the claim form.

After examination of the claim form, please choose which answer best describes the error(s) on the claim form, if any.

    A. ❏ ICD-9 code(s) are incorrect

    B. ❏ CPT code is incorrect

    C. ❏ ICD-9 and CPT code(s) are incorrect

    D. ❏ Claim form is error-free

---

14. DATE OF CURRENT: ILLNESS (First symptom) OR INJURY (Accident) OR PREGNANCY (LMP) MM DD YY 01 20 09	15. IF PATIENT HAS HAD SAME OR SIMILAR ILLNESS GIVE FIRST DATE MM DD YYYY 05 01 06	16. DATES PATIENT UNABLE TO WORK IN CURRENT OCCUPATION FROM MM DD YYYY TO MM DD YYYY
17. NAME OF REFERRING PHYSICIAN OR OTHER SOURCE XXXX XXXXX, M.D.	17a. I.D. NUMBER OF REFERRING PHYSICIAN 40-92XXXXX	18. HOSPITALIZATION DATES RELATED TO CURRENT SERVICES FROM MM DD YYYY TO MM DD YYYY
19. RESERVED FOR LOCAL USE		20. OUTSIDE LAB? ❏YES ☒NO $ CHARGES
21. DIAGNOSIS OR NATURE OF ILLNESS OR INJURY. (RELATE ITEMS 1,2,3 OR 4 TO ITEM 24E BY LINE) 1. V16.3 3. 2. 233.1 4.		22. MEDICAID RESUBMISSION CODE ORIGINAL REF. NO. 23. PRIOR AUTHORIZATION NUMBER 34XXXXXXX

24. A DATE(S) OF SERVICE From MM DD YY To MM DD YY	B Place of Service	C Type of Service	D PROCEDURES, SERVICES, OR SUPPLIES (Explain Unusual Circumstances) CPT/HCPCS MODIFIER	E DIAGNOSIS CODE	F $ CHARGES	G DAYS OR UNITS	H EPSDT Family Plan	I EMG	J COB	K RESERVED FOR LOCAL USE
01 20 09 01 20 09	11	1	99361	1,2	510 00	1				

25. FEDERAL TAX I.D. NUMBER 40-51XXXXX SSN ❏ EIN ☒	26. PATIENT'S ACCOUNT NO. XXX XX	27. ACCEPT ASSIGNMENT? (For govt. claims, see back) ☒YES ❏NO	28. TOTAL CHARGE $ 510 00	29. AMOUNT PAID $ 100 00	30. BALANCE DUE $ 410 00
31. SIGNATURE OF PHYSICIAN OR SUPPLIER INCLUDING DEGREES OR CREDENTIALS (I certify that the statements on the reverse apply to this bill and are made a part thereof) SIGNED XXXX XXXXX DATE XX	32. NAME AND ADDRESS OF FACILITY WHERE SERVICES WERE RENDERED(If other than home or office) XXXX XXXXXX		33. PHYSICIAN'S, SUPPLIER'S BILLING NAME, ADDRESS. ZIP CODE & PHONE# PIN# 40-92XXXXX GRP#		

(APPROVED BY AMA COUNCIL ON MEDICAL SERVICE 8/88)   **PLEASE PRINT OR TYPE**   APPROVED OMB-0938-0008 FROM HCFA-1500 (12-90), FRM RRB-1500. APPROVED OMB-1215-0055 FROM OWCP-1500, APPROVED OMB-0720-0001 (CHAMPUS)

PHYSICIAN OR SUPPLIER INFORMATION

---

25. A 37-year-old male has been experiencing acute exacerbation of narcolepsy with cataplexy and is experiencing deficits with activities of daily living. The patient is now afflicted with paraplegia, which requires the insertion of a simple, indwelling, temporary Foley catheter. The physician ordered a home-health care aid to come in twice per week for a catheter change. The physician also ordered physical therapy for safety instruction and gait training with a walker and cane for 2 hours per week.

Please review the claim form and decide if there is incorrect information on the claim form.

After examination of the claim form, please choose which answers best describes the error(s) on the claim form, if any.

    A. ❏ ICD-9 code(s) are incorrect

    B. ❏ CPT code is incorrect

    C. ❏ ICD-9 and CPT code(s) are wrong

    D. ❏ Claim form is error-free

14. DATE OF CURRENT:	ILLNESS (First symptom) OR INJURY (Accident) OR PREGNANCY (LMP)	15. IF PATIENT HAS HAD SAME OR SIMILAR ILLNESS GIVE FIRST DATE	16. DATES PATIENT UNABLE TO WORK IN CURRENT OCCUPATION
MM DD YY 2 11 09		MM DD YYYY 2 14 08	FROM MM DD YYYY 2 11 09 TO MM DD YYYY 2 14 09

17. NAME OF REFERRING PHYSICIAN OR OTHER SOURCE	17a. I.D. NUMBER OF REFERRING PHYSICIAN	18. HOSPITALIZATION DATES RELATED TO CURRENT SERVICES
XXXX XXXXX	52-31XXXXY	FROM MM DD YYYY ___ TO MM DD YYYY ___

19. RESERVED FOR LOCAL USE	20. OUTSIDE LAB? $ CHARGES
	☐ YES ☒ NO

21. DIAGNOSIS OR NATURE OF ILLNESS OR INJURY. (RELATE ITEMS 1,2,3 OR 4 TO ITEM 24E BY LINE)	22. MEDICAID RESUBMISSION CODE ORIGINAL REF. NO.
1. 347.01 3. ___	
2. 344.1 4. ___	23. PRIOR AUTHORIZATION NIMBER

24. A DATE(S) OF SERVICE		B Place of Service	C Type of Service	D PROCEDURES, SERVICES, OR SUPPLIES (Explain Unusual Circumstances)		E DIAGNOSIS CODE	F $ CHARGES	G DAYS OR UNITS	H EPSDT Family Plan	I EMG	J COB	K RESERVED FOR LOCAL USE
From MM DD YY	To MM DD YY			CPT/HCPCS	MODIFIER							
2 11 09	2 11 09	11	1	51701		1,2	450 00	1	—	—	—	——
2 18 09	2 18 09	12	1	99501		2	325 00	1	—	—	—	——
2 21 09	2 21 09	22	1	97116		2	1800 00	8	—	—	—	——

25. FEDERAL TAX I.D. NUMBER	SSN EIN	26. PATIENT'S ACCOUNT NO.	27. ACCEPT ASSIGNMENT? (For govt. claims, see back)	28. TOTAL CHARGE	29. AMOUNT PAID	30. BALANCE DUE
41-23XXXXX	☐ ☒	XXX XX	☒ YES ☐ NO	$ 2515 00	$ 0	$ 2515 00

31. SIGNATURE OF PHYSICIAN OR SUPPLIER INCLUDING DEGREES OR CREDENTIALS (I certify that the statements on the reverse apply to this bill and are made a part thereof)	32. NAME AND ADDRESS OF FACILITY WHERE SERVICECS WERE RENDERED(If other than home or office)	33. PHYSICIAN'S, SUPPLIER'S BILLING NAME, ADDRESS. ZIP CODE & PHONE#
SIGNED XXXX-XXXX DATE 2-24-09	XXXX - XXXXX	PIN# 41-23XXXXXX GRP#

(APPROVED BY AMA COUNCIL ON MEDICAL SERVICE 8/88)   **PLEASE PRINT OR TYPE**

APPROVED OMB-0938-0008 FROM HCFA-1500 (12-90), FRM RRB-1500,
APPROVED OMB-1215-0055 FROM OWCP-1500, APPROVED OMB-0720-0001 (CHAMPUS)

PHYSICIAN OR SUPPLIER INFORMATION

Practice Coding Examination

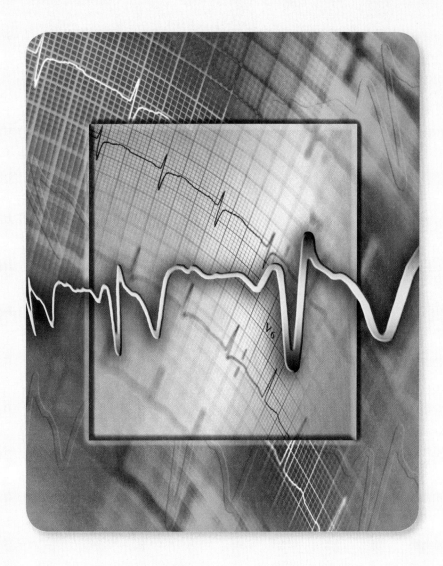

Chapter 14: Practice Examination

Practice Examination

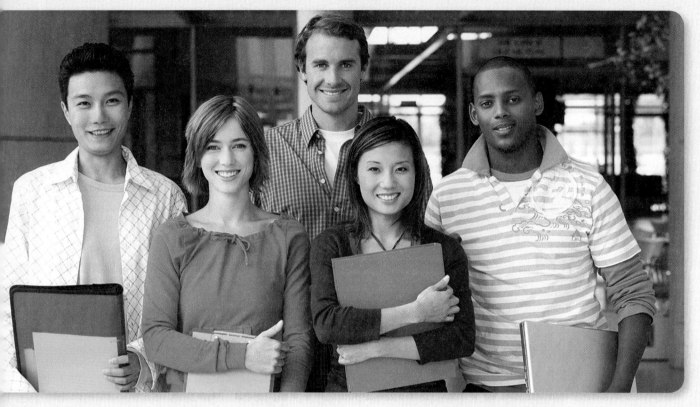

Learning Objectives

- The student will evaluate his or her preparedness for a national coding examination.

- The student will investigate areas of weakness and strengths that need more practice before taking a national coding examination.

- The student will gain an understanding of how the examinations are set up and orientate practice accordingly.

- The student will understand the importance of being thorough and correct when choosing coding assignments to be as accurate as possible.

- The student will use appropriate and up-to-date reference materials while taking the examination.

- The student will gauge his or her knowledge of regulatory guidelines, data quality, and legal issues along with all coding conventions, standards, and guidelines.

From the Author...

"Now you are ready for your final challenge, your mock examination for national coding certification. You have reviewed and studied anatomy and physiology, medical terminology, all coding standards and guidelines, CPT-4, ICD-9-CM, HCPCS coding, HIPAA, and data quality, which prepares you to take this mock examination. Remember to think in a logical and sequential manner when choosing the correct coding assignment. Check your answers if you finish early and don't be too quick to change your answer. Think it through and arrive at coding decisions that are based on the information presented and not a hunch. Please refer to Chapter 1 for test-taking skills and tips for better preparation. Relax, think logically, and create the state of mind you need to "Think Like A Coder!""

Directions

You have exactly 5 hours to complete this examination. If you are not in a formal education setting in which an instructor will be administering the examination, please find someone to help "proctor" your examination. You may take two 5-minute breaks that are not included in the 5-hour time limit. When time is up, please turn your test into your instructor or proctor. Once your instructor or proctor has graded your examination, please review all of your incorrect answers. Appendix A provides answers and rationales for all questions in this textbook, including this mock examination. Remember, understanding the rationale of an incorrect coding assignment is one of the best methods for learning medical coding. Make note of any one section that contains more incorrect answers than most. This is your key to understanding your strengths and weaknesses for professional coding. Once you have assessed your strengths and weaknesses, set up a study plan to concentrate on areas that are more difficult for you than others. Soon you will be ready to tackle the CPC or CCS-P examination!

Please do not skip questions without answering them. Do not spend too much time on one problem or question; move along at a consistent pace. If you are unsure of an answer, go with your first instinct. If you complete the examination before the allotted time, check your answers for accuracy.

Medical Terminology

1. The exchange of gases within the cells of the body is known as _____ respiration.
   A. External
   B. Internal
   C. Diffusion
   D. Adducted

2. The combining form for eardrum is:
   A. opt/o
   B. kerat/o
   C. myring/o
   D. ophthalm/o

3. Which combining form means vertebra or vertebral column?
   A. spondyl/o
   B. splen/o
   C. cephal/o
   D. percuss/o

4. Which of the following terms means movement away from the body?
   A. Adduction
   B. Abduction
   C. Flexion
   D. Extension

5. Which of the following terms is commonly known as "itching"?
   A. Cyanosis
   B. Strabismus
   C. Pruritus
   D. Gastroptosis

6. Which of the following medical terms is commonly known as "heart attack"?
   A. Myocardial infarction
   B. Angina pectoris
   C. Myelopathy
   D. Arteriosclerosis

7. The combining form aden/o means:
   A. Adrenal glands
   B. Bound to
   C. Relationship to the male
   D. Gland

8. The region between the vaginal orifice and the anus is known as the:
   A. Vulva
   B. Perineum
   C. Cervix
   D. Labia minora

9. The suffix –pexy means:
   A. Tube
   B. Fixation
   C. To flow
   D. Pyramid shaped

10. The term meaning the administration of medication by injection is:
    A. Percutaneous
    B. Perfusion
    C. Buccal
    D. Parenteral

Anatomy and Physiology

11. A chronic inflammatory disease characterized by silvery patches on the skin is known as:
    A. Acne vulgaris
    B. Psoriasis
    C. Seborrhea
    D. Eczema

12. The bone of the arm located on the thumb side is known as:
    A. Radius
    B. Ulna

C. Metatarsal

D. Metacarpal

13. What muscle flexes and rotates the thigh leg?

   A. Gluteus maximus

   B. Sartorius

   C. Soleus

   D. Triceps brachii

14. The nervous system that consists of 12 pairs of cranial nerves and 31 pairs of spinal nerves is the:

   A. Autonomic

   B. Central

   C. Peripheral

   D. Limbic

15. The main symptom of Meniere's disease is:

   A. Syncope

   B. Hypertension

   C. Pruritis

   D. Vertigo

16. The oversecretion of cortisol of the adrenal gland is known as:

   A. Diabetes insipidus

   B. Padget's disease

   C. Cushing's syndrome

   D. Crohn's disease

17. Prothrombin is a plasma protein made in the:

   A. Liver

   B. Common bile duct

   C. Pancreas

   D. Thyroglossal duct

18. The outer layer of the heart is:

   A. Myocardium

   B. Superior vena cava

   C. Epicardium

   D. Pericardium

19. The function of the lymph nodes is to produce:

   A. Immune globulin

   B. Lymph fluid

   C. Erythrocytes

   D. Lymphocytes

20. The structure at the end of the bronchial tree where the exchange of carbon dioxide and oxygen take place is the:

   A. Nares

   B. Alveoli

   C. Bronchioles

   D. Venules

Health Information Management

21. Using the SOAP style of documenting progress notes, choose the "subjective" statement from the following:

   A. The patient suffered lower right quadrant stomach pain.

   B. Microscopic examination revealed bacteria in the urine.

   C. Upon palpation the patient was "guarded" on the lower right quadrant of the stomach.

   D. The patient's temperature was 102.4 and his respirations were at 26.

22. If you were designing health record forms, the first resource that you should consider before design would be:

   A. HCFA

   B. UHDDS

   C. AHA

   D. UACDS

23. The quickest and most efficient way to retrieve and report information about a cancer registr's quarterly case load would be to use:

   A. Patient records

   B. Disease index

   C. Physician index

   D. Accession register

24. What would be the best method of protecting the security of data contained in a computer software system?

   A. Monitor the access codes to all terminals on a semiweekly basis.

   B. Create protocol that includes different levels of security for different types of information.

   C. Hire individuals to handle this information who have passed a thorough security check.

   D. Have information technologists create system protocols.

25. Abbreviation and symbols are to be used in the patient record only when:

   A. They should never be used.

   B. They can be found in the CPT-4 code book.

   C. They are approved by the AMA.

   D. They are part of published criteria for the medical facility.

26. Fraud includes all of the following except:

   A. Coding to a higher level of service than is justifiable on the patient record.

   B. Abuse of a child or the elderly.

C. Billing services that were never provided.

D. Listing diagnoses that are not valid.

27. Resource-Based Relative Value Scale (RBRVS) calculates the amount to be paid for a code using the relative value unit of the:

A. Geographical location only

B. Service only

C. Service, geographical location, and conversion factor

D. Service and geographical location

28. A new patient is:

A. One who has not visited the physician is more than 6 months.

B. One who has not visited the physician in more than 3 years.

C. Determined by the physician and staff.

D. Determined by a third-party payer.

29. A covered entity may disclose PHI to facilitate treatment, payment, or health care operations or:

A. If the covered entity has obtained authorization from the individual.

B. If the covered entity is entered into an accession registry.

C. If the covered entity is located in a specific geographical location.

D. If the covered entity is registered in the Physician Index.

30. The fundamental reason for patient-care goals in an acute care setting is:

A. Legal purposes

B. Follow-up of patient care plans

C. JCAHO compliance

D. Advanced directives

Reimbursement

31. There are _____ major diagnostic categories in the DRG system.

A. 35

B. 25

C. 50

D. 15

32. The Correct Coding Initiative (CCI) was developed by _____ to eliminate _____ .

A. Health Care Financing Administration (HCFA); Medicare expenditures

B. Centers for Medicaid and Medicare Service (CMS); improper coding

C. Payment Error and Prevention Program (PEPP); Medicaid expenditures

D. Department of Justice (DOJ); improper coding

33. The Resource-Based Relative Value Scale (RBRVS) system is referred to as:

A. Payment Error and Prevention Program (PEPP)

B. Programs of All-Inclusive Care for the Elderly (PACE)

C. Home Health Resource Groups (HHRG)

D. Medicare Physician Fee Schedule (MPFS)

34. What standard published by HIPAA safeguards protected health information (HPI) that is collected?

A. The Security Rule

B. The Unique Identifiers Rule

C. The Enforcement Rule

D. The Privacy Rule

35. Which statement sent by the payer to the covered individual contains reimbursement amounts and an explanation in an easy-to-read format?

A. Remittance Advice

B. UB-04

C. CMS 1500

D. Explanation of Benefits

36. The patient xxx xxx was admitted to hospital 1 where he underwent skull-base surgery and stayed for 3 days. He was subsequently transferred to nearby hospital 2 where he recuperated for 9 days, receiving physical therapy. Both of the hospitals are short-term acute prospective payment system hospitals with the same DRGs. The PPS amount is $8,500 for hospital 1 and $15,000 for hospital 2. The geometric mean LOS for the DRG is 6.4. Hospital 1 should receive a reimbursement of:

A. $3,500

B. $3,984.50

C. $5,312.50

D. $7,500

37. A patient underwent a thyroidectomy and has already met her deductible. Her physician is a Medicare participating provider. The physician's standard fee for services rendered is $1,800, and the Medicare's PAR fee is $950. How much reimbursement will the physician receive from Medicare?

A. $950

B. $760

C. $1,440

D. $360

38. What is the term used to describe the difference between what a patient is charged and what is paid to the provider?

A. Write-off

B. Reimbursement

C. Fee schedule

D. Contractual allowance

39. Each CPT and HCPCS level II code is assigned a _____ as a payment indicator to identify how each code is paid or not paid under the OPPS.

A. DRG code

B. Status indicator

C. Profile indicator

D. HCPCS code

40. A revenue code is a four-digit:

A. ICD-9 code

B. Relative value unit

C. UB-04 code

D. Morphology code

Data Quality

41. What is the best place in the medical record to locate information on the number of pregnancies and number of living children for each OB patient from a month's worth of obstetrical records?

A. Discharge summaries

B. Growth and development record

C. Recovery room record

D. Antepartum record

42. A patient received a repair of a recurrent incisional, reducible hernia. The coder assigned code 49566. What is wrong with this coding assignment?

A. Nothing, the coding assignment is correct

B. The code assigned should be 49560

C. The code assigned includes incarcerated, which is not mentioned

D. The code assigned should be 49565

43. A patient was diagnosed with human T-cell lymphotrophic virus, type II. The coder assigned ICD-9 code 079.82. What is wrong with this coding assignment?

A. Nothing, the coding assignment is correct

B. The coding assignment is correct; however code 042 should accompany 079.82

C. The correct ICD-9 code is 079.52

D. The coding assignment should be 079.53, 042

44. On a qualitative review audit, what portion of the record for infants and children should be included in the?

A. Medicare EOBs

B. Compliance/non-compliance with physicians

C. Development and growth records

D. Antepartum record

45. Which one of the following statements would be found on a radiology report?

A. Temporary transcutaneous pacing

B. Intermediate proton treatment delivery was administered by using 2 ports with one block

C. Protein, total, by refractometry; serum

D. Nerve repair; with synthetic conduit

46. What is the format used in most hospitals for patient records?

A. SOAP

B. Chronological

C. Source oriented

D. There is no particular format

47. Which test is not included in a metabolic panel?

A. Chloride

B. Urea nitrogen

C. Creatinine

D. Albumin

48. A patient underwent a bilateral vasectomy including postoperative semen examination. Code for the anesthesiologist.

A. 00921

B. 00865

C. 00921–50

D. 00920, 00921

49. A 7-year-old female was seen for a well-child check up for first grade. Her father returned 2 weeks later with her for a removal of a nose ring that became lodged when she tried to insert it in her nose. The father's attempt to retrieve it exacerbated her symptoms. The physician removed the nose ring from the child's nose in the office without anesthesia. The coder assigned codes 99212, 30310, 932. What is incorrect with the coding assignment?

A. Nothing is wrong with the coding assignment

B. Code 30310 should be code 30300

C. There is no need for code 99212, and code 30310 should be 30300

D. There is no need for code 99212, and code 932 should be 930.9

50. The Correct Coding Initiative (CCI) has been established to:

A. Ensure proper coding and billing of health care service

B. Collect data for registries

C. Protect PHI

D. Introduce new treatment procedure to HCFA

ICD-9-CM Coding

51. A 74-year-old male afflicted with Alzheimer's disease wandered off from his daughter's home where he resides. The daughter stated that his dementia had gotten worse over the last several months, and she was afraid for his safety. A search was conducted by neighbors and local authorities and the elderly man was found. Upon admission to the hospital, he was disoriented and suffered a laceration on his right forearm, which required ten stitches. What codes would be reported in this case?

A. 331.82, 294.10, 880.03, 86.59

B. 331.0, 294.11, 881.00, 86.59

C. 331.0, 881.00, 86.59

D. 331.82, 294.11, 881.00, 86.59

52. A 10-month old infant was admitted for surgery for a right-sided, incomplete cleft lip and palate. The infant underwent surgery for both deformities. What codes would be reported in this case?

A. 749.01, 749.12, 27.62, 27.54

B. 749.20, 27.62, 27.54

C. 749.22, 750.0, 27.59

D. 749.22, 27.62, 27.54

53. A 37-year-old female presented with swelling of the neck and lethargy for over 1 month. The physician suspected lymphoma, and a biopsy was scheduled. A large hollow core needle was passed into the thyroid, and a specimen was taken and sent to histopathology for examination. A diagnosis of lymphoma was confirmed. The patient was sent to oncology for consultation. What codes would be reported in this case?

A. 202.01, 10021

B. 201.41, 10021

C. 202.01, 60100

D. 201.41, 60100

54. What is the five-digit code for diabetes with neurological manifestations for a patient with type II uncontrolled diabetes?

A. 250.60

B. There is no fifth digit

C. 250.62

D. 250.63

55. In what volume of the ICD-9-CM manual will you find procedures?

A. Volume I

B. Volume II

C. Volume III

D. You will not find procedures in the ICD-9-CM manual

56. What code would you assign, specifically the fifth digit, for chest pain caused by acute myocardial infarction of the inferolateral wall 5 weeks after the initial diagnosis?

A. 410.42

B. 410.22

C. 410.41

D. 410.32

57. A 56-year-old female was admitted to the hospital for a large pelvic mass located on the lower right quadrant in the pelvic region. After an exploratory laparotomy, pathology confirmed carcinoma of the right ovary with metastasis to the omentum. A total, radical abdominal hysterectomy and total omenectomy was performed with a bilateral salpingo-oopherectomy. What codes would be reported in this case?

A. 158.8, 198.6, 68.6, 65.61

B. 183.8, 198.6, 68.61, 54.4

C. 233.3, 158.8, 68.6, 65.61, 54.4

D. 183.0, 197.6, 68.6, 65.61, 54.4

58. A 27-year-old male patient with AIDS and Kaposi's sarcoma of the skin was admitted to the hospital for the closed fracture of four ribs. The patient received an application of pressure dressing and was referred to an infectious disease specialist. What codes would be reported in this case?

A. 807.14, 176.0, 93.56

B. 807.04, 042, 176.0, 93.56

C. 807.14, 042, 176, 93.58

D. 807.4, 176.1, 042, 93.58

59. A 41-year-old obese female was diagnosed with chronic kidney disease, stage III, resulting from malignant hypertension and type II diabetes mellitus. What codes would be reported in this case?

A. 403.90, 250.41, 585.9

B. 403.00, 250.40, 585.3

C. 403.00, 250.40

D. 403.90, 401.0, 250.40, 585.3

60. Code the following statement: A 30-year-old female with moderate mental retardation as a result of Edward's disease is being evaluated today for her paraplegia, which was caused by a spinal cord injury she suffered 4 years ago.

A. 344.00, 905.1, 318.0

B. 342.90, 905.1, 318.1, 758.0

C. 344.1, 907.2, 318.0, 758.2

D. 344.1, 905.9, 317, 758.0

HCPCS Codes

61. What code would you assign for the topical anesthetic for dialysis?

A. A4737

B. A4740

C. A4736

D. A4725

62. What code would you assign for a sterile syringe with needle, 5 cc?

A. A4206

B. A4210

C. A4209

D. A4208

63. CPT codes are considered HCPCS _____ codes.

A. Level II

B. Level III

C. Level I

D. They are not considered HCPCS codes

64. What HCPCS modifier would you assign for items furnished in conjunction with a urological, ostomy, or tracheostomy supply?

A. AU

B. AW

C. BA

D. AV

65. A 25-year-old male was fitted for a short-arm fiberglass cast after the physician diagnosed him with a fracture. The casting was performed in part by a resident under the direction of the physician. What code would be reported in this case?

A. Q4013 GE

B. Q4009 GC

C. Q4010 GC

D. Q4006 GC

66. A gel-like pressure pad was provided to a patient whose mattress was standard length and width. What code would be reported in this case?

A. E0182

B. E0185

C. E0188

D. E0196

67. A physician provided an 81-year-old male an oxygen concentrator, dual delivery port, capable of delivering 85% or greater oxygen concentration at the prescribed level in an area of the country where physicians are scarce or not present at all. What code would be reported in this case?

A. E1390 AQ

B. E1390 AR

C. E1391 AR

D. E1392 AT

68. An 89-year-old female high-risk patient underwent a glaucoma screening by an optometrist. What code would be reported in this case?

A. GO117

B. G0118

C. G0123

D. G0122

69. A physician documented that a 41-year-old male patient with coronary artery disease was not an eligible candidate for low-density lipoprotein measure. What code would be reported in this case?

A. G8039

B. G8053

C. G8041

D. G8040

70. A physician fitted a semirigid cervical plastic collar on a 59-year-old male who suffered whiplash during a car accident. What code would be reported in this case?

A. L0130

B. L0120

C. L0140

D. L0170

Evaluation and Management Codes

71. What are the three key components of an E&M code?

A. Examination, coordination of care, medical decision making

B. History, examination, medical decision making

C. History, nature of presenting problem, coordination of care

D. Nature of presenting problem, examination, coordination of care

72. An expanded problem-focused examination is:

A. A general multisystem examination or a complete examination of a single organ system.

B. A limited examination of the affected body area or organ system and other symptomatic or related organ system(s).

C. An extended examination of the affected body area(s) and other symptomatic or related organ system(s).

D. A limited examination of the affected body area or organ system.

73. The following is a history and physical examination for a 91-year-old male established patient. Choose the correct E&M code based on the information provided.

PATIENT: xxx xxxx

CHART NUMBER: xxx-xx

HISTORY OF PRESENT ILLNESS: A pleasant, 91-year-old male who lives independently presents with symptoms of shortness of breath, confusion and congestion. Patient denies fever or cough. Patient has a recent history of COPD. Current medications include prednisone and Colace.

PAST HISTORY: The patient's past medical history includes cholecystectomy × 30 years ago. Patient denies any other hospitalization. Patient says that he has been in relatively good health all of his life, with the exception of a recent diagnosis of COPD.

SOCIAL HISTORY: He is retired 30 years ago, widowed for 15 years. No smoking, no ETOH, no known allergies. Denies caffeine and any illicit drug use.

FAMILY HISTORY: Unremarkable.

PHYSICAL EXAMINATION: Vital Signs: Temp: 99.2, Pulse: 64, Respirations: 26, Blood Pressure: 92/50. HEENT: Normocephalic, with post surgical eyes. Neck: No jugular venous distention. No carotid bruits. Skin: Poor turgor and texture. Lungs: Bilateral bibasilar crackles. Liver: Not palpably enlarged. Heart: S1 and S2 present, no S3. Abdomen: Soft and non-tender. Extremities: Bilateral leg edema. Neurological: No deficits, alert × 3, alert to orientation, place and time.

INTERPRETATION: Laboratory data was negative with the exception of elevation white blood cell count. A chest x-ray revealed congestive heart failure and pneumonia.

TREATMENT: The patient was admitted to the hospital as a result of this service and prescribed tobramycin for the pneumonia and Lasix for the congestive heart failure.

A. 99214-57

B. 99214

C. 99215-25

D. 99215

74. Physician #1 sent a 72-year-old female cancer patient to observation at the local hospital following his visit to the patient's nursing care facility. The patient was admitted to observation to rule out CVA (cardiovascular accident) and multisystem organ failure due to a change in her physical status. The next day, Physician #1 became ill, and Physician #2 took over the patient's care. Physician # 2 admitted the patient to the hospital because of a dramatic worsening of symptoms.

Later that day the patient expired. Assuming the patient's status was of high severity, how would the E&M services for the two physicians be coded?

A. Physician #1: 99223; Physician #2: 99219

B. Physician #1: 99223, 99219; no codes would be assigned for Physician #2

C. Physician #1: 99220; Physician #2: 99236

D. Physician #1: 99220; Physician #2: 99217

75. Documentation in history of the use of caffeine, smoking, illicit drug use, sexual preference, and alcohol use is considered part of:

A. Nature of presenting illness

B. Past medical history

C. Social history

D. Occupational history

76. The physician on the following case provided care during and after the helicopter transport of a 29-year-old male who was critically injured during a car crash in an isolated area. The patient was also exposed to the outside elements for more than 24 hours. Choose the correct code(s) based on the information provided.

A 29-year-old male patient was admitted to the critical care unit after his car crashed on an icy, mountainous road and was exposed to freezing temperatures for over 2 days. The patient was wearing a seatbelt, however sustained a skull fracture, subdural hematoma, and frostbite on portion of his feet and hands. The patient was unconscious at the scene and upon examination had respirations of 6, pulse 50, temperature of 97.2, and blood pressure of 82/40. The right pupil was blown, fixed, and dilated, indicating the intracranial injury. Hypoxemia and brain swelling were noted. The patient experienced increasing periods of apnea and dyspnea and was placed on a ventilator 3 hours later after endotracheal intubation. The patient had open fractures of the left tibia and right femur, a closed fracture of the left wrist, and four fractured ribs. Brain wave monitoring showed little functioning, and his family was called. The care provided by the physician included the interpretation of cardiac output measurements, pulse oximetry, blood gases, endotracheal intubation, ventilatory management, and brain wave functions. The total time the physician spent with the patient was about 3 hours.

A. 99289 × 1, 99290 × 4

B. 99291 × 1, 99292 × 5

C. 99292

D. 99291 × 1, 99292 × 4

77. A 37-year-old female presented in the emergency department with shortness of breath, lethargy, and cough with blood in the sputum for 3 days; an expanded problem-focused history was taken.

BRIEF HISTORY: On examination, her skin was warm, moist, and pale. She stated she had been coughing up blood and had been short of breath with fever for more than 3 days. Upon admission, her temperature was 102.6, respirations were 28, pulse 130, and blood pressure 162/92. She appeared very lethargic.

PHYSICAL FINDINGS: The patient's heart was tachycardiac. The patient had decreased breath sounds in the left lower lobe with a line of consolidation about halfway up. No friction rub was heard. PMI was at the mid-clavicular line, and a regular rhythm was noted. No significant murmur or gallop. Abdomen was soft and tender, with no organomegaly, bowel sounds active. Extremities showed no edema, clubbing, or cyanosis.

LABORATORY FINDINGS: Gram stain of sputum showed Gram-positive cocci in clusters and polymorphonuclear cells. Blood and urine cultures showed no growth. Chest x-ray revealed consolidation of the basal segments of the left lower lobe. Hematocrit was 40. Sed rate was 98 mm per hour. WBC was 14,000. PT and PTT were negative. Blood sugar was 150, BUN 20.

IMPRESSION: Lobar pneumonia caused by pneumococcus.

What code would be reported in this case?

A. 99234
B. 99283
C. 99284
D. 99221

78. An elderly 82-year-old deaf male, new patient, presented in the office with dehydration, lethargy, bluish discoloration around the eyes, confusion, and shortness of breath. The patient's caregiver stated that he had not seen a physician in more than 15 years. It was very difficult for the physician to communicate with the patient because of his deafness and confusion, and the caregiver did not speak fluent English. The physician was able to complete a detailed history and a comprehensive examination, and the medical decision making was of moderate complexity. The physician took an extra hour to write down and provide instructions to the caregiver and to coordinate the care of this patient. What codes would be reported in this case?

A. 99204-21, 99354
B. 99203, 99354
C. 99205
D. 99203-21, 99354

79. An established 61-year-old female patient came into the office for a follow-up visit after the removal of pituitary tumor as a result of being diagnosed with non-small adenocarcinoma of the lung.

HISTORY: The patient is a 61-year female with a large pituitary tumor found after lymph node biopsy that demonstrated lung cancer. The patient has a long history of asthma and chronic obstructive pulmonary disease. The patient's social and family history is on record.

PHYSICAL EXAM: Vital Signs: Temp: 98.2. Pulse: 66. Respirations: 12. BP: 98/46. HEENT: Normocephalic. Skin: Carbuncle was noted on left shoulder. PERRLA. Throat unremarkable. Neck: Supple. Heart: Irregular in rate without any murmurs heard. Abdomen: soft and benign without any gross organomegaly; positive bowel sounds. Extremities: Negative, no edema. Neurological: Oriented × 3.

LAB DATA: Not on hand.

ASSESSMENT AND PLAN: Status post resection of the pituitary gland: Patient is to continue on curent medications. Patient is to follow up with oncologist for chemotherapy regime. Follow-up appointment × 4 weeks. Total time spent with patient was about 15 minutes. Later, that same day, the patient returned for a complaint of the boil on her shoulder. The physician lanced and drained the carbuncle and applied a topical antibiotic on the left shoulder area. What code(s) would be reported in this case?

A. 99214-21
B. 99213, 99212-25
C. 99213-24
D. 99214-25

80. The following case involves a 52-year-old male who is encountering subsequent hospital care. Choose the correct code based on the information provided.

HISTORY: A pleasant 52-year-old male patient has returned to the hospital for the E&M of malignant hypertension, diabetes mellitus type II, and congestive heart failure. The patient's new complaints consist of headache, dizziness, shortness of breath, and numbness of the extremities. The patient denies chest pain. The patient has complied with medication regime and monitors his BP daily by visiting a "minute clinic" at the local pharmacy.

EXAMINATION: The patient is not in acute distress; however he suffers shortness of breath because of the congestive heart failure. PERRLA. Neck: Distended neck veins. Skin: Turgor fair. Heart: A hyperactive carotid pulse is present. The heart has an atrial regular rhythm with some periods of irregularity. Chest: Slight congestion is noted along with atelectasis on the right base. VITAL SIGNS: Temp: 99.2. Pulse: 94. Respirations: 18. BP: 168/98. Abdomen: Soft and nontender. Bowels: Positive bowel sounds are noted. Extremities: Edema is noted in both calves.

ASSESSMENT: Patient not responding to BP meds, and a medication change is ordered; congestive heart failure, malignant hypertension, possible pneumonia.

PLAN: The physician orders a chest radiograph and begins Procardia 20 mm b.i.d.

A. 99233
B. 99232
C. 99234
D. 99213

Anesthesia

81. Physical status modifier P3 is documented for:

A. A normal healthy patient

B. A patient with severe systemic disease that is a constant threat to life

C. A moribund patient who is not expected to survive without the operation

D. A patient with severe systemic disease

82. A 78-year-old male patient underwent a popliteal thromboendarterectomy with patch graft for severe carotid artery stenosis. The patient, afflicted with atrial fibrillation, recently had a pacemaker implantation. What codes would be reported in this case?

A. 01444, P2, 99100

B. 01442, P3, 99100

C. 01274, P3

D. 01430, P4, 99140

83. A 2-day-old infant is brought to the operating room for a repair of an interventricular septal defect with pump oxygenator and hypothermic circulatory arrest. The infant is in critical condition and will not survive without the operation. What codes would be reported in this case?

A. 745.4, 00563, P5, 99100

B. 429.71, 00563, P5, 99100

C. 745.5, 00561, P5, 99100

D. 429.71, 00561, P5

84. OPERATIVE REPORT

PREOPERATIVE DIAGNOSIS: Carcinoma of the skin: scrotum, left side

PROCEDURE: Excision of a 3-cm lesion on skin: scrotum

ANESTHETIC: General

CLINICAL HISTORY: The 61-year-old male had a biopsy of the lesion on the left side of the scrotum to confirm findings of squamous cell carcinoma of the scrotum.

PROCEDURE: The patient was taken to the operating room and put in the lithotomy position, prepped and draped in the usual manner. The anesthesiologist administered a general anesthetic and monitored for the duration of the procedure. An ellipse was taken around the primary lesion with 7-mm margins for excision around the lesion. The lesion was elliptically excised and closed in layers with 4-vicryl. The patient tolerated the procedure well and was given instructions to follow up in the office in 10 days for suture removal. What codes would be reported in this case?

A. 187.3, 11423, 00926

B. 187.3, 11603, 00920

C. 187.7, 11423, 00928

D. 187.7, 11623, 00920

85. In accordance with CPT Guidelines, anesthesia time begins when the anesthesiologist begins to prepare the patient for administration and ends:

A. When the anesthesiologist is no longer in attendance

B. When the patient has been released from recovery

C. When the patient leaves the OR

D. It depends on the OR protocol

86. Code the anesthesia only for the following: Anesthesia for a lumbar laminectomy with fusion and insertion of rods and hooks.

A. 00640

B. 00670

C. 00630

D. 00600

87. OPERATIVE REPORT

PROCEDURE: Sigmoidoscopy

INDICATIONS: The patient was a 43-year-old female with significant changes in bowel patterns and occult blood in stool who was evaluated with a sigmoidoscopy.

ANESTHESIA: Conscious sedation.

PROCEDURE: The patient was given Versed, which was well tolerated. A fleet enema was given 2 hours before the procedure. The video colonoscope was inserted and passed without difficulty to 60 cm. The mucosa were normal. Diverticulosis was noted, as well as several polyps. A biopsy sample was taken and sent to pathology. The patient tolerated the procedure well and was sent to recovery.

What code(s) would be reported in this case?

A. 00904

B. No code is required for conscious sedation

C. 00902

D. 00902, 99148

88. A physician performed a partial hepatectomy and administered the anesthesia for a 37-year-old male prison inmate infected with hepatitis C.

A. 47120-47

B. 00792-47

C. 47010-47

D. 47120-47, 00792

89. What anesthesia code would be assigned for physiological support for harvesting organs(s) from a brain-dead patient?

A. 00580-P6

B. 01990-P6

C. 01999

D. 01990

90. Anesthesia was administered to an 18-year-old male for second- and third-degree burn debridement with skin grafting on the lower right and left legs for a

19% total body surface area burn. What codes would be reported in this case?

A. 01953 × 5

B. 01952, 01953 × 5

C. 01952, 01953 × 2

D. 01953 × 2

Surgery Section

91. OPERATIVE REPORT

PREOPERATIVE DIAGNOSIS: Thrombosed hemorrhoids

POSTOPERATIVE DIAGNOSIS: Same

ANESTHESIA: General

BRIEF HISTORY: A 41-year-old man whose occupation is driving a semi-trailer truck presented in the office 1 week ago with very painful hemorrhoids. He had not had a bowel movement for 10 days as a result of the pain he has recently encountered. The procedure was explained to him for the removal of the hemorrhoid, and his consent was obtained.

PROCEDURE: Induction of general anesthesia was completed and the patient was prepped and draped in the usual manner. The patient was placed in the supine position, and a retractor was placed in the anus. A large external hemorrhoid, partially thrombosed, was identified at 4 o'clock in the lithotomy position. It was grasped with a hemorrhoidal clamp, and a 4-0 chromic stitch was placed at the apex. Electrocautery was used to elliptically excise the hemorrhoid, which was deemed simple, keeping superficial to the sphincter muscle. The hemorrhoid was then passed off to pathology. Bleeding was controlled with electrocautery, and the mucosa was closed with a running stitch. There was no prominent hemorrhoidal tissue remaining. Xeroform wrapped around 4 × 4s was placed in the anus as a dressing, with ABD placed over the top. The patient was then taken to the recovery room. Estimated blood loss was 100 cc. No complications were present. What codes would be reported in this case?

A. 46250, 46940-51

B. 46250

C. 46255

D. 46221, 46940-51

92. The following may be considered _____ if reported separately when performed during the same operative session using the same approach.

58740   Repair: Lysis of adhesions

49320   Laparoscopy, abdomen, peritoneum, and omentum, diagnostic, with or without collection of specimen(s) by brushing or washing

A. Separate procedures

B. Unbundling

C. Add-on codes

D. Diagnostic procedures

93. When would a coder report an unlisted procedure?

A. When a procedure is commonly carried out in addition to the primary procedure

B. When a reduction of services is indicated

C. When a more specific code is not available

D. When the service is greater than usually required for the listed procedure

94. OPERATIVE REPORT

PROCEDURES: 1. Cardiac catheterization 2. Stent to the marginal vein graft

BRIEF HISTORY: The patient was a 52-year-old male with known coronary artery disease who was experiencing recent chest pain, fatigue, hyperhidrosis, and dyspnea. The patient had a history of myocardial infarction followed by a three-vessel coronary artery bypass.

PROCEDURE: The combined right and left heart cardiac catheterization was performed by left ventricular puncture and revealed a sluggish left ventricular function and mild anterior hypokinesis. The left anterior descending had a 60% occlusion in the anterior segment and an 80% occlusion in the distal segment. The left circumflex artery had a 90% occlusion. The first marginal branch had a 100% occlusion, and the second marginal branch also had a 100% occlusion. The right coronary artery had a 50% occlusion. Three grafts were identified. The graft to the left anterior descending to the first marginal and then to the second marginal was 100% occluded at the ostium of the left anterior descending and had a 90 occlusion at the junction of the first marginal. The lesion at the junction of the marginal artery and the saphenous vein graft was successfully stented. Stenosis was reduced to less than 20%. The patient tolerated the procedure well and was taken to recovery.

DISCHARGE MEDICATIONS: Plavix 100 mg t.i.d. for 60 days

Enteric-coated aspirin 100 mg b.i.d.

Combivent 2 puffs t.i.d.

PLAN: Patient to comply with medication treatments. Follow-up care with cardiologist × 2 weeks postop. Patient was instructed to resume normal activities if cleared by cardiologist after follow-up visit. Patient was advised to report recurrent symptoms to PCP or office. What codes would be reported in this case?

A. 93528, 92980-51

B. 93528, 37205, 37206 × 2

C. 93529, 37205-51

D. 93531, 92980-51

95. OPERATIVE REPORT:

PROCEDURE(S): Primary rhinoplasty

BRIEF HISTORY: A 32-year-old female presented with symptoms of nasal airway obstruction that had been chronic for more than 10 years with recent exacerbation. She was concerned about her difficulties and the appearance of her nose. She had a history of tubinectomy and septoplasty to address her airway problems. The patient was well informed concerning the rhinoplasty procedure and elected to proceed. PROCEDURE: The complete rhinoplasty including bony pyramid and lateral and alar cartilages, and elevation of nasal tip was carried out through a columellar chevron incision by the primary surgeon and the minimum assistant surgeon. The nose was infiltrated with 2% lidocaine without epinephrine before incision. The incision was made and carried to bilateral rim incisions. The nasal skin was excised using dissecting scissors. The irregular nasal bones were smoothed with a rasp. Excision of the dorsal nasal bone was then carried out with a straight guarded osteotome. An approximately 2-mm thickness of bone was removed. The cartilaginous nasal dorsum was then smoothed and brought down by using direct shave excision with a #10 blade. Portions of the upper lateral cartilage were also excised. The dorsum was fully straightened; the upper lateral cartilage was resutured to the septum. The nasal fibrofatty tissue between the lower cartilage was excised. The nasal tip was narrowed with interrupted 5-0 PDS sutures. The alar domes were also sharpened with narrowing suture of 5-0 PDS. Dissection was then carried down through the inferior columellar base for a 2.0-cm reconstruction. The caudal septum was excised. The skin was redraped, and closure was carried out by using interrupted 4-0 Prolene for the columellar and stab incisions. Xeroform packs were placed lateral to the nasal splints. The dorsum of the nose was taped, and a dorsal thermoplast spint was also placed. The patient was extubated; she tolerated the procedure well and was sent to recovery. What codes would be reported in this case?

   A. 30400-82
   B. 30410, 13152-82
   C. 30410, 13151-81
   D. 30450, 13151-81

96. A 36-year-old male weightlifter recently ruptured his intervertebral disks at L1-L3. A laminectomy without decompression and disk removal with pedicle fixation anterior instrumentation were performed. What codes would be reported in this case?

   A. 22630, 22632 × 2, 22845
   B. 22630, 22632, 22842
   C. 63017, 22632 × 2, 22845
   D. 63047, 63048 × 3, 22842

97. Code for a free, full-thickness skin graft including direct closure of donor site, neck 11 cm. The surgical preparation of recipient site, 11 cm, was also performed during the same operative session.

   A. 15320, 14041-51
   B. 15004, 13131, 13133 × 2-80
   C. 15240, 13131, 13133 × 2-66
   D. 15240, 15004-51

98. A 4-month-old infant underwent a repair of an initial, incarcerated inguinal hernia with hydrocelectomy, but the repair was discontinued halfway through because of physiological disturbances the infant was experiencing. What code would be reported in this case?

   A. 49496-53, -63, -99
   B. 49492-53
   C. 49492,-53, -63, -99
   D. 49496-53

99. Strabismus surgery including two vertical muscles was performed on a 3-year-old male during which a transposition procedure was also performed to detach and relocate two paretic extraocular muscles next to the paralyzed left eye. What codes would be reported in this case?

   A. 67316, 67320
   B. 67312, 67340
   C. 67318, 67334
   D. 67312, 67320, 67335

100. A 73-year-old female was diagnosed with a myotonic cataract caused by Steinert's disease. An extracapsular cataract removal with insertion of intraocular lens prosthesis, one-stage procedure, by manual technique was performed. What codes would be reported in this case?

   A. 366.13, 275.4, 66983
   B. 366.42, 275.4, 66982
   C. 366.9, 359.2, 66983
   D. 366.43, 359.2, 66984

Radiology

101. Certain procedures are a combination of a physician component and a technical component. When the physician component is reported separately, the service may be identified by adding which modifier?

   A. –22
   B. –26
   C. –62
   D. –82

102. RADIOLOGY REPORT
PATIENT NAME: xxxx xxxxx
BIRTH DATE: xx/xx/xx
STUDY: Chest x-ray, front and lateral
PATIENT HISTORY: Patient is a 45-year-old female with complaints of dyspnea, chest tightness, blood in sputum, congestion, and lethargy × 1 week.
IMPRESSION: Moderate eventration of the anterior portion of the right hemidiaphragm is present. Partial collapse of the right middle lobe is identified, and an unusual spherical density is seen over the apex of the right hemidiaphragm on the PA projection.

PLAN: A follow-up examination is recommended in 1 week.

What code would be reported in this case?

A. 71035

B. 71030

C. 71020

D. 71021

103. A CT scan was performed on a 27-year-old male baseball player who was hit in the face with a baseball during a game. The CT scan was made of the maxillofacial area without contrast material, followed by a scan with contrast material and further sections. A 3-D rendering with interpretation and report of the CT scan, which did not require an independent workstation, was included. What codes would be reported in this case?

A. 70482, 76377

B. 70488, 76376

C. 70487, 76376

D. 70470, 76376

104. RADIOLOGY REPORT

PATIENT NAME: xxxx xxxxx

BIRTH DATE: xx/xx/xx

STUDY: MRI, no contrast material: spine

PATIENT HISTORY: The patient is a 54-year-old female, postmenopausal, who has complaint of chronic back pain for more than 4 years and was diagnosed 3 years ago with degenerative arthritis of the spine. Recent symptoms have exacerbated, and an MRI was indicated.

IMPRESSION:

CERVICAL SPINE: Degenerative disk disease is noted throughout the cervical spine but is most severe from C4 to C6. Marked spur formation is noted to the intervertebral foramina unilaterally at these levels. No fracture or dislocation is identified.

THORACIC SPINE: The vertebral bodies have normal height and alignment, and the disks are or normal width.

LUMBAR SPINE: Progressive degenerative changes have occurred on the left side between the first and third lumbar vertebrae inclusive. No fracture is identified.

What code(s) would be reported in this case?

A. 72159

B. 72141, 72146, 72148

C. 72156, 72157, 72158

D. 72125, 72128, 72131

105. A physician performed an ultrasound on the pregnant uterus of a 21-year-old female, with real-time image documentation; fetal and maternal evaluation was included. The transabdominal approach was used for ultrasound of the first trimester, 12-week-old pregnancy. Code for the physician component only.

A. 76805-26

B. 76816-59

C. 76801-26

D. 76813, 76801-26

106. Code for a red cell survival study with hepatic sequestration and platelet survival study.

A. 78130, 78190

B. 78135, 78191

C. 78135, 78201, 78191

D. 78135, 47505, 78191

107. What scan implies a one-dimensional ultrasonic measurement procedure with movement of the tract to record amplitude and velocity of moving echo-producing structures?

A. A-mode scan

B. B-scan

C. Real-time scan

D. M-mode scan

108. What code(s) would be assigned for a therapeutic radiology plan that includes three or more converging ports, two separate treatment areas, multiple blocks, or special time-dose constraints?

A. 77262

B. 77285

C. 77261, 77262

D. 77523

109. A 16-year-old female underwent a tumor-imaging PET scan with a concurrently acquired CT for attenuation correction and anatomical localization from skull base to midthigh. What codes would be reported in this case?

A. 78812, 70450

B. 78812, 70450, 70470

C. 78815

D. 78608, 70470

110. RADIOLOGY REPORT

PATIENT NAME: xxxx xxxxx

BIRTH DATE: xx/xx/xx

STUDY: X-ray; wrist

PATIENT HISTORY: The patient is a 13-year-old male with a history of wrist soreness, stiffness, intermittent swelling, and erythema. The patient states that he hurt his right wrist last month playing basketball but did not tell his coach or parents.

IMPRESSION: The four views showed an ill-defined 2.0-mm bony fragment on the dorsal aspect of the right wrist, which could represent a small avulsion fracture from either the capitate or lunate bone. No evidence of any joint disease is noted.

What code(s) would be reported in this case?

A. 73115

B. 73110

C. 73721

D. 73100, 73110

Pathology and Laboratory

111. When pathology and laboratory tests are performed on the same date of service to obtain multiple results, what modifier should be used?

    A. −51

    B. −91

    C. −90

    D. −56

112. PATHOLOGY REPORT

    NAME: xxxx xxxxx

    BIRTH DATE: xx/xx/xx

    HISTORY: A 55-year-old male with a history of transurethral resection of the bladder for grade II TCC with miroinvasion; multiple tumors.

    GROSS DESCRIPTION: The specimen is labeled "biopsy bladder tumor" and consists of multiple fragments of gray-brown tissue that appear slightly hemorrhagic. They are submitted for processing.

    MICROSCOPIC DESCRIPTION: Section of the bladder contains areas of transitional cell carcinoma. No area of invasion can be identified. A marked acute and chronic inflammatory reaction with eosinophils is noted, with some necrosis.

    DIAGNOSIS: Papillary transitional cell carcinoma, grade II, bladder biopsy.

    What code(s) would be reported in this case?

    A. 88305

    B. 88309

    C. 88305, 88307

    D. 88307

113. A routine venipuncture was performed on a 29-year-old female. Quantitative therapeutic drug assays were performed for haloperidol and phenobarbital. What codes would be reported in this case?

    A. 80173, 80184

    B. 36410, 80173, 80184

    C. 36415, 80173, 80184

    D. 80103, 36410, 80173, 80184

114. What code would you assign for the sweat collection by iontophoresis?

    A. 82438

    B. 89230

    C. 89240

    D. 88189

115. Code for elevation and pH of blood gases CO_2, pCO_2 and HCO_3.

    A. 82810

    B. 82803

    C. 82800, 82820

    D. 82805

116. PATHOLOGY REPORT

    NAME: xxxx xxxxx

    BIRTH DATE: xx/xx/xx

    HISTORY: The patient was a 17-year-old male experiencing RLQ pain for the previous 12 hours with recent exacerbation. Radiology report showed inflamed appendix.

    GROSS DESCRIPTION: The specimen was labeled appendix and was received in formalin. The specimen consisted of an appendix that measured $5 \times 1 \times 1$ cm in greatest dimension.

    MICROSCOPIC DESCRIPTION: The serosa surface had some white fibrinoid material attached to it across it and on a cross-section necrosis was noted. The representations were submitted.

    DIAGNOSIS: Acute appendicitis

    What codes would be reported in this case?

    A. 540.0, 88300

    B. 540.9, 88302

    C. 540.9, 88304

    D. 543.9, 88304

117. Which is the study of diseased tissues?

    A. Cytology

    B. Histology

    C. Cytopathology

    D. Hematology

118. Code for the qualitative analysis of organic acids, 2 specimens.

    A. 83919 × 2-91

    B. 83918, 83919-51

    C. 83921 × 2-91

    D. 83918 × 2-91

119. Code for a qualitative urinalysis for a bacteriuria screen.

    A. 81000, 86609

    B. 81002, 86609

    C. 81007

    D. 81007, 86609

120. A pathology consultation during surgery was performed for three tissue blocks with frozen sections. What codes would be reported in this case?

    A. 88329, 88331, 88332 × 2

    B. 88329, 88332 × 2

    C. 88331 × 3

    D. 88331, 88332 × 2

Medicine

121. A physician who specializes in the study of electromyography and nerve conduction tests is a(n):

- A. Immunologist
- B. Internist
- C. Cardiologist
- D. Neurologist

122. Which code(s) would be correct for the 8-channel EEG monitoring for identification and lateralization of cerebral seizure focus, with electroencephalographic recording and interpretation for 48 hours?

- A. 95951 × 2
- B. 95950 × 2
- C. 95813
- D. 95812, 95950

123. A 54-year-old female went into the hospital for chemotherapy administration by intravenous infusion technique for three hours. What code(s) would be reported in this case?

- A. 96401
- B. 96405, 96411 × 2
- C. 96413, 96415 × 2
- D. 96420, 96423 × 2

124. Which code(s) would you assign for a home visit for a homebound, elderly patient who needs stoma care and colostomy maintenance?

- A. 99505
- B. 50810, 99505
- C. 99504
- D. 99505, 99507

125. Mild sedation services were rendered to a 4-year-old male who underwent repair (12 sutures) in the left forearm as a result of a complex wound he received from a dog bite. The same physician who repaired the wound also provided the sedation support, which also required a trained observer to assist in the monitoring of the patient's level of consciousness and physiological status for 45 minutes. What codes would be reported in this case?

- A. 99143, 99144
- B. 99148, 99150
- C. 99143, 99145
- D. 99148, 99149

126. A 61-year-old female with disorganized schizophrenia who is an inpatient at a mental ward took part in individual psychotherapy, insight oriented with a behavior-modifying focus. The physician spent 80 minutes face-to-face with the patient. What code would be reported in this case?

- A. 90821
- B. 90814
- C. 90808
- D. 90828

127. In what subsection in the Medicine section of the CPT manual would you find comprehensive computer-based motion analysis by video taping and 3-D kinetics?

- A. Functional Brain Mapping
- B. Neurostimulators, Analysis Programming
- C. Evoked Potentials and Reflex Testing
- D. Motion Analysis

128. Code for the determination of maldistribution of inspired gas with multiple breath nitrogen washout curve, including alveolar helium equilibration time.

- A. 94770
- B. 94350
- C. 94250
- D. 94370

129. An 18-year-old male with a history of detached retina of the left eye underwent external ocular slit-lamp photography with interpretation and report for documentation of medical progress on his injury. What code would be reported in this case?

- A. 92230
- B. 92250
- C. 92285
- D. 92020

130. What codes would be assigned to the intravenous hydration for 5 hours for an 11-month-old infant who has RSV and hyperemesis?

- A. 90706, 90761 × 3-63
- B. 90761 × 5-63
- C. 90760, 90761 × 4
- D. 90765, 90766 × 4

Miscellaneous

131. The exchange of oxygen and carbon dioxide between the body and the air we breathe in is called:

- A. External respiration
- B. Cellular respiration
- C. Internal respiration
- D. Active transport

132. A high level of _____ in the body is indicative of Cushing's disease.

  A. Lymphocytes
  B. Trigylcerides
  C. Cortisol
  D. Digoxin

133. The following is an office visit for a new patient, a 69-year-old male with no prior cardiac history who is now referred for cardiac catheterization to evaluate chest pain. Choose the correct codes based on the information provided.

  HISTORY OF PRESENT ILLNESS: The patient gives a several-month history of left anterior chest and throat "burning and tightness," occurring with exertion associated with mild shortness of breath and improving with rest after several minutes. He denies radiation of pain, nausea, vomiting, diaphoresis, and palpitations. He provides no history of othopnea.

  PAST MEDICAL HISTORY: Hyptertension, hypercholesterolemia, prostate cancer, and arthritis.

  MEDICATIONS: Celebrex® 150 mg p.o. t.i.d.
  Lipitor® 20 mg p.o. t.i.d.
  Aspirin 325 mg p.o. q.d.

  ALLERGIES: No known drug allergies.

  FAMILY HISTORY: Positive for coronary artery disease, sister and mother had bypass surgery at uncertain age, brother underwent stenting in his 50s.

  SOCIAL HISTORY: The patient is married with three grown children. He is a retired professor, and he denies tobacco, alcohol, and illicit drug use.

  REVIEW OF SYSTEM: The patient describes occasional lower left leg pain. He acknowledges he is hard of hearing.

  PHYSICAL EXAMINATION: Alert and oriented, comfortable-appearing male. Vital signs: Temp: 98.6. Pulse: 82. Respirations: 20. BP: 182/100.

  HEENT: PERRLA. Neck: Supple. No adenopathy or carotid bruits. Heart: Regular rate and rhythm. S1 and S2. No murmurs, gallops or rubs. PMI: Normal. Negative jugular distention. Lungs: Clear. Abdomen: Soft, nontender. Positive bowel sounds × 3. Extremities: Warm, with edema left leg. No femoral bruits heard. The physician spends longer than usual to explain the procedure to the patient because of his hearing deficit. IMPRESSION: Angina pectoris unspecified, essential hypertension; benign.

  PLAN: Cardiac catheterization with further management based on findings. The patient is informed of the procedure and provides appropriate consent.

  A. 413.0, 401.9, 99242
  B. 413.9, 401.1, V10.46, 99202-21
  C. 402.10, V10.46, 99242-21
  D. 402.10, V10.46, 99202-21

134. Code for the open dislocation of the shoulder, contusion of the orbital tissue on the left eye, and a crushing injury to the larynx resulting from the patient's bicycle collision with a scooter.

  A. 831.00, 918.0, 925, E825.6
  B. 831.10, 921.2, 925.2, E826.1
  C. 831.11, 920, 929.0, E824.6
  D. 832.00, 921.2, 918.9, 952.2, E826.1

135. A 10-year-old female, ESRD patient underwent dialysis for 21 days. What code(s) would be reported in this case?

  A. 90919
  B. 90922 × 21
  C. 90947, 90923
  D. 90923 × 21

136. A 25-year-old professional football player presents in the emergency room with dehydration, fatigue, syncope, and elevated pulse. The physician performs a history and physical exam and orders an electrolyte panel, a comprehensive metabolic panel, and an automated urinalysis with microscopy. What codes would be reported in this case?

  A. 80051, 80053, 81001
  B. 80051, 80048, 81003
  C. 80050, 81001
  D. 80050, 80048, 81001

137. Patient advocacy is part of the _____ .

  A. Claims management process
  B. Utilization management process
  C. Risk management process
  D. Case management process

138. What is the primary purpose of the medical record?

  A. To provide data for research studies
  B. To provide data for governmental health care agencies
  C. To document the diagnosis and treatment of the patient
  D. To protect the interests of the physician

139. ENDOSCOPY REPORT
  PATIENT: xxxx xxxxx
  DATE: xx/xx/xxxx
  BRIEF HISTORY: The patient is a 77-year-old female with symptoms of dysphagia while eating solids × 2 weeks. Patient has a history of Alzheimer's disease with hypercholesterolemia and arthritis and is in poor health.
  PROCEDURE: Gastroscopy; esophageal dilation
  INDICATIONS: Barium swallow showed a smooth stricture at the LEX. Patient was administered Versed.

Conscious sedation was monitored in the usual manner. The video endoscope was introduced into the esophagus with balloon dilation to 25 mm. A tight stricture was noted at the LES. The stomach to the duodenum was visualized and appeared normal. The scope was withdrawn, and the patient was serially dilated. The patient tolerated the procedure well and was sent to recovery without complications. What code(s) would be reported in this case?

A. 43220

B. 43249

C. 43235, 91040

D. 43235, 43456

140. What fifth digit would you assign for poliovirus type II?

A. 1

B. 2

C. 0

D. 3

141. An 11-year-old boy presented in the office of his pediatrician for the treatment of a 4-cm laceration on his left knee. The physician sutured his knee and administered a tetanus toxoid after realizing the boy was not current on his tetanus immunization. What E&M code would you assign for this case?

A. 99212

B. No E&M code would be assigned

C. 99213

D. 99281

142. A 22-year-old female presented in the ER with multiple lacerations on her body caused by glass breaking in her apartment building. The emergency physician performed the following repairs:
1-cm simple repair of the nose
2.5-cm simple repair of the left ear
7-cm intermediate repair of the scalp
5-cm intermediate repair of the left lower leg
4.2-cm intermediate repair of the left foot
3.7-cm complex repair of the lip
What codes would be reported in this case?

A. 13152, 12035, 12013-51

B. 13131, 12035, 12001, 12011-51

C. 13152, 12042, 12034, 12013-51

D. 13132, 12035, 12001, 12013-51

143. Which one is not an element of a history?

A. Nature of presenting problem

B. Chief complaint

C. System review

D. Social history

144. The following is an operative note for a 46-year-old male who is returning to the operating room for a related heart procedure during his initial postoperative period. Choose the correct codes based on the information provided.

OPERATIVE REPORT

PATIENT: xxxx xxxxx

DATE: xx/xx/xxxx

BRIEF HISTORY: A 46-year-old male was admitted with a diagnosis of acute systolic heart failure complicated by congestive heart failure.

PREOPERATIVE DIAGNOSIS: Acute systolic heart failure; congestive heart failure

POSTOPERATIVE DIAGNOSIS: Same

PROCEDURE: Insertion of permanent pacemaker with transvenous electrodes.

The patient was placed supine on the operating table and was prepped and draped in the usual manner. General anesthesia was administered by an anesthesiologist and was monitored in the usual fashion. A subcutaneous incision was made creating a pocket for the pulse generator. By guide wire, a sheath technique lead was introduced into the subclavian vein and subsequently directed to the right ventricle. The pacemaker was positioned at the threshold 0.5 volts, current 2.0 milliamps and R wave 10. The lead was secured under the clavicle with multiple sutures of 2-0 Vicryl. The pacemaker was programmed at 68 beats per minute. The pulse generator was then anchored in the pocket with a single 2-0 PDS suture. Sterile dressing was applied. The patient tolerated the procedure well and was taken to the recovery room.

A. 428.1, 428.41, 33211

B. 428.31, 428.0, 33208-76

C. 428.21, 33206-78

D. 428.21, 428.0, 33206-78

145. A 31-year-old female, para 2, gravida 3, 31 weeks gestation, underwent a cephalic version under general anesthetic. The patient is a type II diabetic who is also afflicted with Meniere's disease. Code for the anesthesia only.

A. 00902-22, P3

B. 01958, P3

C. 00940, P4

D. 01960-23, P4

146. OPERATIVE NOTE

PATIENT: xxxx xxxxx

DATE: xx/xx/xxxx

BRIEF HISTORY: The patient was a 66-year-old female with chronic hypertension and Parkinson's syndrome, with a unilateral mass on the lung. The patient had lost more than 30 pounds and was experiencing lethargy, anorexia, dyspnea, and bilateral chest pain.

PROCEDURE: Bronchoscopy with washings and brushings

PROCEDURE IN DETAIL: The patient was administered Versed with 10 mg of Fentanyl by an anesthesiologist who remained during the procedure.

The bronchoscope was placed in the right naris and was passed first the right tracheobronchial tree and then to the left where no lesions or bleeding were noted. With the use of fluoroscopic guidance, biopsies of the left upper lobe mass were accomplished with brushings and washings. There was minimal bleeding associated with the biopsies. The patient tolerated the procedure well. Oxygen saturation was 94%, pulse was 88, and BP was 122/76. The patient was taken to the recovery room with no complications. The biopsies were sent to pathology.

What codes would be reported in this case?

A. 31625, 31623-51

B. 31622, 31623, 31625-51

C. 31622, 31625-52

D. 31622, 31625, 31628-51

147. What code would you assign to an intestinal allotransplantation from a living donor?

A. 44120, 44135

B. 44140

C. 44136

D. 44120, 44121

148. Where would you look first to find the code(s) to describe the allergic reaction to an anesthetic agent during surgery?

A. E code index

B. V code index

C. Table of Drugs and Chemicals

D. Index to Procedures

149. Which organization maintains HCPCS Level II codes?

A. World Health Organization

B. Medicare

C. American Medical Association

D. National Hospital Association

150. What code would you assign to indicate that a person is homeless?

A. No code would be used; the circumstance would be documented in the patient's health record

B. E 849.7

C. V60.6

D. V60.0

APPENDIX A

ANSWERS AND RATIONALE BY CHAPTER TO "THINK LIKE A CODER" AND "APPLYING CODING TO THEORY PRACTICE" AND ANSWERS TO THE MOCK EXAMINATON

Chapter 1 Test-Taking Skills

Answers to Think Like A Coder, Chapter 1

1.1 Answer is in the body of the text under "Time Management." It was an exercise to gauge how long it takes for the student to code
1.2 No answer needed.
1.3 No answer needed
1.4 No answer needed
1.5 No answer needed
1.6 No answer needed

Answers to Apply Theory to Practice

1. The answer can be neither right or wrong.
2. Try to answer the question anyway.
3. You should re-read the material again.
4. Motivation
5. No one can, you must decide for yourself after reading this chapter.
6. No, all elements in the Daily Life Schedule need to be included to keep a well-balanced life.
7. Test anxiety is a type of performance anxiety. Some of the symptoms includes sweating, a feeling of being overwhelmed and difficult or fast breathing.
8. The "alternative" the choices of answers presented in the question.
9. Answers could be: peruse the Code Books, read all of the notes in each section, decide how many procedure or diagnoses might be assigned to each problem, look at colors and symbols and try to remember what their meaning are and note the level of complexity of each problem.
10. Go back and review all of your answers as time allows. Make sure all "blanks" are filled in!

Chapter 2 Anatomy and Physiology Review

Answers to Think Like A Coder

2.1. COPD
2.2. Surgery; male genital system
2.3. Gastrojejunostomy
2.4. Strabismus
2.5. Cerebrum
2.6. Thyroglossal duct; cyst

Answers to Applying Coding Theory to Practice

1. C. Coccyx
2. A. Tendons
3. B. Gout
4. C. Voluntary muscle
5. A. Diaphragm
6. C. Meningitis
7. D. The central nervous system
8. C. Pupil
9. A. Hyperopia
10. B. Surgical incision into the middle ear
11. B. Taste
12. D. Diabetes insipidus
13. D. Red blood cell
14. B. Too many red blood cells
15. C. Balloon surgery
16. C. Traveling blood clot
17. B. Scleroderma
18. B. Tuberculosis
19. A. Pharyngitis
20. C. Cholecystectomy
21. A. Urination
22. C. Femur
23. C. Perineum
24. C. Epididymis
25. A. More than one fracture and bone is splintered or crushed

Chapter 3 Medical Terminology and Pathophysiology Review

Answers to Think Like A Coder

3.5. Trachea
3.6. 49520
3.7. Uterus
3.8. Hemoglobin

Answers to Applying Coding Theory to Practice: Prefixes

1. without, not; two
2. three; move from one part to another
3. excessive, beyond; four
4. back, again; below, under
5. away; around

Answers to Applying Coding Theory Practice: Suffixes

1. surgical puncture; pertaining to
2. using instrument to view; enlargement
3. tumor; mass; process
4. medical treatment; disease
5. surgical excision, removal; process of recording

Answers to Applying Coding Theory to Practice: Medical Terms

1. A. Skin
2. B. Surgical puncture of the chest wall with a needle
3. D. Lithotomy
4. C. Removal of waste products from the blood
5. D. Scrotum
6. D. Fallopian tube
7. B. Endocardium
8. B. Process of engulfing and swallowing

9. B. Bile; gall
10. B. Tears
11. C. Surgical correction of middle ear
12. D. Metatarsal bones
13. C. Voluntary muscle
14. C. Central nervous system
15. D. Sugar

Chapter 4 CPT Guidelines Review

Answers to Applying Coding Theory to Practice

1. B. Guidelines
2. B. Foraccurate coding
3. D. Alteration of a procedure or service
4. + Add-on codes
    ▲ Revised code
    ● New procedure
5. Stand-alone code contains full description of code. Indented code contains subordinate clause that separates one code from another and contains all information that the stand-alone code contains prior to the semicolon.
6. Evaluation and Management, Anesthesia, Surgery, Radiology, Pathology and Laboratory, and Medicine, Category II Codes, Category III Codes.
7. The semicolon is used to separate the main and subordinate clause in code descriptions.
8. A procedure that is so new that no definite description or code has been assigned. Unlisted procedures are found in the section guidelines and at the end of every subheading in a section.
9. Summary of deletions, revisions, and additions to codes
10. A. Revision of a code
11. C. Modifier 21
12. B. Modifier 50
13. C. Appendix D
14. A. New and revised text
15. D. Medicine
16. B. Appendix H
17. D. Appendix F
18. C. Category III codes
19. C. Special report
20. A. True

Chapter 5 Evaluation and Management Review

Answers to Think Like A Coder

5.3.   99204
5.5.   99203
5.6.1. 99219
5.6.2. 99220
5.7.   99218-99220 and 99221-99223
5.8.   99254
5.9.   99291, 99292 × 4 Rationale: Codes 99291 and 99292 are for critical care services. Using the chart for Critical Care Services code combination 99291 and 99292 × 4 equates to 165–194 minutes of time. The problem called for 2 hours and 45 minutes, which equals 165 minutes.
5.10. 99328
5.11. 99366
5.12. 99403

Answers to Applying Coding Theory to Practice

1. B. 99232 Rationale: Hospital Inpatient Services, Subsequent Hospital Care. An expanded problem focused history and examination was performed. The descriptor of the code indicates at least two of the three key components must be met.
2. B. 99213, 99212 -25 Rationale: Office or Other Outpatient Services 99213–: Established patient with expanded problem-focused history and exam that requires at least two of the three key components. The descriptor of the code indicates at least two of the three key components must be met. Code 99212 -25 is used to describe the exam for the wrist. Modifier -25 indicates a significant, separately identifiable E&M service by the same physician on the same day of the procedure or other service.
3. B. 99241 Rationale: Consultations, Office or Other Outpatient Consultations. Detailed history and examination were performed. Medical decision making was of low complexity.
4. A. 99288 Rationale: Other Emergency Services. Code 99288 describes physician direction of emergency medical systems emergency care, advanced life support via helicopter.
5. A. 99282 Rationale: Emergency Department Services, New or Established Patient. The descriptor with code 99282 includes text that says, "usually the presenting problems are of low to moderate severity."
6. C. -25 See appendix "A"
7. C. 99214 Rationale: Office or Other Outpatient Services, Established Patient. History and examination were detailed and medical decision making was of low complexity. The descriptor requires at least two of the three key components.
8. B. 99381 Rationale: Preventive Medicine Services, New Patient. Age-appropriate code assignment.
9. C. 99349 Rationale: Home Services, Established Patient. Detailed interval history, detailed examination, and medical decision making was of moderate complexity. Time element, 40 minutes.
10. B. 99431 Rationale: Newborn Care. Code 99431's descriptor indicates history and examination of a newborn in a hospital setting.
11. D. 99284, 99291, 99292 × 4 Rationale: Emergency Department Services, Other Emergency Services. Code 99288 descriptor indicates physician services provided during life transport to a critical care unit. Critical Care Services include 180 minutes of time spent in critical care. Codes 99291 and 99292 accurately describe the amount of time the service covered.
12. B. 99334 Rationale: Domiciliary, Rest Home, Established Patient. Descriptor includes text that states, "Usually, the presenting problem(s) are self-limited or minor."
13. C. 99295 × 5 Rationale: Inpatient Neonatal Critical Care. Code 99295 includes inpatient neonatal critical care, per day. Patient stay was for 5 days.
14. B. 99360 × 2 Rationale: Physician Standby Service. Code descriptor reads physician standby each for 30 minutes. Code 99360 accurately codes for time spent on standby.
15. D. 99404 Rationale: Counseling and/or Risk Factor Reduction Intervention, Preventive Medicine, Individual Counseling. Code 99404 is accurate code to describe amount of time services were provided.
16. B. 99239 Rationale: Hospital Discharge Services. Code 99239 covers the amount of time spent with hospital discharge services.

17. B. 99236 Rationale: Observation or Inpatient Care Services (including Admission and Discharge Service). Code 99236's descriptor includes text, usually the presenting problem requiring admission is of high severity.

18. A. 99298 × 2 Rationale: Intensive (Non-Critical) Low Birth Weight Services. Code 99298 covers services per day.

19. C. Unrelated E&M service by the same physician during a postoperative period. Rationale: See Appendix A in the CPT manual.

20. B. 99375 Rationale: Care Plan Oversight Services. Code 99375 includes time element of 30 minutes or more.

21. B. 99363, 99364 Rationale: Anticoagulant Management. Code 99363 indicates the management of the warfarin and INR testing for the initial 90 days. Code 99364 indicates each subsequent 90 days of therapy thereafter.

22. A. 99309 Rationale: Subsequent Nursing Facility Care. History was detailed interval, examination was comprehensive, and medical decision making was of moderate complexity.

23. C. 99436 Rationale: Newborn Care Services. Code descriptor includes initial stabilization of newborn by physician other than delivering physician.

24. B. 99236 Rationale: Observation or Inpatient Care Services (including Admission and Discharge Service). Code 99236's descriptor includes text, "usually the presenting problem requiring admission is of high severity."

25. B. 99239 Rationale: Hospital Discharge Services. Code 99239 covers the amount of time spent with hospital discharge services.

Chapter 6 Anesthesia Review

Answers to Think Like A Coder

6.3 P5 Rationale: Physical status modifier P5 is assigned for a patient who is not expected to survive without the operation.

6.4. 99135 Rationale: Qualifying circumstance code 99135 is assigned for a patient whose condition is complicated by hypotension.

Answers to Applying Coding Theory to Practice

1. C. 00866 Rationale: Only anesthesia code would be assigned and would be found in the index under anesthesia; adrenalectomy.

2. B. 00580, P5 Rationale: Only the anesthesia code would be assigned, and the physical status modifier P5 is appropriate for a patient who is moribund and is not expected to live without the operation.

3. D. 00797 Rationale: Only anesthesia code would be assigned. To index, begin with "anesthesia"; stomach; restriction for obesity. A qualifying circumstance code would be assigned because of the extreme age of the patient.

4. A. 00212, 99100 Rationale: Only anesthesia code would be assigned. To index, begin with "anesthesia" > "skull, 00190" > to "subdural taps." A qualifying circumstance code would also be assigned because of the extreme age of the patient.

5. B. 13132, 99144 Rationale: Anesthesia code would not be used since the physician performing the surgery administered the conscious sedation. In Anesthesia Guidelines for conscious sedation, codes 99143-99145 are to be used in conjunction with the procedure that was performed.

6. C. 01961, P2 Rationale: Code only for the anesthesia. Index "anesthesia." "Cesarean delivery." Physical status modifier P2 would also be assigned because of the mild systemic disease.

7. D. 01951 Rationale: Code only for anesthesia. Index "anesthesia," "burn excisions or debridement." Code for less than 4% of total body surface.

8. D. 01400 Rationale: Code only for anesthesia. Index "anesthesia," "knee."

9. A. 00540, P3, 99100 Rationale: Index, "anesthesia, intrathoracic." Assign P3 for 2 systemic diseases considered greater than mild, and assign qualifying circumstance code for the extreme age of the patient.

10. C. 01462 -23 Rationale: Code for basic service due to "unusual anesthesia" that was administered to an extremely anxious patient who otherwise would not require general anesthesia. Modifier -23 indicates "unusual anesthesia" procedures.

11. C. 00921 Rationale: Index, "anesthesia, perineum," and choose code 00921.

12. D. 01996 Rationale: Index, "anesthesia, other procedures." Choose 01996 for the daily hospital management of an epidural.

13. A. 00404 Rationale: Index, "anesthesia, thorax; chest wall." Choose 00404 for radical or modified radical procedures on breast. Code 00406 would not be used due to the "simple" mastectomy that was performed.

14. C. 00214 Rationale: Index, "anesthesia, burr holes." Choose 00214 for burr holes with ventriculography.

15. D. 00320 Rationale: Index: "anesthesia, larynx." Choose code 00320; patient is more than 1 year of age.

Chapter 7 Surgery Review

Answers to Think Like A Coder

7.1. No. Rationale: The phrase "separate procedure" comes after the semicolon, signifying that not all indented codes of the main code are to be billed as separate.

7.3. 11624 Rationale: Excision of a malignant lesion, measurement range 3.1 cm to 4.0 cm.

7.4.1. 12015, 12001 -51 Rationale: Coder must add lengths of like repairs, 4.5-cm face wound and 3.2-cm lip wound, to sum 7.7 cm for code assignment 12015. Code 12001 is for the simple repair of a wound 2.5 cm or less. Subsection notes instruct coder to use -51 for more than one classification of wound.

7.4.2. 11057 Rationale: Code 11057 is assigned for more than 4 lesions.

7.5.1. 22630, 22632 Rational: Code 22630 is the primary procedure, and code 22632 (add-on code) lists each additional interspace in the lumbar region.

7.5.2. 29075 Rationale: Charges would apply since the same physician is reapplying the cast (short arm cast; elbow to finger).

7.6.1. 31643 Rationale: Code 31643 includes placement of catheter for intracavitary radiolement application. Only one code is needed.

7.6.2. 31255, 31256 -51 Rationale: You must add code 31256 with modifier -51; code 31255 does not include maxillary antrostomy.

7.7.1. 33511, 33508 -80 Rationale: Code 33508 is used for the surgical vascular endoscopy and used in conjunction with codes 33510-33523. The modifier -80 is used because a surgical assistant performed the graft procurement. (This info is in a "note" under subheading "Venous Grafting Only for Coronary Artery Bypass")

7.7.2. 37185 Rationale: Code 37185 includes all procedures; descriptor directs the coder to not use codes 76000 or 76100 in conjunction with code 37185.

7.8.1. 41105, 41250 -51 Rationale: Code 41250 must be reported in addition to the primary code 41105. Modifier -51 is used to show multiple procedure during same operative session by same physician.

7.8.2. 47630, 74327 Rationale: Code 74327 needs to reported in addition to 47630 because of the radiological supervision and interpretation.

7.9. 50780 -50 Rationale: Modifier -50 must be used in conjunction with code 50780 to report a bilateral anastomosis.

7.10.1. 54690, 54800 -51 Rationale: Surgical laparoscopy includes diagnostic laparoscopy. Code 54800 is assigned to indicate the needle biopsy of the epididymis. Modifier -51 is reported for multiple procedures by same physician in same operative session.

7.10.2. 58292 Rationale: Code 58292 is inclusive of all procedures performed by surgeon. Laparoscope was not used.

7.11. Physician 1: 61590, 61605 -51, Physician 2: 61618 Rationale: Physician 1 performed the approach procedure and the definitive procedure during same operative session, so modifier -51 needs to be reported. Physician 2 performed only the reconstruction procedure, which is reported by him using code 61618; no modifier -62 is necessary since neither physician was "primary."

7.12.1. 67314, 67335 Rationale: Code 67314 instructs to report code 67335 for adjustable sutures.

7.12.2. 69644 Rationale: Code 69644 includes all procedures described in problem.

Answers to Applying Coding Theory to Practice

1. A. 12035, 13152 -51 Rationale: Coder must add the length of like repairs, 12.4 cm and 6.1 cm, to sum 18.5 cm, for code assignment 12035. Code 13152 is for the complex repair of the eyelid measuring 3.5 cm. Modifier -51 is assigned for multiple procedures during the same operative session.

2. C. 27759 Rationale: Code 27759 includes fibular fracture with or without cerclage.

3. B. 31625, 32480 -51 Rationale: Code 31625 includes rigid bronchoscopy with fluoroscopic guidance, and code 32480 is reported for the single lobectomy. Modifier -51 is used to report multiple procedures during same operative session.

4. D. 33233, 33212 Rationale: Both codes must be reported for removal and insertion of the pacemaker pulse generator replacement. A third code would not be used unless physician performed lead placements during the operative session. Pacemaker pulse generator was a dual chamber.

5. B. 10022, Radiology: 77012 Rationale: Code 10022 encompasses imaging guidance for fine needle aspiration. Code 77012 is reported for the CT guidance code.

6. D. 69424 -50 Rationale: Code 69424 encompasses entire surgery including general anesthesia. Modifier -50 is reported to include bilateral procedure.

7. A. 55250 Rationale: Code 55250 includes semen examinations. It is not required to code twice for multiple semen examinations.

8. C. 63016, 63020 -51 Rationale: Code 63016 includes laminectomy and more than two thoracic segments. Code 63020 includes laminotomy with one cervical interspace. Modifier -51 is used to report multiple procedures during same operative session.

9. B. 27100 -78 Rationale: Code 27100 encompasses entire procedure. Modifier 78 must be reported to include a return to the operating room during postoperative period for a related procedure.

10. C. 31380 -53 Rationale: Hemilaryngectomy (partial laryngectomy) was performed anterovertically. Modifier -53 is reported to indicate that the procedure was discontinued.

11. A. Physician 2 Rationale: The note for Mohs Micrographic Surgery indicates that the physician who is delegated the responsibilities of these services should report the codes.

12. A. 50382 -50 Rationale: Code 50382 includes the removal and replacement of the ureteral stent and radiologic supervision and interpretation. Modifier -50 is reported for a bilateral procedure.

13. A. 34900, 34825 -51, 75954 Rationale: Code 34900 includes the iliac repair and graft. Code 34825 is reported for placement of the prosthesis, and code 75954 is used for radiological supervision and interpretation.

14. C. -58 Rationale: Modifier -58 clearly indicates stage or related procedure by the same physician during the postoperative period.

15. B. 59001 Rationale: Problem only described the therapeutic amniocentesis. No other procedure should be reported.

16. B. 65772 Rationale: Code 65772 is used to describe the corneal relaxing incision for correction of surgically induced astigmatism.

17. D. 69436 -50 Rationale: Code 69436 -50 is assigned to describe the bilateral tympanostomy with insertion of tubes. Modifier -50 is assigned to indicate bilateral procedure. An anesthesia code should not be assigned as the descriptor for code 69436 indicates that general anesthesia is included in the service.

18. B. 66984 Rationale: Code 66984 is assigned to indicate the unilateral cataract removal by phacoemulsification. Modifier -50 should not be assigned since only one eye was indicated in the procedure.

19. 15823 -50 Rationale: Code 15823 is assigned to indicate that the patient underwent blepharoplasty of the upper eyelid. The statement, "Previously outlined excessive skin, weighing down both lids of both the right and left upper eyelid, was excised with blunt dissection," would indicate the use of code 15823 instead of code 15822 due to excessive skin weighing down the eyelid. Modifier -50 should be assigned to indicate a bilateral procedure was performed.

20. 11626, 14021 Rationale: Code 11626 is assigned to indicate the excision of a malignant lesion of the scalp that is 6 cm in diameter. Code 14021 is assigned to indicate that an advancement flap closure was performed on the scalp. The note under Adjacent Tissue Transfer or Rearrangement" instructs the coder to measure the primary defect (tumor itself) and the secondary defect (area surrounding) together, which would equal 30 sq cm in total. Therefore, code 14021 should be assigned.

Chapter 8 Radiology Review

Answers to Think Like A Coder

8.1. Intrathecally, intra-articularly, and intravascularly Rationale: All three routes of administration are used, and the information can be found in the Radiology Guidelines of the CPT manual.

8.2.1. 74470 -26 Rationale: Code 74470 is diagnostic radiology, not angiography. Modifier -26 is used to report technical component only.

8.2.2. 76813 -26 Code 76813 best describes this real time ultrasound. Modifier -26 is used when the physician component is reported separately.

Answers to Applying Coding Theory to Practice

1. B. 70482 Rationale: Procedure was a computed tomography scan with and without contrast of the inner ear and further sections.
2. C. 47630, 74327 Rationale: Both codes would be reported since the physician performed the primary procedure and the radiology procedure.
3. C. 78707 Rationale: Code 78707 includes vascular flow, single study without pharmacological intervention. Multiple codes should not be used.
4. B. 78813 -22 Rationale: Code 78813 reports a whole body PET scan. Modifier -22 should be reported because of the unusual and lengthened time involved in the procedure. A special report should also be attached.
5. D. 74247 Rationale: Radiology report consists of upper GI series with KUB and delayed films. Modifier -26 should not be reported because the supervision and interpretation was part of the procedure.
6. C. 75660 Rationale: The review of available codes for angiography, code 75660 best describes the procedure performed.
7. A. 70110 -26 Rationale: Code 70110 describes more than four views of the mandible. Modifier -26 is used to report only the professional component of the service.
8. A. 99283, 71022 Rationale: Code 99283 is reported for the evaluation and management of emergency department services. Code 71022 best describes the radiological procedure performed.
9. D. 78216 Rationale: Code 78185 directs the coder to use codes 78215 or 78216 if spleen imaging is combined with liver study. To report both 78185 and 78201 would be considered "unbundling."
10. C. 78460, 93015 Rationale: Code 78460 is reported for the perfusion imaging, and code 93015 is reported for the cardiovascular stress test with supervision, interpretation and report. The subheading "Cardiovascular System" under Nuclear Medicine contains a note that instructs the coder to use these codes in combination for reporting.
11. B. 77328 Rationale: Code 77328 indicates complex brachytherapy isodose plan and best describes the procedure performed.
12. C. 79005 Rationale: Code 79005, found under the subsection "Nuclear Medicine" and subheading "Therapeutic," best describes this procedure.
13. D. 43215, 74235 Rationale: Code 43215 best describes the esophagoscopy with removal of foreign body. The note under code 43215 directs the coder to use code 74235 for supervision and interpretation of procedure.
14. C. Physician A: 75940 Physician B: 37620 Rationale: Code 75940 should be reported for the radiological supervision and interpretation of the procedure. Code 37620 best describes the procedure performed by physician B. To find code 75940, index "Placement" and "IVC filter."
15. D. 70491, 76377 Rationale: Code 70491 best describes the CT scan, and the note below refers the coder to use codes 76376-76377 for 3D rendering. Code 76377 was reported because the procedure called for image postprocessing on an independent workstation.

16. B. 73620 Rationale: Code 73620 best describes the radiology procedure in the report. Code 73718 calls for MRI of the lower extremity.
17. C. 75960–TC Rationale: Code 75960 best describes the radiology procedure. The modifier "TC" must be added to indicate technical component only.
18. D. 72052–26, 72070–26 Rationale: Code 72052 is assigned to indicate that a radiological examination of the cervical spine (neck) was performed. Modifier -26 would be assigned to indicate the professional component only.
19. B. 73530 Rationale: Code 73530 is assigned to indicate that an x-ray for the hip was performed during the operative procedure. Code 73500 should not be used because the descriptor does not indicate "during the operative procedure." No modifier is needed if the procedure was global.
20. A. 75560 -26 Rationale: Code 75560 is assigned to indicate a cardiac MRI without contrast material with performance of velocity quantification and stress. Modifier -26 indicates supervision and interpretation only. Code 75564 should not be assigned because the descriptor includes, "without contrast material, followed by contrast material."

Chapter 9 Pathology and Laboratory Review

Answers to Think Like A Coder

9.1.1. 80406 Rationale: This code includes ACTH stimulation panel and is for 3 beta-hydroxydehydrogenase deficiency. Index: ACTH
9.1.2. 80050 Rationale: The other individual procedure codes are NOT reported separately in addition to the general health panel code 80050.
9.2. -86001 × 4 Rationale: Code 86001 best describes this procedure. It is necessary to report the code 4 times since the descriptor calls for "each allergen."
9.3. 88307 Rationale: Code 88307 best describes this procedure. Code 88305 includes traumatic amputation of the extremity. The procedure code for the amputation is not coded.

Answers to Applying Coding to Theory Practice

1. C. 81001 Rationale: Code 81001 best describes this procedure. You should not separately report codes for the various constituents.
2. A. 88332 × 3 Rationale: Code 88332 best describes this procedure that is a pathology consultation during surgery. The code should be reported three times since the descriptor includes, "each additional block with frozen section(s)."
3. C. 88304 Rationale: The pathology report indicates that surgical pathology, gross and microscopic examination, was required. The coding assignment indicates surgical pathology at Level III since the appendectomy was not incidental.
4. B. 82805 Rationale: Code 82805 includes all of the analytes in problem 4 as well as 0_2 saturation by direct measurement except pulse oximetry.
5. B. 83002 -91, 83727 Rationale: Code 83002 best describes the procedure, and the note under code 83002 instructs the coder to assign code 83727 for luteinizing releasing factor. Modifier -91 should be assigned for a repeat diagnostic laboratory test.
6. A. 83890, 83901 × 4 Rationale: Code 83901 instructs the coder to use this code in addition to the primary code (83890). The code descriptor also specifies "each additional nucleic acid sequence," which call for code 83901 to be reported four times.

7. C. Evaluation and Management section Rationale: The note under subsection Evocative/Suppression Testing informs the coder to use E&M codes to report physician attendance and monitoring.

8. C. 87110 Rationale: Code 87110 describes a *Chlamydia* culture and best describes this procedure.

9. D. 88025 -90Rationale: Code 88025 describes a gross and microscopic autopsy of the brain. Modifier -90 should be assigned because an outside laboratory performed the procedure.

10. C. 88174 Rationale: Index: cytopathology > cervical. Code 88174 best describes this procedure. No modifier is needed.

11. B. 89264, 89310 Rationale: Both 89264 and 89310 should be reported to best describe these procedures.

12. B. 88305 Rationale: Pathology report indicated gross examination of breast mass. Code 88305 best describes this procedure.

13. D. 88262 Rationale: Code 88262 includes the count of cells within the chromosomes are up to 20 and 2 karotypes with banding.

14. A. 84443, 84479 Rationale: Code 84443 should be reported for the TSH, and code 84479 should be reported for T3 uptake.

15. A. 82139 Rationale: Code 82139 is reported for only one specimen for six or more amino acids and is quantitative not qualitative. This code should be reported only one time unless there is more than one specimen.

16. C. 85290 Rationale: Code 85290 is reported for clotting factor XIII with fibrin stabilizing. Only one code should be assigned.

17. B. 86301 Rationale: Code 86301 is reported for an immunoassay for tumor antigen; quantitative; CA 19–9.

18. D. 87390 -90 Rationale: Code 87390 is reported to describe the infectious agent being tested by enzyme immunoassay technique; semiquantitative for HIV-1. Modifier -90 is assigned to indicate that an outside laboratory performed the test and obtained the results.

19. B. 89272 Rationale: Code 89272 indicates cultures on embryo(s) for a range of 4 to 7 days. This code should be reported only one time.

20. C. 86200 Rationale: CCP is the abbreviation for cyclic citrullinated peptide; code 86200 best describes this antibody test.

21. C. 88307 Rationale: Code 88307 best describes the surgical pathology, gross and microscopic, for the transurethral resection of the bladder (Urinary bladder, TUR). Code 88305 indicates a bladder biopsy, and code 88309 indicates total or partial resection of the bladder.

22. D. 88309, 88302 Rationale: Code 88309 best describes the surgical pathology of the stomach, which was resection due to a tumor. Code 88307 would not be coded because of the descriptor's phrase, "other than for tumor." Code 88302 should be assigned for the surgical pathology of the vagus nerve.

23. C. 86813, 86816, 86821 Rationale: Code 86813 indicates the HLA typing, code 86816 indicates the DR/DQ, single antigen, and code 86821 indicates the mixed lymphocyte culture that was ordered.

24. A. 82550, 82552, 82553 Rationale: Code 82550 indicates a total creatine kinase, code 82552 indicates the analyte isoenzymes, and code 82553 indicates MB fraction only.

25. B. 80173 Rationale: Code 80173 indicates that haloperidol was assayed by drawing bloBod levels. The note under

Therapeutic Drug Assays indicates that the material for examination may be from any source and that the examination was quantitative, not qualitative.

Chapter 10 Medicine Section Review

Answers to Think Like A Coder

10.1. 90465, 90702 Rationale: Code 90465 is indicated because of the child's age and the counsel provided by the physician to the parents. The problem did not indicate "psychotherapy." Code 90702 is indicated because it best describes the immunization administered to the child.

10.2.1. 90827 Rationale: Code 90827 best describes the psychotherapy for the child. A separate E&M code would not be assigned since the code descriptor includes "with medical evaluation and management services."

10.2.2. 90865 Rationale: Code 90865 best describes this procedure and can be indexed under "psychiatric treatment" > "narcosynthesis analysis."

10.3. 92602, 92626 Rationale: Code 92602 best describes the analysis of the cochlear implant for a child under 7 years of age. Code 9262 must be reported for evaluation of rehabilitation status.

10.4.1. 95145 Rationale: There was only one stinging insect in the problem. Code 95145 is assigned for a "single stinging insect venom."

10.4.2. 780.51, 95806 Rationale: Code 780.51 is assigned to describe the insomnia with sleep apnea (absence of breathing) unspecified. Code 95806 is assigned to describe the sleep study that was unattended by a technician.

10.5. 95863 Rationale: Code 95863 includes three extremities and related paraspinal areas. Modifier -50 should not be used because the code descriptor indicates "three extremities."

10.6.1. Obstetrical care, date of visit, and LMP Rationale: Category II code 0500F's descriptor includes all of these services.

10.6.2. 1035f Rationale: Category II code 1035F best describes the indication.

10.7.1. 00081T Rationale: Category III code 0081T best describes the indication.

10.7.2. 0178T Rationale: Category III code 0178T best describes the procedure of an EKG with 64 leads.

Answers to Applying Coding Theory to Practice

1. A. 90471, 90648 Rationale: Code 90471 must be reported for the administration of the vaccines. Code 90648 best describes the vaccines administered and should be reported only once.

2. C. 98961 × 2 Rationale: Code 98961 best describes the procedure and should be reported twice to include 60 minutes of face-to-face time with physician.

3. A. 98942 Rationale: Code 98942 best describes the procedure. The code 98942 would not be reported five times as that would be considered overcharging. This code is not considered an unusual procedural service.

4. D. Once Rationale: Dialysis subsection notes indicate that dialysis codes are to be reported only once per month.

5. B. 90862 Rationale: Code 90862 best describes the procedure, and no other code should be reported. All services listed in the problem are included in the code descriptor.

6. C. 90815 Rationale: Code 90815 includes individual psychotherapy, interactive and provides a time limit of approximately 75 to 80 minutes. Medical evaluation and management services are also included in the descriptor.

7. D. 92594 Rationale: Code 92594 best describes the procedure; left ear indicates monaural procedure was performed.

8. D. 96004 Rationale: Code 96004 encompasses all tests indicated in the problem. In the Motion Analysis subsection notes, the coder is instructed to report only 96004 once regardless of the number of studies reviewed or interpreted.

9. B. 91133 Rationale: Code 91133 indicates electrogastrography with provocative testing. Subsection heading is Gastric Physiology; the coder would index "electrogastrography."

10. C. 96413, 96415 Rationale: Code 96413 best describes the procedure and indicates that the code 96415 should be used separately for each additional hour.

11. A. 93016 Rationale: Code 93016 best describes the procedure and indicates "physician supervision only, with out interpretation and report."

12. C. 97113 × 3 Rationale: Code 97114 is used to describe aquatic therapy and must be reported three times due to the phrase "each 15 minutes" in the primary procedure code (97110).

13. B. 97802 × 4 Rationale: Code 97892 is specifically directed to medical nutrition therapy. E&M codes must be used for activities conducted by a physician. Code 97802 must be reported four times to indicate 1 hour of service provided.

14. C. 92982, 92973, 92980 Rationale: Code 92973 best describes the procedure, and the note below the code directs the coder to use codes 92980 and 92982 in conjunction with code 92973.

15. D. 95806 -52 Rationale: Code 95806 indicates all services mentioned in the problem including the use of a technician; modifier -52 is indicated because the sleep study was performed in less than 6 hours. This information can be found in the subsection notes under "Sleep Testing."

16. C. Anesthesia Rationale: Qualifying Circumstances for Anesthesia can be found in the Medicine section and refer to particularly difficult circumstances surrounding the administration of anesthesia, such as age and condition of patient (see Chapter 6).

17. A. 96921 Rationale: Code 96921 describes laser treatment of inflammatory skin disease for areas of 250 sq cm to 500 sq cm.

18. C. 99503 Rationale: Code 99503 best describes the home visit that includes respiratory therapy and apnea assessment.

19. B. 99175, 91105 Rationale: Code 99175 describes the administration of a drug that induces vomiting until all poison is removed from the stomach contents. Code 91105 is reported to include the diagnostic gastric lavage treatment. No E&M service should be reported.

20. B. 86890 -52 Rationale: Code 86890 is reported for the service of the patient providing autologous blood for postoperative services if needed. Modifier -52 is used to indicate that the procedure was reduced because it had to be terminated.

Chapter 11 HCPCS Level II Coding Review

Answers to Think Like A Coder

11.1. J9265 Rationale: HCPCS code J9265 is assigned to describe the drug Paclitaxel 30 mg IV. You can find this code in the Table of Drugs under "Paclitaxel," which directs the coder to verify code J9265.

11.2.1. A6210 Rationale: HCPCS code A6210 best describes the medical supply (wound dressing) for this patient.

11.2.2. A4625 Rationale: HCPCS code A4625 best describes the supply of the tracheostomy kit for a new tracheostomy patient. Code A4629 should not be assigned because it indicates that the tracheostomy kit is for an established patient.

11.3.1. D3310 Rationale: HCPCS code D3310 best describes the root canal, anterior, excluding final restoration.

11.3.2. D5520 × 4 Rationale: HCPCS code D5520 best describes the replacement of missing or broken teeth off of a complete denture. The "× 4" indicates each tooth that was missing in the complete denture.

11.4.1. E0148 Rationale: HCPCS code E0148 best describes the heavy-duty walker without wheels.

11.4.2. E0730 Rationale: HCPCS code E0730 best describes the tens unit (transcutaneous electrical nerve stimulation device) for four or more leads for multiple nerve stimulation.

11.5.1. H0013 Rationale: HCPCS code H0013 best describes the alcohol services for acute detoxification outpatient program.

11.5.2. H2019 × 5 Rationale: HCPCS code H2019 best describe the therapeutic behavior services. Code H2019 would be assigned 5 times due to the code descriptor indicating that this code is used for 15 minute increments. The patient had a total of 1 hour and 15 minutes with behavioral services.

11.6.1. L1660 Rationale: HCPCS code L1660 is assigned to describe the hip orthosis with abduction control of the hip joints, static, plastic prefabricated to include fitting and adjustment.

11.6.2. L5976 Rationale: HCPCS code L5976 is assigned to indicate the type (Seattle Carbon Copy II, found in the index) of prosthetic foot used as a replacement foot for patient.

Answers to Applying Coding Theory to Practice

1. D. K0843 Rationale: Code K0843 indicates the wheelchair described in the problem.

2. D. 57170, A4266 Rationale: Code 57170 is assigned to describe the fitting of the diaphragm accompanied by instructions. HCPCS code best describes the diaphragm for contraceptive use.

3. B. A4554 Code A4554 is assigned to describe the disposable underpads, any size.

4. A. J1940 × 2 Rationale: Code J1940 is assigned to describe the injection of the drug furosemide, 40 mg. The code must be assigned twice to indicate the 40 mg.

5. C. A4673 Rationale: Code A4673 is assigned to describe the extension line with easy lock connectors used with dialysis. To index, look under "ESRD."

6. R0076 Rationale: Code R0076 is assigned to indicate that a portable EKG machine was used at a facility.

7. R0076 Rationale: Code R0076 would be used, and the three patient's bill would be prorated.

8. G0204 GG Rationale: Code G0204 is assigned to best describe the mammography, and HCPCS modifier GG is assigned to indicate performance and payment of a screening mammogram and diagnostic mammogram on the same patient, same day.

9. A4570 F3 Code A4570 best describes the application of a splint to the finger. HCPCS modifier F3 indicates the left hand, fourth digit.
10. A6537 Rationale: Code A6537 best describes the type of compression stocking.

Chapter 12 ICD-9-CM Guidelines and Coding Conventions Review, Part I

Answers to Think Like A Coder

12.1.1. Tabular List of Diseases and Tabular List of Procedures
12.1.2. Contains a "use additional codes" note for clarification
12.2.1. V10.3 Rationale: V code V10.3 is assigned for the personal history of malignant neoplasm; breast. Family history of malignant neoplasm of breast is not the correct assignment.
12.2.2. V25.01, V11.0 Rationale: Code V25.01 describes counseling for oral contraceptives, and code V11.0 describes the personal history of schizophrenia.
12.3.1. 883.2, E919.2, E849.3 Rationale: Code 883.2 best describes the wound the patient suffered. Code E919.2 describes how it occurred (accidents caused by machinery; forklift), and code E849.3 describes the place of occurrence (plant, industrial).
12.3.2. E910.2 Rationale: Code E910.2 falls under the category "Accidents Caused by Submersion, Suffocation and Foreign Bodies," for accidental drowning while fishing.
12.4.1. 642.73, 584.9 Rationale: Code 642.73 describes the hypertension with preeclampsia. The fifth digit "3" is used to indicate antepartum condition or complication. Code 584.9 describes the acute renal failure. No fifth digit is required.
12.4.2. 141.3, 198.89 Rationale: Code 141.3 is primary code for malignant cancer of the tongue, no fifth digit required. The neoplasm table instructs the coder to code 198.89 for the secondary site, which is the roof of the mouth. Code 198.89 is assigned for "other specified sites; other."
12.5.1. 188.3, V10.04 Rationale: Code 188.3 describes the malignant neoplasm of the anterior portion of the urinary bladder (primary), and code V10.04 is assigned to describe the personal history of malignant neoplasm of the stomach.
12.5.2. 381.62, 382.9, 20.01, 69436 Rationale: Code 381.62 best describes the intrinsic cartilaginous obstruction of the eustachian tube, indexed under "obstruction" > "eustachian tube." Code 382.9 indicates the assignment of unspecified otitis media. In Volume III of the ICD-9-CM manual, procedure code 20.01 is used to describe the myringotomy and insertion of a tube in the left ear. Procedure code 69436 is assigned to describe the tympanostomy (incision of eardrum) unilateral. 12.6.1. 250.00, 288.00, 287.5 Rationale: Code 250.0 is assigned for diabetes mellitus type II, not stated as uncontrolled (fifth digit 0). Code 288.00 requires a fifth digit, and "0" is assigned to indicate unspecified. Code 287.5 is assigned for thrombocytopenia unspecified.
12.6.2. V56.0, 585.2 Rationale: Code V56.0 is assigned for an encounter for dialysis. Code 585.2 is assigned for chronic kidney disease, stage II.
12.7. 303.91, 291.3 Rationale: Code 303.91 best defines chronic alcoholism; the fifth digit (1) describes the continuous condition of the alcoholism. Code 291.3 best describes alcohol-induced hallucinations.

12.8.1. V07.0, 342.91, 907.2 Rationale: Code V07.0 is assigned to indicate need for isolation to protect the patient from his surroundings. Code 342.91 is assigned to indicate the hemiplegia on the patient's dominant side. Code 907.2 is assigned to indicate the late effects of spinal cord injury.
12.8.2. 211.3, 88305 Rationale: Code 211.3 is assigned to describe the benign colonic polyp. Code 88305 is assigned to describe the microscopic examination of the colonic polyp.
12.9.1. 491.21 Rationale: Code 491.21 completes the description of the diagnosis. The fifth digit (1) describes the "acute exacerbation."
12.9.2. 466.11, 472.1 Rationale: Code 466.19 best describes the acute bronchiolitis resulting from RSV. There is no need to assign 079.6 when assigning code 466.19. Code 472.1 best describes the chronic pharyngitis.
12.10.1. Stress Rationale: The symptom code for fatigue is designated the principal diagnosis, with the additional code for stress and hypothyroidism.
12.10.2. Encephalitis and encephalomyelitis Rationale: Two or more diagnoses equally meet the definition for the principal diagnosis.

Answers to Applying Coding to Theory Practice

1. B. 284.8 Rationale: Code 284.8 best describes this condition. V58.11 should not be assigned because the note below code V58.11 excludes chemotherapy for nonneoplastic conditions and says to code to condition.
2. A. V30.0, 99435 Rationale: V Code V30.0 describes the live-born infant that was born in a hospital. CPT code 99435 is assigned to indicate newborn care of the infant with a history and examination and that the newborn was assessed and discharged on the same date.
3. C. 007.1, 008.45 Rationale: Code 007.1 best describes *Giardia lamblia,* and code 008.45 best describes *Clostridium difficile.* Both codes must be assigned.
4. D. 282.62, 517.3, 518.81 Rationale: Code 282.62 best describes the sickle-cell disease with crisis. Code 517.3 best describes the acute chest syndrome and instructs the coder to code first the underlying sickle-cell disease. Code 518.81 indicates the acute respiratory failure that is not otherwise specified.
5. B. Secondary malignancy Rationale: The secondary malignancy of cancer of the prostate should be considered primary in this case because the patient was admitted for treatment of the secondary cancer.
6. A. 304.70, 307.43, 292.12 Rationale: Code 304.70 best describes the addiction of the opioid type drugs. The fifth digit "0" is assigned to describe unspecified to classification. Code 307.43 is assigned to describe the transient insomnia and the inability of the patient to maintain wakefulness. Code 292.12 best describes the drug-induced psychotic disorder accompanied by hallucinations.
7. B. 256.31, 627.2 Rationale: Code 256.31 best describes the patient's premature menopause due to the fact that the patient was under 40 years of age. The coder is instructed to use additional code for state associated with natural menopause. Code 627.2 best describes the symptomatic menopausal state.
8. E950.8 Rationale: This E code can be found in the Tabular List of Diseases under, "Suicide and Self-Inflicted Injury." Code E950.8 best describes self-inflicted arsenic poisoning.

9. V22.0, V27.4 Rationale: Code V22.0 is assigned to describe the supervision of a normal first pregnancy. Code V27.4, outcome of delivery, best describes twins who were stillborn.

10. C. 150.0, 230.0 Rationale: Code 150.0 best describes the primary cancer of the cervical esophagus. This code must be assigned first since it is the primary cancer. Code 230.0 is assigned to indicate the secondary cancer of carcinoma in situ of the epiglottis at the anterior aspect. Code 231.0 should not be assigned because it does not completely describe where the cancer in situ is located on the epiglottis.

11. B. 434.11, 428.0, V15.07 Rationale: Code 434.11 is assigned to describe the CVA with embolism. Code 428.0 is assigned to describe the CHF, unspecified. V code V15.07 was assigned to describe the personal history of latex allergy.

12. 250.51, 369.08 Rationale: Code 250.51 best describes type I diabetes mellitus with ophthalmic manifestations. Code 369.08 best describes the profound impairment of both eyes.

13. B. 042 Rationale: When a patient has been diagnosed with AIDS, the primary diagnosis is always 042. The coder is instructed to use additional codes to identify all manifestations of HIV/AIDS.

14. B. No set time

15. D. 569.85, 562.11 Rationale: Code 569.85 is assigned to describe angiodysplasia of the intestine with hemorrhage. Code 562.11 is assigned to describe the diverticulitis of the colon that does not include hemorrhage.

Chapter 13 ICD-9-CM Guidelines and Coding Conventions Review, Part II

Answers to Think Like A Coder

13.1.1. 532.01, E930.4 Rationale: Code 532.01 describes the acute duodenal ulcer with hemorrhage and obstruction. No other code should be used in conjunction with the diagnosis of the ulcer. Code, E930.4 describes the drugs causing adverse effects in therapeutic use for doxycycline.

13.1.2. 573.1, 075 Rationale: Code 573.1 best describes hepatitis in viral diseases. The coder is instructed to also code the underlying viral disease, which is mononucleosis, code 075.

13.2.1. 600.91, 788.64 Rationale: Code 600.91 best describes the hyperplasia of prostate with obstruction. The coder is directed to use additional code to identify further urinary symptoms such as "hesitancy," which is the 788.64 code assignment for symptoms, signs, and ill-defined conditions.

13.2.2. 616.10, 041.4, 611.2 Rationale: Code 616.10 best describes unspecified vaginitis and vulvovaginitis and directs the coder to use an additional code to specify the organism, which is *Escherichia coli* (E coli), code 041.4. Code 611.2 describes the fissure on the nipple of the left breast.

13.3.1. 634.32 Rationale: Code 634.32 best describes the spontaneous abortion complicated by renal failure. The fifth digit "2" describes the "complete" spontaneous abortion. Code 639.3 would not be assigned because (1) the complication itself did not require an episode of medical care and (2) the patient did not suffer from an ectopic or molar pregnancy.

13.3.2. 633.10, 639.0, 041.04 Rationale: Code 633.13 best describes the tubal pregnancy without intrauterine pregnancy. Code 639.0 is assigned to describe the complications of the ectopic pregnancy which is salpingitis. Code 041.04 is assigned to describe the infectious organism.

13.4.1. 682.2, 942.4, 041.10 Rationale: Code 682.2 best describes the cellulitis as the fourth digit specifies the site. Code 942.4 best describes the type of second-degree burn the patient suffered. The fourth digit describes the degree of burn, and the fifth digit describes the anatomical site of the burn. Code 041.10 is assigned to describe the infectious organism involved in the cellulitis.

13.4.2. 707.07, 707.03, 707.01 Rationale: Category 707.0 is assigned to decubitus ulcer, or "pressure ulcers." The fifth digits describe the anatomical sites.

13.5.1. False

13.5.2. 732.4, 733.16, 268.2 Rationale: Code 732.4 describes the juvenile osteochrondosis of the tibia. Code 733.16 describes the pathological fracture of the fibula due to osteomalacia, code 268.2. Fracture codes from category 823 would not be used since the fracture was not due to an injury rather a disease (pathological condition).

13.6.1. Code only a V Code (V10–V15) to indicate personal history of the individual

13.6.2. 741.01 Rationale: Code 741.01 best describes the spina bifida with hydrocephalus (Arnold-Chiari syndrome type II). There is no need to also assign code 742.3.

13.7.1. Time of birth up to 28 days after the birth Rationale: This information can be found in the Official ICD-9-CM Coding Guidelines.

13.7.2. V30.00, 771.81, 041.5 Rationale: Code V30.00 describes the live-born birth in the hospital with no mention of cesarean section. Code 771.81 describes the septicemia of newborn, and code 041.5 describes the infectious organism hemophilus influenzae. Code V30.00 is used only for the newborn's chart. Code V27 is used only for the mother's chart.

13.8. 795.02, 795.6 Rationale: Code 795.02 describes the abnormal Pap smear, and code 795.6 describes the false-positive serological test for syphilis.

13.9.1. Degree and site

13.9.2. 960.0, 787.03, E856 Rationale: The poisoning code 960.0 is listed first, and code 787.03 describes the symptom of severe vomiting followed by the E code to describe the accidental overdose.

13.10. Diagnosis and procedure code are incorrect Rationale: The correct procedure codes are 17000, 17003. The coder must assign 17000 for the first lesion and 17003 for the second through 14 lesion. The correct diagnosis code is 702.0 to indicate "other dermatoses," > actinic keratosis.

Answers to Applying Coding Theory to Practice

1. B. 820.31, 920, E881.0, E849.3 Rationale: Code 8201.31 describes the open intertrochanteric fracture of the femur. Code 920 best describes the contusions on the face and scalp. E codes need to be assigned to explain the injuries. Code E881.0 is assigned to describe the fall from a ladder, and code E849.3 describes the place of occurrence, which is an industrial place, "building under construction."

2. D. 005.1 Rationale: Code 005.1 is assigned to describe the food poisoning due to botulism. There is no need to code the symptom of nausea.

3. B. 205.00 Rationale: Code 205.00 is assigned to describe the acute promyelocytic leukemia. The fifth digit "0" is used to describe unspecified site.

4. B. Type I Rationale: Official ICD-9-CM Coding Guidelines indicate that type I is always insulin dependent.

5. C. 280.0, 531.40 Rationale: Code 280.0 describes the chronic blood loss which is secondary to the chronic ulcer. Code 531.40 describes the chronic gastric ulcer and the fifth digit "0" is assigned to indicate without mention of obstruction.

6. B. 303.1, 291.1, 291.0 Rationale: Code 303 indicates alcohol dependence, and the fourth digit "1" describes the continuous classification. Code 291.1 is used to describe Korsakoff's psychosis, and code 291.0 is used to indicate delirium tremens associated with Korsakoff's syndrome. Code 291.3 should not be assigned as code 291.0 excludes this code.

7. B. 337.22 Rationale: Code 337.22 best describes the reflex sympathetic dystrophy of the lower limb. Code 338.21 is excluded for code 337.22 and should not be assigned.

8. C. V17.3, 410.90, 427.60 Rationale: Code V17.3 is assigned to describe the family history of ischemic heart disease. Code 410.90 describes the AMI; the fifth digit "0" is assigned for episode of care unspecified. Code 427.60 is assigned to describe the extrasystolic arrhythmia.

9. A. 477.2, 474.02 Rationale: Code 477.2 was assigned to describe allergic rhinitis due to animal dander. Code 474.02 describes the chronic tonsillitis and adenoiditis.

10. C. 524.62, 520.5 Rationale: Code 524.62 best describes the arthralgia of the temporomandibular joint, and code 520.5 describes the odontogenesis.

11. C. 584.6, V10.51, 189.0 Rationale: Code 584.6 indicates acute renal failure, with the fourth digit describing the site of the lesion. Code V10.51 indicates the personal history of malignant neoplasm of the bladder. Code 189.0 indicates primary malignant neoplasm of the kidney parenchyma.

12. D. Antepartum Rationale: Perperium is the time period before and after childbirth.

13. c. 644.21, 656.41, 651.01, V27.4 Rationale: Code 644.21 indicates the premature birth, and the fifth digit describes "without mention of antepartum condition." Code 656.41 indicates an intrauterine death took place, with the fifth digit meaning "without mention of antepartum condition." Code 651.01 indicates twin pregnancy, with the fifth digit meaning "without mention of antepartum condition." Code V27.4 indicates the outcome of delivery of twins, both stillborn.

14. B. 706.1, 680.0 Rationale: Code 706.1 is indicated for "other acne" > "acne vulgaris." Code 680.0 indicates carbuncle on the face, any part except the eye.

15. D. 252.00, 713.0, 737.11, V10.81 Rationale: Code 252.00 best describes the hyperparathyroidism unspecified. Code 713.0 indicates the arthropathy that directs the coder to "code first underlying disease," which is code 252.00. Code 737.11 is indicated for kyphosis due to radiation. V10.81 is assigned to indicate the personal history of the bone cancer (malignant neoplasm of the bone).

16. B. 963.0, E858.1 Rationale: Code 963.0 is assigned to indicate poisoning by anti-allergic drug (antihistamine). E code E858.1 is assigned to indicate accidental poisoning by primarily systemic agents.

17. A. V30.00, 747.63, 744.01, 389.01 Rationale: Code V30.00 indicates live-born birth in hospital (fourth digit "0") with mention of cesarean section (fifth digit "0"). Code 747.63 is assigned to indicate the congenital anomaly of upper limb vessel. Code 744.01 is assigned to indicate the congenital anomaly of the absence of the external ear canal. Code 389.01 is assigned to indicate the type of conductive hearing loss the infant had.

18. B. A. E958.0 B. E916 Rationale: Code E958.0 can be found in the E code index under, "Suicide and self-inflicted injuries by other and unspecified means." Coe E916 can be found in the E code index under "Other Accidents" > "Struck accidentally by falling object."

19. C. V code Rationale: A V code would be assigned to record the admission to the hospital for renal dialysis. The code can be indexed under "Admission for" > "dialysis" > "renal."

20. B. 451.0 Rationale: Code 451.0 can be indexed under "phlebitis," > "leg." Code 451.0 best describes the superficial phlebitis.

21. B. 174.8 and 88307 were assigned incorrectly. Rationale: The correct coding assignment should be 174.3, malignant (primary) neoplasm of the lower-inner quadrant of the breast. Code 19306 is assigned to describe the procedure for Urban type radical mastectomy, unilateral. Code 88309 is assigned as a Level VI gross and microscopic examination of the specimen from the breast.

22. B. 525 Rationale: The three-digit code for "Other diseases and conditions of the teeth and supporting structures" is 525.

23. A. 438.84 Rationale: The late effect for the CVA is ataxia, assigned to code 438.84.

24. C. ICD-9 and CPT codes are incorrect Rationale: Code V16.3 is a family history of breast cancer and not a personal history of breast cancer (V10.3). Carcinoma insitu of the uterus, unspecified is code 233.2 and not code 233.1. Code 99361 has been deleted. Time spent with the medical team conference was 65 minutes; code 99367 should be assigned.

25. B. CPT code is incorrect Rationale: All ICD-9 codes are correct. Code 51701 indicates the insertion of nonindwelling bladder catheter, which is incorrect. Code 51702 is the correct CPT code and indicates a temporary, indwelling catheter such as a "Foley." CPT code 99507 indicates a home visit for care and maintenance of a catheter. CPT code 97116 × 8 indicates therapeutic procedure, one of more areas, each 15 minutes.

Chapter 14 Practice Examination

Answers to Medical Terminology

1. B. Internal
2. C. myring/o
3. A. spondyl/o
4. B. Abduction
5. C. Pruritis
6. A. Myocardial infarction
7. D. Gland
8. B. Perineum
9. B. Fixation
10. D. Parenteral

Answers to Anatomy and Physiology

11. B. Psoriasis
12. A. Radius
13. B. Sartorius
14. C. Peripheral
15. D. Vertigo
16. C. Cushing's syndrome
17. A. Liver

18. C. Epicardium
19. D. Lymphocytes
20. B. Alveoli

Answers to Health Information Management

21. A. The patient suffered lower right quadrant stomach pain
22. B. UHDDS (Uniform Hospital Discharge Data Set)
23. D. Accession register Rationale: The accession register is a permanent database of all cases entered into the database.
24. B. Create protocol that includes different levels of security for different types of information Rationale: Computer-based systems are better controlled if different levels of security are defined.
25. D. They are part of published criteria for the medical facility—Rationale: All abbreviations must first be approved by medical staff and then published in a proper manner.
26. B. Abuse of a child or the elderly
27. C. Service, geographical location, and conversion factor
28. B. One who has not visited the physician in more than 3 years
29. A. If the covered entity has obtained authorization from the individual
30. B. Follow up of patient care plans

Answers to Reimbursement

31. B. 25 32. b. Centers for Medicaid and Medicare Service (CMS); improper coding
33. D. Medicare Physician Fee Schedule (MPFS)
34. A. The Security Rule
35. D. Explanation of Benefits
36. C. $5,312.50 Rationale: LOS + 1 at transferring hospital, multiplied by the PPS amount, divided by geometric mean length of stay.

$$\frac{(3+1) \times 8500}{6.4} = \$5,312$$

37. A. $950 Rationale: The physician receives 80% of the MPFS amount ($760) and 20% ($190) is paid to the physician by the patient. Total amount equals $950.
38. D. Contractual allowance
39. B. Status indicator
40. C. UB-04 code

Answers to Data Quality

41. D. Antepartum record
42. D. The code assigned should be 49565 Rationale: Code 49565 is the best code to describe the repair of the incision hernia without mention of incarcerated or strangulated.
43. C. The correct ICD-9 code is 079.52 Rationale: Code 079.52 best describes the human T-cell lymphotrophic virus type II found under category 079.5 "Retrovirus."
44. C. Development and growth records
45. B. Intermediate proton treatment delivery was administered by means of two ports with one block. This would be found in the CPT manual under "Radiology" > "Proton Beam Treatment Delivery."
46. C. Source oriented
47. D. Albumin Rationale: Code 80048, basic metabolic panel, does not include albumin.
48. A. 00921 Rationale: Code 00921 best describes the anesthesiologists code. Modifier -50 would not be used because code 00921 includes unilateral and bilateral vasectomy.

Code 00920 is not necessary to assign in conjunction with code 00921.
49. C. There is no need for code 99212, and code 30310 should be 30300 Rationale: There is no need for code 99212 because the patient was in the office only 2 weeks ago. The only procedure is the removal of the foreign body in the nose code 30300. Code 932 is the correct diagnosis code for a foreign body in the nose and not unspecified site.
50. A Ensure proper coding and billing of health care service

Answers to ICD-9-CM

51. B. 331.0, 294.11, 881.00, 86.59 Rationale: Code 331.0 is assigned to describe the Alzheimer's disease. Code 294.11 is assigned to describe the dementia with behavior disturbance (becoming lost). Code 881.00 is used to describe the laceration he received on the forearm without mention of complication. Code 86.59 is used to describe the suturing of the forearm.
52. D. 749.22, 27.62, 27.54 Rationale: Code 749.22 is assigned to describe the unilateral cleft palate with cleft lip. Procedure codes 27.62 (cleft palate) and 27.54 (cleft lip) are assigned to describe the repair of the cleft palate and cleft lip.
53. C. 202.01, 60100 Rationale: Code 202.01 is assigned to describe the malignant neoplasm; nodular lymphoma. The fifth-digit describes the site of the neoplasm, which was in the neck. Code 60100 is assigned to describe the thyroid biopsy performed by a percutaneous core needle, not fine needle aspiration.
54. C. 250.62 Rationale: The fifth digit subclassifications instruct the coder to use the fifth digit "2" for type II diabetes stated as uncontrolled.
55. B. Volume III
56. B. 410.22 Rationale: Code 410.22 best describes the acute myocardial infarction of the inferolateral wall. The fifth-digit "2" is assigned to describe the subsequent episode of care following the initial episode that is still less than 8 weeks old.
57. D. 183.0, 197.6, 68.6, 65.61, 54.4 Rationale: Code 183.0 is assigned to describe the carcinoma of the ovary (primary). Code 197.6 is assigned to describe the carcinoma of the omentum (secondary). Procedure code 68.6 is assigned to describe the radical abdominal hysterectomy and the coder is instructed to code also any synchronous which is the bilateral salpingo ooperectomy, code 65.61. Code 54.4 is necessary to assign to indicate the excision of the omentum.
58. B. 807.04, 042, 176.0, 93.56 Rationale: Code 807.04 was assigned to describe the closed fracture of 4 ribs. The fifth digit indicates how many ribs were fractured. Code 042 indicates that the patient has AIDS. Code 176.0 is assigned to indicate the Kaposi's sarcoma of the skin. Procedure code 93.56 is assigned for the application of a pressure bandage for the fractured ribs.
59. B. 403.00, 250.40, 585.3 Rationale: Code 403.00 is assign to describe the hypertensive chronic kidney disease; the fifth digit "0" indicates stages I-IV. Code 250.40 is assigned to indicate diabetes with renal manifestations; the fifth digit indicates type II diabetes not stated as uncontrolled. Code 250.4 instructs the coder to use additional code to identify the manifestation which is code 585.3. Code 585.3 is assigned to indicate chronic kidney disease, stage III moderate.
60. C. 344.1, 907.2, 318.0, 758.2 Rationale: Code 344.1 is assigned to describe the paraplegia. Code 907.2 is assigned to

describe the late effect of the spinal cord injury. Code 318.0 is assigned to describe the moderate mental retardation and code 758.2 is indicated for the Edward's syndrome or trisomy 18.

Answers to HCPCS Coding

61. C. A4736 Rationale: Code A4736 is assigned to describe the topical anesthetic for dialysis, not injectable.
62. C. A4209 Rationale: Code A4209 best describes the type of sterile syringe needle used, 5 cc.
63. C. Level I
64. A. AU
65. C. Q4010 GC Rationale: Code Q4010 best describes the application for an individual over 11 years of age for a short arm, fiberglass cast. Modifier GC is assigned to indicate that a resident, under the supervision of a physician, took part in the procedure.
66. B. E0185 Rationale: Code E0185 best describes the durable equipment.
67. C. E1391 AR Rationale: Code E1391 best describes the oxygen equipments. Modifier AR is assigned to describe the physician scarcity in the patient's demographic area.
68. A. GO117 Rationale: Code G0117 best describes the glaucoma screening for the high-risk patient by an optometrist.
69. C. G8041 Rationale: Code G8041 best describes the documentation that the patient is not a candidate for low-density lipoprotein measure.
70. C. L0140 Rationale: Code L0140 best describes the adjustable semirigid plastic cervical collar.

Answers to Evaluation and Management Coding

71. B. History, examination and medical decision making Rationale: This information can be found in the Evaluation and Management Services Guidelines in the CPT-4 manual.
72. B. A limited examination of the affected body area or organ system and other symptomatic or related organ system(s). Rationale: This information can be found in the Evaluation and Management Services Guidelines in the CPT-4 manual.
73. D. 99215 Rationale: The patient was established and the service rendered was in the physician's office. E&M code 99215 would be assigned to indicate that two of the three key components in this service were met. The history and examination were comprehensive; however, the medical decision making was of moderate complexity, as indicated by the data provided.
74. C. Physician #1 -99220, Physician #2 -99236 Rationale: Code 99219 would be assigned for Physician #1 for initial observation of the patient and the severity of the patient's condition. Because Physician #1 was no longer evaluating the patient, Physician #2 was allowed the assignment of code 99236. Code 99236 is assigned for observation or inpatient care services (including admission and discharge service) with presenting problems of high severity. Code 99217 for Physician #2 should not be assigned because the patient was not discharged from observation until the next day.
75. C. Social history Rationale: This information can be found in the Evaluation and Management Services Guidelines in the CPT-4 manual.
76. D. 99291 × 1, 99292 × 4 Rationale: The patient was provided critical care by the physician (codes 99291 and 99292) for over three hours. To document the service and time spent with the patient for critical care services is to assign code 99291 once and code 99292 four times to allow a time span of 3 hours.

77. B. 99283 Rationale: Code 99283 (emergency department services) is assigned to indicate the presenting problem was of moderate severity. An expanded problem focused history and examination were present.
78. B. 99203, 99354 Rationale: Code 99203 is assigned because of the requirements that include three key components. Even though the exam and medical decision making was more comprehensive than described in code 99203, the history was not, and all three key components must be met. Code 99354 is assigned to describe the prolonged physician service that last for 1 hour face to face. A modifier would not be assigned in conjunction with code 99354.
79. 99213, 99212–25 Rationale: Code 99213 should be assigned to describe the established patient office visit and the time spent with the patient. Code 99212 should be assigned to indicate the second E&M service on the same day, same physician, different encounter. Modifier -25 should be assigned to describe the significant, separately identifiable E&M service by the same physician on the same day of the procedure or other service.
80. B. 99232 Rationale: Category is "subsequent hospital care," and code 99232 is indicated because of the expanded problem-focused history and examination. The medical decision making was of moderate complexity.

Answers to Anesthesia

81. D. A patient with severe systemic disease Rationale: This information can be found in the Anesthesia Guidelines in the CPT-4 manual.
82. B. 01442, P3, 99100 Rationale: Code 01442 is indicated for the procedure of a popliteal thromboendarterectomy. Physical status modifier P3 indicates the patient's severe systemic disease, and code 99100 indicates the extreme age of the patient (more than 70 years of age).
83. A. 745.4, 00563, P5, 99100 Rationale: Code 745.4 best describes the interventricular septal defect. Code 00563 is assigned to describe the anesthesia services. The physical status modifier P5 describes the moribund patient who is not expected to live without the surgery. Code 99100 is assigned to describe the extreme age of the infant (less than 1 year of age). The coder cannot report anesthesia code 00561 in conjunction with code 99100.
84. D. 187.7, 11623, 00920 Rationale: Code 187.7 is assigned to describe the primary cancer of the skin of the scrotum. Code 11623 is assigned to describe the excision of a malignant lesion on the genitalia. Code 00920 is the code for the anesthesia, "Anesthesia for procedures on male genitalia, not otherwise specified."
85. A. When the anesthesiologist is no longer in attendance Rationale: Please see Anesthesia Guidelines in the CPT manual.
86. B. 00670 Rationale: Code 00670 is assigned to describe the extensive spine and spinal cord procedures involving rods and hooks.
87. C. 00902 Rationale: Code 00902 was assigned to describe the anesthesia for a sigmoidoscopy (anorectal procedure). The anesthesia code is required for conscious sedation. Code 99148 is not assigned.
88. A. 47120 -47 Rationale: Code 47120 is assigned to describe the partial excision of the liver along with modifier -47 to indicate that the same physician that performed the surgery also performed the administration of the anesthesia. The use modifier -47 in conjunction with anesthesia procedures is not indicated.

89. B. 01990 -P6 Rationale: Code 01990 is indicated for the physiological support for the harvesting of organ(s) from a brain-dead patient along with physical status modifier P6 to indicate the same.

90. C. 01952, 01953 × 2 Rationale: Code 01952 is assigned to indicate the first 9% of TBSA for debridement, and code 01953 is assigned to indicate each additional 9% of the total body surface area the second and thereof 9% of TBSA.

Answers to Surgery

91. B. 46250 Rationale: Code 46250 is assigned to indicate a hemorrhoidectomy, external, simple. The cauterization should not be coded.

92. B. Unbundling Rationale: Please refer to the CPT manual for Surgery Standards and Guidelines.

93. C. When a more specific code is not available Rationale: Please refer to the CPT manual for Surgery Standards and Guidelines.

94. A. 93528, 92980 -51 Rationale: Code 93528 is assigned to indicate the combined right heart catheterization with left ventricular puncture. Code 92980 is assigned to indicate the placement of a coronary stent. Modifier -51 should be assigned to indicate multiple procedures were performed. Code 37205 is for the placement of an intravascular stent that excludes coronary and therefore should not be assigned.

95. C. 30410, 13151 -81 Rationale: Code 30410 best describes the procedure of a complete primary rhinoplasty including bony pyramid, lateral, and alar cartilages and the elevation of the nasal tip. Code 13151 is assigned to indicate the 2.0-cm columellar reconstruction. Modifier -81 is assigned to indicate the presence of a minimum assistant surgeon during the procedure.

96. B. 22630, 22632, 22842 Rationale: Code 22630 is assigned to indicate the laminectomy at the lumbar spaces without decompression. In the index under "laminectomy," the coder should refer to "lumbar" to find the correct code (22632). Code 22632 should also be assigned to indicate each additional interspace. If three vertebrae were involved, then only 2 interspaces would be coded. Code 22842 is assigned to indicate the pedicle fixation.

97. D. 15240, 15004 -51 Rationale: Code 15240 is assigned to indicate the full-thickness graft, free, including direct closure of donor site, neck under 20 sq cm. Code 15004 is assigned to indicate the surgical preparation of the recipient site for the neck, less than 100 sq cm. Modifier -51 is used to indicate multiple procedures during the same operative session. No assistant surgeon or surgical team is indicated in the problem or in the coding descriptors.

98. D. 49496 -53 Rationale: Code 49496 is assigned to indicate the repair of an incarcerated initial inguinal hernia of an infant less than six months of age. Modifier -53 is indicated for the discontinuance of the procedure because of difficulties. Modifier -63 cannot be used in conjunction with code 49496, as indicated by the note directly below code 49496.

99. A. 67316, 67320 Rationale: Code 67316 is assigned to indicate the strabismus surgery on two or more vertical muscles. Code 67320 should be used in conjunction with code 67316 and is assigned to indicate the transposition procedure.

100. D. 366.43, 359.2, 66984 Rationale: Code 366.43 is assigned to describe the myotonic cataract; the code instructs the coder to code first underlying disease, 359.2, which indicates Steinert's disease. Code 66984 is assigned to describe the cataract removal and insertion of intraocular lens prosthesis by manual technique.

Answers to Radiology

101. B. -26 Rationale: Description of modifier -26 can be found in the Appendix A "Modifiers" in the CPT manual.

102. C. 71020 Rationale: Code 71020 is assigned to describe the radiological examination of the chest, two views, frontal and lateral.

103. B. 70488, 76376 Rationale: Code 70488 is assigned to indicate the CT scan of the maxillofacial area without contrast material followed by contrast material and further sections. Code 76376 is assigned for the 3-D rendering of the CT scan not requiring an independent workstation.

104. B. 72141, 72146, 72148 Rationale: Code 72141 is assigned to indicate the MRI without contrast material for the cervical spine. Code 72146 is assigned to indicate the MRI without contrast material for the thoracic spine. Code 72148 is assigned to indicate the MRI without contrast material for the lumbar spine.

105. C. 76801 -26 Rationale: Code 76801 is assigned to indicate the ultrasound of a pregnant uterus, no more than 14 weeks gestation, transabdominal approach, single gestation. Modifier -26 is assigned to indicate the physician component only.

106. B. 78135, 78191 Rationale: Code 78135 is assigned to describe the red cell survival study with hepatic sequestration. Code 78191 is assigned to describe the platelet survival study.

107. D. M-mode scan Rationale: This information can be found in the Radiology section under subsection "Diagnostic Ultrasound" notes. Under the note, please see the highlighted word "definitions" in which you will find the definition of "mode scans"

108. A. 77262 Rationale: Code 77262 is assigned to describe the clinical treatment plan for therapeutic radiology treatment planning. This series of codes can be found in the Radiology section under "Clinical Treatment Planning."

109. C. 78815 Rationale: Code 78815 is assigned to describe the tumor imaging by PET with concurrently acquired CT scan for attenuation correction and anatomical localization for skull base to midthigh. No other coded would be used in conjunction with this code.

110. B. 73110 Rationale: Code 73110 is assigned to describe the radiological examination of the wrist, minimum of three views.

Answers to Pathophysiology and Laboratory

111. B. -91 Rationale: The description of modifier -91 can be found in Appendix A of the CPT manual.

112. D. 88307 Rationale: Code 88307 is assigned to describe the TUR of the bladder and the gross and microscopic examination. No other surgical pathology code should be assigned.

113. C. 36415, 80173, 80184 Rationale: Code 36415 is assigned to describe the routine venipuncture that was performed. Codes 80173 (haloperidol) and 80184 (phenobarbital) are assigned to describe the quantitative therapeutic drug assays.

114. B. 89230 Rationale: Code 89230 can be found in the index under "sweat collection."

115. B. 82803 Rationale: Code 82803 is assigned to describe the blood gases with any combination of the elements listed in the problem. Two or more must be listed to use code 82803.

116. C. 540.9, 88304 Rationale: Code 540.9 is assigned to describe the acute appendicitis, and code 88304 is assigned to describe the gross examination of the appendix other than incidental.

117. B. Histology
118. A. 83919 × 2 -91 Rationale: Code 81919 should be assigned twice to indicate the qualitative analysis of organic acids. Modifier -91 should be assigned to indicate a repeat clinical diagnostic test took place on the same day to obtain multiple results.
119. 81007 Urinalysis for the screening of bacteria in the urine.
120. D. 88331, 88332 × 2 Rationale: Code 88331 is assigned to indicate the pathology consultation during surgery for the first frozen block with frozen section; code 88332 is indicated twice to describe each additional frozen block with frozen sections.

Answers to Medicine

121. D. Neurologist
122. B. 95950 × 2 Rationale: Code 95950 is assigned to describe the eight-channel EEG recoding and interpretation for 24 hours each. Code 95950 would be assigned twice to indicate 48 hours of recording and monitoring.
123. C. 96413, 96415 × 2 Rationale: Code 96413 is used to describe the first hour of chemotherapy administration by intravenous infusion. Code 96415 is assigned twice to indicate each additional hour of chemotherapy infusion.
124. A. 99505 Code 99505 should be assigned to indicate a home visit for stoma care and maintenance for colostomy.
125. C. 99143, 99145 Rationale: Code 99143 is assigned to describe the moderate sedation services rendered by the physician and trained observer for a child younger than 5 years of age. Code 99145 is assigned to indicate each additional 15 minutes of intraservice time in addition to the first 30 minutes allocated in code 99143.
126. A. 90821 Rationale: Code 90821 is assigned to describe the individual psychotherapy, insight oriented and behavior modifying for 80 minutes face-to-face.
127. D. Motion Analysis
128. B. 94350 Rationale: Code 94350 is assigned to describe the determination of maldistribution of inspired gas. Code 94350 can be found under "Pulmonology" > "Maldistribution of inspired gas."
129. C. 92285 Rationale: Code 92285 is assigned to describe the slit-lamp photography with interpretation and report.
130. C. 90760, 90761 × 4 Rationale: Code 90760 is assigned to describe the intravenous infusion for the first hour, and code 90761 × 4 is assigned to describe the additional 4 hours of infusion.

Answers to Miscellaneous

131. C. Internal respiration
132. C. Cortisol
133. B. 413.9, 401.1, V10.46, 99202 -21 Rationale: Code 413.9 is assigned to describe the angina pectoris. Code 401.1 is assigned to describe the essential hyptertension that is benign. V10.46 is assigned to acknowledge the personal history of malignant neoplasm of the prostate. E&M code 99202 is assigned to describe the level of E&M service provided to the patient. Modifier -21 is assigned to describe the prolonged evaluation and management service.
134. B. 831.10, 921.2, 925.2, E826.1 Rationale: Code 831.10 is assigned to describe the open dislocation of the shoulder; the fifth digit describes shoulder unspecified. Code 921.2 is assigned to describe the contusion of the orbital tissue,

and code 925.2 is assigned to describe the crushing of the larynx. E code E826.1 is assigned to describe how the injuries occurred. Code E826.1 includes accidents involving other road vehicles being used in recreational activities.
135. D. 90923 × 21 Rationale: Code 90923 is assigned 21 times to describe the dialysis' services rendered for the 10-year-old patient for a total of 21 days.
136. A. 80051, 80053, 81001 Rationale: Code 80051 is assigned to describe the electrolyte panel, code 80053 is assigned to describe the metabolic panel, and code 80051 is assigned to describe the automated urinalysis with microscopy.
137. C. Risk management process
138. C. To document the diagnosis and treatment of the patient
139. B. 43249 Rationale: Code 43249 is assigned to describe the upper gastrointestinal endoscopy that included the esophagus to the duodenum and the balloon dilation of the esophagus of less than 30 mm. Code 43456 should not be coded because the balloon dilation is included in code 43249.
140. B. 2
141. B. No E&M code would be assigned Rationale: No documentation supports the use of an E&M code.
142. C. 13152, 12042, 12034, 12013 -51 Rationale: Code the most complex repair first. Code 13152 is assigned to describe the complex repair of the lip, 3.7 cm. Code 12042 is for the intermediate repair of the left foot, 4.2 cm. Code 12034 is assigned for the intermediate repair of the 7-cm scalp wound and 5-cm leg wound (add together), for a total of 12 cm. Code 12031 is assigned to describe the simple repair of the 1-cm nose and 2.5-cm ear wounds(add together), for a total of 3.5 cm. Modifier -51 is assigned to indicate that multiple procedures were performed. See notes under "Repair" (Closure) in subsection Integumentary of the Surgery section in the CPT manual.
143. A. Nature of presenting problem Rationale: This information can be found in the Evaluation and Management Guidelines in the CPT manual.
144. D. 428.21, 428.0, 33206 -78 Rationale: Code 428.21 is assigned to describe the acute systolic heart failure. Code 428.0 is assigned to describe the CHF unspecified. Code 33206 is assigned to describe the insertion of the pacemaker with transvenous electrodes.
145. B. 01958, P3 Rationale: Code 01958 is assigned to describe the anesthesia for the "cephalic version." This can be indexed under "Anesthesia," > "Childbirth" > "external cephalic version" Physical status modifier P3 describes the severe systemic disease.
146. A. 31625, 31623 -51 Rationale: Code 31625 is used to describe the bronchoscopy with or without fluoroscopic guidance with multiple biopsies. Code 31623 should also be assigned to indicate that brushings and washing (protected brushings) were also performed. Modifier -51 should be assigned to indicate multiple procedures were performed.
147. C. 44136 Rationale: Code 44136 can be found in the Index under "Allotransplantation," > "intestines".
148. C. Table of Drugs and Chemicals
149. C. American Medical Association
150. D. V60.0 Rationale: Code V60.0 can be found under "Persons Encountering Health Services in Other Circumstances" in the V code section of the ICD-9-CM manual.

THE FOLLOWING ARE COMMON ABBREVIATIONS TYPICALLY USED IN MEDICAL CODING:

Abbreviation	Term
AAA	abdominal aortic aneurysm
AAT	activity as tolerated
ABD	abdomen
ABX	antibiotics
a.c.	before food
ACE	angiotensin-converting enzyme
ACI	autologous chondrocyte implantation
ACTH	adrenocorticotropic hormone
AFB	acid-fast bacilli
AHG	antihemophilic globulin
ALA	aminolevulinic acid
ALT	alanine transferase
AMP	adenosine monophosphate
ANA	antinuclear antibodies
AP	abdominal voiding pressure
ARB	angiotensin receptor blocker
ART	automated regain test
AV	arteriovenous
BAL	blood alcohol level
BCG	bacilli Calmette-Guerin
BMT	bone marrow transplant
BUN	blood urea nitrogen
BV	bacterial vaginosis
Bx	biopsy
CABG	coronary artery bypass graft
CAD	coronary artery disease
CA	carcinoma
Ca	calcium
CAP	community-acquired bacterial pneumonia
CAT	computed axial tomography
CBC	complete blood count
CCF	congestive cardiac failure
CCU	critical care unit
CEA	carcinoembryonic antigen
CF	cystic fibrosis
CK	creatine kinase
CKD	chronic kidney disease
CMG	cystometrogram
CMRI	cardiac magnetic resonance imaging
CMV	cytomegalovirus
CNPB	continuous negative pressure breathing
CNS	central nervous system
COPD	chronic obstructive pulmonary disease
CP	cerebral palsy
CPAP	continuous positive airway pressure
CPK	creatine phosphokinase
CPR	cardiopulmonary resuscitation
CRF	corticotropic-releasing factor
CRH	corticotropic-releasing hormone
CS	cesarean section
CSF	cerebrospinal fluid
CT	computed tomography
CVA	cerebrovascular accident
CVC	central venous catheter
CVD	chorionic villus sampling
CVID	common variable immunodeficiency
DA	dopamine
DBP	diastolic blood pressure
D&C	dilation and curettage
DCM	dilated cardiomyopathy
DDD	daily defined doses
D&E	dilation and evacuation
DHEA	dehydroepiandrosterone
DHT	dihydrotestosterone
DIC	disseminated intravascular coagulation
DJD	degenerative joint disease
DM	diabetes mellitus
DNA	deoxyribonucleic acid
DNI	do not intubate
DNR	do not resuscitate
DOA	dead on arrival
DRIL	distal revascularization and interval
DT	diphtheria and tetanus toxoid
DTaP	diphtheria, tetanus toxoid, and acellular pertussis
DTaP-Hib	diphtheria, tetanus toxoid, and acellullar pertussis plus hemophilus influenza b
DTP	diphtheria, tetanus toxoid, and pertussis
DVT	deep vein thrombosis
Cx	diagnosis
EMB	evidenced-based medicine
ECG	electrocardiogram
ECMO	extracorporeal membrane oxygenation
ED	emergency department/erectile dysfunction

EDC	estimated date of confinement	GMP	guanosine monophosphate
EDD	estimated date of delivery	GU	genitourinary
EEG	electroencephalography	GvHD	graft-versus-host disease
EGF	epidermal growth factor	HAA	hepatitis-associated antigen
EKG	electrocardiogram	HAAb	hepatitis A antibody
ELISA	enzyme-linked immunosorbent assay	HAD	HIV-associated dementia
EMG	electromyography	HAI	hemagglutination inhibition
ENT	ear, nose, throat	HAST	high altitude simulation test
ePTFE	expanded polyetra fluoroethylene	HAV	hepatitis A virus
ERCP	endoscopic retrograde cholangiopancreatography	Hb	hemoglobin
		HBcAb	hepatitis B core antibody
ESL	extracorporeal shockwave lithotripsy	HBcAg	hepatitis B core antigen
ESRD	end-stage renal disease	HBeAb	hepatitis Be antibody
ESBL	extended spectrum beta-lactamase	HBeAg	hepatitis Be antigen
ESR	erythrocyte sedimentation rate	HBsAb	hepatitis B surface antibody
ETOH	ethanol/ethanol alcohol	HBsAg	hepatitis B surface antigen
FBC	full blood count	HDL	high-density lipoprotein
FBE	full blood exam	HEENT	head, eyes, ears, nose and throat
FBG	fasting blood sugar	HF	heart failure
F/C	fever, chills	Hgb	hemoglobin
FDP	fibrin degradation products	hGH	human growth hormone
Fe	iron	HIAA	hydroxyindoleacetic acid
FEV	forced expiratory value	Hib	hemophilus influenza b
FFA	free fatty acids	HIV	human immunodeficiency virus
FFP	fresh frozen plasma	HLA	human leukocyte antigen
FHR	fetal heart rate	H&P	history and physical
FHT	fetal heart tones	HP	hapatoglobin
FHx	family history	HPI	history of present illness
FISH	fluorescent in situ hybridization	hPL	human placental lactogen
FPG	fasting plasma glucose	H.S.	at bedtime
FSE	fetal scalp electrode	HTN	hypertension
FSF	fibrin stabilizing factor	HTLV	human T-lymphocyte virus
FSH	follicle-stimulating hormone	HVA	homovanillic acid
FT-4	free thyroxine	Hx	history of
FVC	forced vital capacity	IBD	inflammatory bowel disease
FWB	full weight bearing	IBS	irritable bowel syndrome
Fx	fracture	ICD	implantable cardioverter-defibrillator
G-CSF	granulocyte colony stimulating factors	ICF	intermediate care facilities
G	gravida	ICP	intracranial pressure
GA	general anesthesia	ICU	intensive care unit
GABA	gamma-aminobutyric acid	I&D	incision and drainage
GCA	giant cell arteritis	IDC	indwelling catheter
GERD	gastroesophageal reflux disease	IDDM	insulin-dependent diabetes mellitus
GFR	glomerular filtration rate	IDH	isocitric dehydrogenase
GH	growth hormone	IDL	intermediate-density lipoprotein
GIFT	gamete intrafallopian transfer	Ig	immunoglobulin
GORD	gastroesophageal reflux disease	I&O	inputs and outputs
GM-CSF	granulocyte macrophage colony stimulating factors	IOL	intraocular lens
		IPPB	intermittent positive pressure breathing

IPPV	intermittent positive pressure ventilation		MSH	melanocyte-stimulating hormone
IPV	inactive polio virus		MSLT	multiple sleep latency testing
ISH	in situ hybridization		MSU	midstream urine sample
i.s.q.	no change		MTMS	medication therapy management services
IUD	intrauterine device		MTX	methotrexate
IV	intravenous		MUGA	multiple-gated acquisition
IVC	intravenous cholangiography/inferior vena cava		MVPS	mitral valve prolapse syndrome
IVF	in vitro fertilization		NAD	no apparent distress
IVP	intravenous pyelogram		NCV	nerve conduction volume
IVU	intravenous urogram		NE	norepinephrine
JVD	jugular vein distention		NGU	nongonococcal urethritis
KOH	potassium hydroxide		NHL	non-Hodgkin lymphoma
KUB	kidney, ureter, bladder		NIDDM	non–insulin-dependent diabetes mellitus
LATS	long-acting thyroid-stimulating hormone		NKA	no known allergies
LAP	leukocyte alkaline phosphatase		NMR	nuclear magnetic resonance
LD	lactic dehydrogenase		NPO	nothing by mouth
LDH	lactate dehydrogenase		NREM	non–rapid eye movement
L-DOPA	dihydroxyphenylalanine		NSAID	nonsteroidal anti-inflammatory drug
LES	lower esophageal sphincter		NSR	normal sinus rhythm
LDL	low-density lipoproteins		NTD	nitroblue tetrazolium dye test
LEEP	loop electrode excision procedure		N&V	nausea and vomiting
LH	luteinizing hormone		NVD	normal vaginal delivery
LHR	leukocyte histamine release test		O_2	oxygen
LIA	lysine iron agar		OA	osteoarthritis
LLL	lower left lobe		OBGYN	obstetrics and gynecology
LMP	last menstrual period		OCD	obsessive compulsive disorder
LRH	luteinizing releasing factor		OD	ocular dexter (right eye)/overdose
LSD	lysergic acid diethylamide		OGTT	oral glucose tolerance test
LUL	left lower lobe		OS	ocular sinister (left eye)
LUQ	left upper quadrant		OSA	obstructive sleep apnea
LVF	left ventricular function		OTC	over the counter
LVSD	left ventricular systolic dysfunction		OU	ocular uterque
MAO-I	monoamine oxidase inhibitor		PA	posterior-anterior/pulmonary artery
MCHC	mean cell hemoglobin concentration		PAPP-A	pregnancy-associated plasma protein-A
MCH	mean cell hemoglobin		PAD	peripheral arterial disease
MCV	mean cell volume		PAF	platelet-activating factor/paroxysmal atrial fibrillation
MEG	magnetoencephalography		PAH	pulmonary arterial hypertension
MER	microelectrode recording		PAP	Papanicolaou smear
MI	myocardial infarction		PAT	paroxysmal atrial tachycardia
MIC	minimum inhibitory concentration		p.c.	after food
MIF	migration inhibitory factor		PCP	phencyclidine
MLC	mixed lymphocyte culture		PCR	polymerase chain reaction
MMR	measles, mumps, and rubella		PDT	photodynamic therapy
MPV	mean platelet volume		PEEP	positive end-expiratory pressure
MR	mitral regurgitation		PEF	peak expiratory flow
MRA	magnetic resonance angiography		PERRLA	pupils equal and reactive to light and accommodation
MRI	magnetic resonance imaging			
MRSA	methicillin-resistant *Staphylococcus aureus*		PET	positive emission tomography
			pH	hydrogen ion concentration

PICC	peripherally inserted central venous catheter		RVF	right ventricular failure
PID	pelvic inflammatory disease		RVSP	right ventricular systolic pressure
PIH	pregnancy-induced hypertension		Rx	prescription
PKD	polycystic kidney disease		SAH	subarachnoid hemorrhage
PKU	phenylketonuria		SARS	severe acute respiratory syndrome
PD	purified protein derivative		SBP	systolic blood pressure
PMD	postmenopausal bleeding		SCC	squamous cell carcinoma
PMH	past medical history		SCID	severe combined immunodeficiency
p.o.	by mouth		SD	standard deviation
prn	as necessary		SGOT	serum glutamic oxaloacetic
PSA	prostatic specific antigen		SGPT	serum glutamic pyruvate
PT	prothrombin time		SH	social history
PTA	percutaneous transluminal angioplasty		SHx	surgical history
PTCA	percutaneous transluminal coronary angioplasty		SIDS	sudden infant death syndrome
			SIS	saline infusion sonohysterography
PTM	pulmonary tuberculosis		SISI	short increment sensitivity index
PTx	pneumothorax		SLAP	superior labral anterior posterior
PUVA	psoralen and ultraviolet A		SLE	systemic lupus erythematosus
PVD	peripheral vascular disease		SOB	shortness of breath
PVR	pulmonary vascular resistance		SPECT	single-photon emission computed tomography
PWP	pulmonary wedge pressure			
Px	physical examination/prognosis		SROM	spontaneous rupture of membranes
q	each/every		SRS	stereotactic radiosurgery
q.AM	every morning		SSRI	selective serotonin reuptake inhibitor
q.d.	every day		STD	sexually transmitted disease
q.d.s.	four times each day		STH	somatotropic hormone
q.h.	each hour		STS	serologic test for syphilis
q.i.d.	four times each day		SVI	systemic viral infection
q.o.d.	every other day		SVR	systemic vascular resistance
RA	rheumatoid arthritis		T&A	tonsillectomy and adenoidectomy
RAI	radioactive iodine		TAH/BSO	total abdominal hysterectomy/bilateral salpingo-oopherectomy
RBBB	right bundle branch block			
RBC	red blood cell		TB	tuberculosis
RCA	right coronary artery		TBG	thyroxine-binding globulin
RCT	randomized controlled trial		TBI	total body irradiation
REM	rapid eye movement		t.d.s	three times a day
RF	rheumatoid factor		TBSA	total body surface area
RFA	radiofrequency ablation		TENS	transcutaneous electrical nerve
RFT	renal function test		TFT	thyroid function test
Rh	rhesus factor		TG	triglycerides
RhF	rheumatoid factor		Tg	thyroglobulin
Rho (D)	red cell antigen		TGA	transposition of great arteries
RLQ	right lower quadrant		THR	total hip replacement
RNA	ribonucleic acid		TIA	transient ischemic attack
ROM	range of motion		TIBC	total iron-binding capacity
ROS	review of symptoms		t.i.d.	three times a day
RPR	rapid plasma regain		TIPS	transvenous intrahepatic portosystemic shunt
RSV	respiratory syncytial virus			
RUQ	right upper quadrant		TKR	total hip replacement
			TLC	thin-layered chromatography/total lung capacity

TMJ	temporomandibular joint
TNF	tumor necrosis factor
TORCH	toxoplasmosis, rubella, cytomegalovirus, and herpes virus serology
TORP	total ossicular replacement prosthesis
TRF	transfer
TRH	thyrotropin-releasing hormone
TSH	thyroid-stimulating hormone
TSI	thyroid-stimulating immumoglobin
TT	thrombin time
TTS	transdermal therapeutic system
TUR	transurethral resection
TURP	transurethral resection of the prostate
Tx	treatment
UBT	urea breath test
UC	ulcerative colitis
UFE	uterine fibroid embolization
UFR	uroflowmetry
UPP	urethral pressure profile
URI	upper respiratory infection
USG	ultrasonography
UTI	urinary tract infection
VA	visual acuity
V-BAC	vaginal birth after cesarean
VC	vital capacity
VD	vaginal delivery
VE	vaginal examination
VEP	visual evoked potential
VF	ventricular fibrillation
VIP	vasoactive intestinal peptide
VLDL	very-low-density lipoprotein
VMA	vanillylmandelic acid
VOD	volume of distribution
VP	voiding pressure
VRE	vancomycin-resistant enterococci
VSD	ventricular septal defect
VT	ventricular tachycardia
WAT	white adipose tissue
WBC	white blood cell
WDWN	well developed, well nourished
WNL	within normal limits

CORRELATIONS TO THE CPC, CCS, AND CCS-P PROFESSIONAL CODING EXAMINATIONS

CPC Examination Correlations

This appendix begins with the correlations of the CPC (American Academy of Professional Coders) National Examination's content categories to *"Coding Review for National Certification: Passing the CPC and CCS-P Exams"* textbook. Table 1.1 provides the correlations of the CPC examination by category and referenced by unit/chapter.

Table 1.1 Correlations to the CPC Examination (American Academy of Professional Coders) AAPC

Content Category	Examination Type	Unit/Chapter
Medical Terminology	CPC	Unit 1, Chapters 3, 2 Unit 4, Chapter 13
Anatomy and Physiology	CPC	Unit 1, Chapter 2, 3 Unit 4, Chapter 13
ICD-9 Coding Concepts	CPC	Unit 3, Chapter 12 Part I and Part II Unit 4, Chapter 13
CPT Coding Concepts	CPC	Unit 2, Chapter 4 Unit 2, Chapters 5, 6, 7, 8, 9, 10 Unit 4, Chapter 13
HCPCS Coding Concepts	CPC	Unit 2, Chapter 11 Unit 4, Chapter 13
Anesthesia Coding Concepts	CPC	Unit 2 Chapter 6 Unit 4, Chapter 13
Surgical Coding Concepts	CPC	Unit 2, Chapter 7 Unit 3, Chapter 12 Part I and Part II Unit 4, Chapter 13
E/M Coding Concepts	CPC	Unit 2, Chapter 5 Unit 3, Chapter 12 Part I and Part II Unit 4, Chapter 13
Use of Modifiers	CPC	Unit 2, Chapters 4, 5, 6, 7, 8, 9, 10, 11 Unit 4, Chapter 13

CCS-P Examination Correlations

The final section of this appendix outlines the correlations of the CCS-P National Examinations to *"Coding Review for National Certification: Passing the CPC and CCS-P Exams"* textbook. The CCS and CCS-P national examinations have been established through the American Health Information Management Association (AHIMA). Table 1.2 outlines the CCS-P examination domains with content that correlate with this review textbook.

Table 1.2 CCS-P Examination Domain/Content Correlations

Domain/Content	Examination Type	Unit/Chapter
Domain 1: Health Information Documentation		
1. Interpret health record documentation to identify diagnoses and conditions for code assignment	CCS-P	Unit 3, Chapter 12 Part I and Part II Unit 4, Chapters 13
2. Interpreted health record documentation to identify procedures or services for code assignment	CCS-P	Unit 2, Chapters 4, 5, 6, 7, 8, 9, 10, 11 Unit 4, Chapter 13
3. Determine if sufficient clinical information is available to assign one or more diagnosis codes	CCS-P	Unit 3, Chapter 12 Part I and Part II Unit 4, Chapter 14
4. Determine if sufficient clinical information is available to assign one or more procedure or service codes	CCS-P	Unit 2, Chapters 4, 5, 6, 7, 8, 9, 10, 11 Unit 4, Chapter 13
5. Consult with physicians or other healthcare providers when additional information is needed for coding and/or to clarify conflicting or ambiguous information	CCS-P	Unit 3, Chapter 12 Part I Unit 4, Chapter 13
6. Consult reference materials to facilitate code assignment	CCS-P	Unit 2 Chapters, 4, 5, 6, 7, 8, 9, 10, 11 Unit 3, Chapter 12 Part I and Part II Unit 4, Chapter 13
7. Identify the etiology and manifestation(s) of clinical conditions	CCS-P	Unit 1, Chapter 3 Unit 1, Chapter 2
Domain 2: Coding		
1. Assign ICD-9-CM code by applying "Diagnostic Coding and Reporting Guidelines for Outpatient (Hospital-Based and Physician Office)"	CCS-P	Unit 3, Chapter 12 Part I and Part II Unit 4, Chapter 13
2. Interpret ICD-9-CM conventions, formats instructional notations, etc.	CCS-P	Unit 3, Chapter 12 Part I and Part II Unit 4, Chapter 13
3. Interpret CPT and HCPCS II guidelines, format, and instructional notes to select services, procedures, and supplies that require coding	CCS-P	Unit 2, Chapters 4, 5, 6, 7, 8, 9, 10, 11 Unit 4, Chapter 13
4. Assign CPT codes for procedures and/or services rendered during encounter	CCS-P	Unit 2, Chapters 4, 5, 6, 7, 8, 9, 10, 11 Unit 4, Chapter 13
5. Assign codes to identify E/M services	CCS-P	Unit 2, Chapter 5 Unit 4, Chapter 13
6. Recognize if an unlisted must be assigned	CCS-P	Unit 2, Chapters 4, 5, 6, 7, 8, 9, 10, 11 Unit 4, Chapter 13
7. Exclude from coding those procedures that are component parts of another reported procedure code	CCS-P	Unit 2, Chapters 4, 5, 6, 7, 8, 9, 10, 11 Unit 4, Chapter 13

(continued)

Table 1.2 Continued

Domain/Content	Examination Type	Unit/Chapter
8. Code for the professional vs. technical component when applicable	CCS-P	Unit 2, Chapters 4, 7, 8, 9
9. Assign HCPCS Level II codes	CCS-P	Unit 2, Chapter 11
10. Append modifiers to procedure or service codes when applicable	CCS-P	Unit 2, Chapters 4, 5, 6, 7, 8, 9, 10, 11 Unit 4, Chapter 13
Domain 3: Reimbursement Methods and Regulatory Guidelines		
1. Apply global surgical package concept to surgical procedure	CCS-P	Unit 2, Chapters 4, 5, 6, 7, 8, 9, 10, 11 Unit 4, Chapter 13
2. Apply bundling an unbundling guidelines	CCS-P	Unit 2, Chapters 4, 5, 6, 7, 8, 9, 10, 11 Unit 4, Chapter 13
3. Interpret health record documentation to identify diagnoses and conditions for code assignment	CCS-P	Unit 3, Chapter 12 Part I and Part II Unit 3, Chapter 12 Part I and Part II Unit 4, Chapter 13
4. Apply reimbursement methods for billing or reporting	CCS-P	Unit 3, Chapter 12 Part I and Part II Unit 4, Chapter 13
5. Link diagnosis code to the associated procedure code for billing or reporting	CCS-P	Unit 2, Chapters 4, 5, 6, 7, 8, 9, 10, 11 Unit 3, Chapter 12 Part I and Part II Unit 4, Chapter 13
6. Evaluate payer remittance or payment reports for reimbursement or denials	CCS-P	Unit 3, Chapter 12 Part I and Part II
7. Interpret Local Medical Review Policies to determine coverage	CCS-P	Unit 2, Chapter 11
8. Process claim denials and/or appeals	CCS-P	Unit 4, Chapter 13
Domain 4: Data Quality		
1. Validate assigned diagnosis and procedure codes supported by health record documentation	CCS-P	Unit 2, Chapters 4, 5, 6, 7, 8, 9, 10, 11 Unit 3, Chapter 12 Part I and Part II Unit 4, Chapter 13
2. Validate assigned E/M codes based on health record documentation using E/M guidelines	CCS-P	Unit 2, Chapter 5 Unit 4, Chapter 13

(continued)

Table 1.2 Continued

Domain/Content	Examination Type	Unit/Chapter
3. Assess the quality of coding and billing using routinely generated reports	CCS-P	Unit 2, Chapters 6, 7, 8, 9, 10 Unit 4, Chapter 13
4. Verify that the data on the claim form correctly reflect the services provided	CCS-P	Unit 2, Chapters 4, 5, 6, 7, 8, 9, 10, 11 Unit 4, Chapter 13
5. Verify that the data on the claim form correctly reflect the conditions managed or treated during the encounter	CCS-P	Unit 3, Chapter 12 Part I and Part II Unit 4, Chapter 13
6. Validate the accuracy of the required data elements on the claim form	CCS-P	Unit 3, Chapter 12 Part I and Part II
7. Conduct coding and billing audits for compliance and trending	CCS-P	Unit 2, Chapter 4 Unit 3, Chapter 12 Part I
8. Determine educational needs for physicians and staff on reimbursement and documentation rules and regulations related to coding	CCS-P	
9. Participate in the development of coding and billing policies and procedures for reporting professional services	CCS-P	
10. Evaluate payer remittance or payment	CCS-P	Unit 3 Chapter 12 Part I and Part II

GLOSSARY

A

achalasia   The failure of muscle to relax.

acronym   A word that is formed from the initials of several words.

adenopathy   Disease of a gland or lymph node.

adjuvant   Something that helps or assists.

adrenaline   Hormone secreted by the adrenal gland that increases physical reactions.

antepartum   The period of time before a baby is delivered.

antibody   A protein that fights infection, produced by B cells in the body in response to an antigen.

antigen   A substance that stimulates the production of an antibody.

aneurysm   A bulge in the artery that can weaken the wall of the artery.

aponeurosis   A membrane that connects muscle to bone.

arthrodesis   The surgical immobilization of a joint.

arthrography   The radiography of a joint.

atrium   An upper chamber of the heart in which blood is pumped from the veins into ventricles.

B

bifurcated   Divided in two; split into two parts.

bilateral   Two-sided.

C

capsulotomy   To make a surgical incision into a capsule surrounding a body part.

carcinoma   A malignant tumor located in the surface layer of the epithelium or an organ or other body part.

cellulitis   An inflammation of the connective tissue that can be caused by a bacteria infection, usually *Streptococcus* or *Staphylococcus.*

cholecystectomy   Surgical removal of the gallbladder.

cirrhosis   A chronic and progressive disease of the liver characterized by scar tissue.

conjunctivitis   Inflammation of the conjunctiva, also known as *pink eye.*

contusion   A bruise; an injury to the body in which the tissue is damaged, causing a bruise.

conventions   Accepted standards and norm.

co-payment   A provision in an insurance policy requiring the policyholder to pay a specific payment for each medical service or claim.

correlation   A relationship between two or more things.

craniectomy   Surgical removal of part of the cranium.

cranioplasty   Surgery involving using plastic on the skull.

curettement   Removal of growths from the wall cavity or other surface.

D

debridement   The removal of dead or contaminated tissue from a wound; treatment for burns.

decubitus ulcer   Bedsore.

dementia   The progressive deterioration of intellectual functions.

diagnostic   Identifying the nature or cause of an illness, condition, or injury.

dialysis   The medical filtering of accumulated waste product from the blood of a patient with nonfunctioning kidneys.

disseminate   To spread or distribute something.

domiciliary   Relating to a home; a rest home for older adults.

dosimetry   The act of measuring the amount of radiation absorbed by something.

E

embolus   A mass of undissolved matter (clot) that moves through the bloodstream until it is caught or lodged.

endocardium   The thin membranous lining of the heart's cavities.

enucleation   The surgical removal of something from its capsule; the removal of an eyeball.

etiology   The cause and origin of disease.

evocative   Suggestive; reminiscent.

exacerbate   To make something worse; to worsen symptoms.

exanthem   A skin rash appearing as a sign of an infection such as chickenpox.

explanation of benefits   A statement from the insurance company that explains how the amount of reimbursement was disbursed to the company and the provider.

F

furuncle   A boil on the skin.

G

gallbladder   The small organ on the inferior surface of the liver that serves as a storage unit for bile until needed for digestion.

glomerulus   A round structure in the kidney that removes body waste to be excreted as urine.

gonads   A reproductive organ that produces reproductive cells; ovaries or testes.

H

hydration   The provision of water to something or someone.

hyperkeratosis   The excessive thickening of the skin.

hypertension   High blood pressure.

hypertrophy   Enlargement of an organ as a result of the increase in cell growth.

hysterectomy   Surgical removal of the uterus in the female body.

I

idiopathic   Without apparent cause or etiology.

immunoglobulin   A protein capable of acting as an antibody to help fight infection.

infiltrate   To pass through a substance by filtration.

infusion   The introduction of a solution such as a drug or chemical into the body.

insulin   A hormone that regulates glucose level in the blood.

intravascular   Situated or occurring within blood vessels.

intravenous   Within a vein.

iridectomy   The surgical removal of the iris of the eye.

L

lacrimal gland   The tear duct of the eye.

laminectomy   Surgery involving the removal of the rear arches of spinal vertebrae to gain access to the spinal cord or spinal nerve roots.

large intestine   The last section of the digestive tract, extending from the ileum to the anus.

larynx   The voice box, situated between the level of the tongue and the top of the trachea.

late effect   A symptom, condition, or disease that occurs as a result of the primary illness, e.g. paralysis after stroke.

lesion   A wound; a term sometimes used interchangeably with tumor.

lidocaine   Anesthethic drug; local.

lymphadenectomy   Surgical removal of the lymph glands or nodes.

M

maladaptive   Poorly adapting to; unable to adapt to a particular situation, function, or purpose.

manifestation   One of the first signs of a disease.

mastectomy   Surgical removal of the breast.

meconium   The first feces of a newborn baby.

Medicaid   A government-funded program that pays medical expenses for people who are unable to pay their own expenses.

medulla oblongata   The lower part of the brain that controls involuntary functions, such as of the heart and lungs.

menses   Menstruation and the period of time it lasts.

microorganism   A tiny organism such as bacteria, virus, or protozoan that can only be seen with the use of a microscope.

misadventure   An unfortunate event, occurrence, or situation.

morbidity   The presence of illness, health condition, or injury.

moribund   Dying; becoming obsolete.

morphology   The study of the structure of organisms and their interdependent parts.

mortality   The condition of certain death.

myringotomy   A surgical incision into the middle ear.

N

necrotizing   Causing or undergoing cell death.

neonate   Newborn infant.

neoplasm   A tumor; an abnormal growth of tissue.

nephrons   The small tubes in the kidneys that filter and excrete waste from the blood and produce urine.

neuron   A functional cell of the nervous system that contains fibers called dendrites that carry messages to the cell body.

normocephalic   Referring to normal functioning brain activity relating to the senses.

nystagmus   Involuntary movement of the eyeball, usually from side-to-side, caused by illness that affects the nerves of the eyes.

O

opacification   Becoming opaque; making so that images cannot be seen through something.

ophthalmologist   A physician who studies the diseases of the eye.

orthotics   The science of design and fitting of medical devices in the treatment of orthopedic disorders.

osteomalacia   A condition in which, through the deficiency of vitamin D, bones become soft, brittle and deformed.

otorhinolaryngological   Pertaining to the ears, nose, and throat.

otosclerosis   Abnormal hardening of the stapes of the ear caused by unusual bone development.

P

papilloma   A benign skin tumor.

pathology   The study of disease; process of a disease.

percutaneous skeletal fixation   Fracture fixation/pins placed through the skin across the fracture after closed reduction.

peruse   To read something carefully; to examine carefully and thoroughly.

pharynx   The throat, situated between the mouth and the esophagus.

phimosis   Stenosis (narrowing) of the preputial orifice so that the foreskin cannot be pushed back over the penis. Narrowness or closure of the vaginal orifice.

polysomnography   The continuous measuring of physiological activity during sleep for diagnostic purposes.

postoperative   The time period after an operation, usually six weeks.

procurement   The act of acquiring something.

prognosis   A medical opinion regarding the outcome of a disease, condition, or injury.

prophylactic   Protecting against disease or infection.

prothrombin   Protein essential for the clotting of blood.

protocol   The customary way in which things are done.

psychogenic   Coming from mental or emotional processes.

psychotherapy   The psychological treatment of mental disorders.

puerperium   The period immediately following childbirth, usually lasting six weeks.

pustulent   An agent that produces the formation of pustules.

Q

qualitative   Relating to the quality or character of something.

quantitative   Relating to the quantity or the amount of something.

R

receptor   A nerve ending that converts stimuli into nerve impulses.

S

sarcoma   A malignant tumor that begins growing in connective tissue such as bone or cartilage.

septicemia   The presence of toxic microorganisms in the bloodstream, causing illness.

sequela   A condition following and resulting from a disease.

sialoadenitis   Inflammation of the salivary gland.

sigmoidoscopy   A surgical instrument inserted in the anus for visual inspection of the interior of the rectum and colon.

solvent   A substance that dissolves something.

spirometry   A medical device used for measuring lung capacity.

stapes   A small, stirrup-shaped bone in the innermost part of the middle ear that transmits vibration to the inner ear.

stereotaxis   Surgery involving the insertion of delicate instruments by using dimensional scanning techniques.

stratum corneum   The outermost horny layer of the skin.

subcutaneous   Beneath the skin; third layer of the skin.

superlative   The highest degree in comparison to something.

symbology   The study of symbols; interpretation of symbols.

synthesize   To combine various components into a new whole.

systemic   Relating to or affecting a body system as a whole.

T

tangential   With only slight relevance to the current subject; almost irrelevant.

thoracotomy   Incision in the chest wall.

thrombectomy   The surgical removal of a thrombus.

toxoid   A toxin that has been treated to destroy its toxicity but is still capable of inducing formation of antibodies on injection.

tracheostomy   The surgical procedure of cutting a hole in the trachea to ensure an open airway.

U

urodynamics   The functioning of the urinary system.

V

vascular   Pertaining to fluid-carrying vessels.

Z

zoonitic   Coming from an animal.

INDEX

Bold page references indicate definitions of key terms; page numbers followed by *f* indicate figures; page numbers followed by *t* indicate tables.

Symbols
: (colon), 167
; (semicolon), 65
⊙ (conscious sedation), 94, 152
☼ (moderate sedation), 69
* (neoplasm), 175
• (new procedure), 69
() (parentheses), 166–167
+ (plus), 67, 102, 143
ζ (vaccines pending FDA approval), 69
∅ (modifier 51 exempt), 69, 105, 107
↻ (revised description), 69
⌐◄ (new and revised text), 69
[ ] (brackets), 166
[ ] (slanted brackets), 166

A

A codes, 158
AAPC (American Academy of Professional Coders), CPC exam, 5–6, 8, 164, 255
Abbreviations, 250–254
  drug administration routes, 159*t*
  ICD-9-CM codes, 166
Abdominal hernia, 49*t*
Abduction, 53*t*
Ablation procedures, 110, 148*t*
Abnormal reaction, to medical or surgical procedures, 173
Abortion, 199–200
Abscess, 200
Abuse
  child, 173
  drug, 160
  health care, 187–188
Accidental intent, 173
Acetylcholine, 24
Achalasia, **193**
Acromegaly, 58*t*
Acronyms, 65, **131**
Actinic keratosis, 201
Acupuncture, 151
Acute myocardial infarction (AMI), 184–185
ADA (American Dental Association), 160
Add-on codes, 67
  medicine, 143
  surgery, 102–103, 107
Addison disease, 58*t*
Adenoiditis, 37*t*
Adenomyosis, 43*t*
Adenopathy, **82**
Adhesiolysis, 116
Adhesive capsulitis, 202
Adipose, 35*t*
Adjuvant, 109*t*, 136
Administrative examination V codes, 171
Administrative safeguards (HIPAA), 188
Adrenal gland, 26, 57, 57*t*
Adrenaline (epinephrine), **9**, 24
Adverse effects, 173, 209–210
Aftercare visit codes, 170
Agglutinate, 46*t*
Agranulocytosis, 180
AHIMA (American Health Information Management

Association), CCS-P exam, 5–6, 8, 164, 255–258
Alcohol abuse treatment services, 160
Alimentary canal, 48
Allowed charges, 210
Alphabetic indexes
  CPT, 64, 64*f*
  ICD-9-CM
    to Diseases, 165, 168, 206
    to External Causes of Injury or Poisoning, 171
    to Procedures, 166, 168
Alphanumerical codes; *see* HCPCS Level II codes
Alveolar ducts, 15
Alveolus, 15, 36*t*
Alzheimer's disease, 57*t*, 182
AMA (American Medical Association), 63, 158
Amenorrhea, 43*t*, 196
American Academy of Professional Coders (AAPC), CPC exam, 5–6, 8, 164, 255
American Dental Association (ADA), 160
American Health Information Management Association (AHIMA), CCS-P exam, 5–6, 8, 164, 255–258
American Medical Association (AMA), 63, 158
American Psychiatric Association, 180
American Society of Anesthesiologists, 93
AMI (acute myocardial infarction), 184–185
Amniotic, 42*t*
Anal fissure, 194
Anastomosis, **114**
Anatomical position, 13, 13*f*
Anatomical site, fifth digit subclassifications, 202
Anatomy
  defined, 13
  overview, 13–26
And (note), 167*t*
Anemia, 46*t*, 180, 180*t*
  aplastic, 47*t*
Anencephaly, 203
Anesthesia
  administration routes, 95*f*
  local, 94, 94*t*, 144, 150
  by surgeon, 93
  types of, 94, 94*t*
Anesthesia section (CPT), 91–97
  how to locate codes in, 94–95
  materials supplied by physician, 92
  modifiers, 92–93, 93*t*
  qualifying circumstances, 93, 94*t*
  special report, 92
Aneurysm, **67**
Angina pectoris, 184
Angiography, 125*f*, 125–126, 148
Angioma, 46*t*
Ankle bones, 22*f*, 23
Ankylosis, 54*t*
Antepartum services, 114, 197
Anterior, 13
Antibodies, **131**, 136
Antigens, **131**, 136
Anxiety, test, 9–10

Aorta, 18, 18*f*
  endovascular repair of, 110–111
  radiological procedures, 125*f*, 125–126
Aortic semilunar valve, 18, 18*f*
Aphakia, 50*t*
Aplastic anemia, 47*t*
Aponeurosis, **23**, 23*f*
Appendices
  CPT, 69
    A, 69
    B, 69
    C, 77
    D, 67
    G, 151
    H, 153
  ICD-9-CM, 165
Appendicitis, 49*t*, 193
Appendicular skeleton, 22*f*, 22–23
Arachnoid membrane, 56*t*
Areolar, 42*t*
Arm bones, 22, 22*f*, 53*t*
Arrector pili muscle, 14, 35*t*
Arrhythmias, 109, 109*f*, 148
  induction of, 148*t*
Arterial grafting, for coronary artery bypass, 110
Arterial-venous grafting, for coronary artery bypass, 110
Arteries, radiological procedures, 125*f*, 125–126
Arteriosclerosis, 46*t*
Arthritis, 55*t*, 202, 203*f*
Arthrodesis, **23, 105**, 107
Arthrography, **123**, 124–125
Arthropathy, 201–202
Articulation, 53*t*
Aspiration, 116
Assisted living facilities, 84
Asthma, 185–186, 186*f*
Atrial septal defect, 203
Atrioventricular (AV) node, 19, 19*f*, 44*t*
Atrioventricular valve, 18, 18*f*
Atrium, 18, 18*f*, **44*t***
Attitude, toward coding examination, 7
Audiological function tests, 148
Auditory nerve, 51*t*
Auditory system; *see* Ears
Automated testing
  blood, 135
  urinalysis, 134
Autonomic function tests, 150*t*
AV (atrioventricular) node, 19, 19*f*, 44*t*
Axial skeleton, 21–22, 22*f*
Axons, 23

B

B codes, 158
Backbench work
  heart/lung, 111
  intestinal, 112
  lung, 107
  renal, 113
Bacterial meningitis, 182, 183*f*
Bacteriology, 136
Balance, 20–21, 147–148
Basal cell carcinoma, 36*t*
Basic metabolic panel, 133, 133*f*
Battery, pacemaker, 109
Bedsores, 201
Behavioral disturbances, 145–146

Bell's palsy, 57*t*
Benign hypertension, 175
Benign lesions, 103, 104*f*
Benign neoplasms, 174–175, 177*f*, 177–178, 178*t*
Benign prostatic hyperplasia, 41*t*
Bethesda System, 136
Bicuspid valve, 18, 18*f*, 44*t*
Bifurcated, **111**
Bilateral, **68**
Bile, 48*t*
Biological substances, adverse effects of, 173
Biopsy
  breast, 105
  skin, 103
Bladder, urinary, 16, 16*f*, 38
Bladder catheterization, 113, 113*f*
Bleeding; *see* Hemorrhage
Blood-forming organs, diseases of, 180, 180*t*
Blood pressure
  high (*see* Hypertension)
  measurement of, 183, 183*f*, 184
Blood system, 18*f*, 18–19
  disorders, 47*t*–48*t*, 180, 180*t*
  hemodialysis, 146, 147*f*
  terminology review, 46, 46*t*–47*t*
Blood testing, 135, 135*f*
Body areas
  chiropractic regions, 151
  directional terms, 13, 13*f*
  extent of examination by, 79
  finding codes by, 64, 95
Body surface, burns classified by, 208–209, 209*f*
Body systems; *see* Organ systems; *specific system*
Bone, 21–23, 22*f*
  terminology review, 52, 53*t*
Bone fractures, 52, 105, 105*t*, 106*f*, 107, 201, 202, 207
Bone grafting, 105
Bowman's capsule, 39*t*
Brachytherapy, 127*f*, 128
Brain
  disorders, 57*t*, 204, 204*f*
  functional mapping, 150*t*
  structure, 24–25, 183*f*
  terminology review, 56*t*
Brainstem, 24–25
Breast biopsy, 105
Breast cancer, 127*f*
Breast excision, 105
Bronchi, 15, 15*f*
Bronchial, 36*t*
Bronchial tree, 15, 15*f*
Bronchioles, 15, 15*f*
Bronchitis, 185–186, 186*f*
Bulbourethral glands (Cowper's glands), 16*f*, 17, 40*t*
Bundle of His, 19, 19*f*, 44*t*
Burns, 206, 207–209, 209*f*, 210

C

C codes, 158
Cachexia, 207
Cadaver donor
  cardiectomy, 111
  enterectomy, 112

nephrectomy, 113
pneumonectomy, 107
Cancer; *see also* Neoplasm(s)
   bone, 55*t*
   breast, 127*f*
   radiation therapy, 127–128
   testicular, 41*t*
Canthus, 50*t*
Capsulotomy, **101**
Carbuncle, 200
Carcinoma, **174**
Cardiac catheterization, 148
Cardiac muscle, 23
Cardiectomy, cadaver donor, 111
Cardiovascular system, 18*f,* 18–19
   disorders, 46*t,* 182–185, 184*t*
   procedure codes, 148
   surgery codes, 19, 108*t*–109*t,* 108–111
   terminology review, 44, 44*t*–45*t,* 184
Cardioverter-defibrillator, 108–109
Care plan oversight services, 85–86
Carpal bones, 22, 22*f,* 53*t*
Case management services, 85–86
Cast(s), 107
Cast removals, **107**
Category II codes, 152–153
   modifiers, 153, 153*t*
Category III codes, 153–154
Catheterization
   bladder, 113, 113*f*
   cardiac, 148
   indwelling, 144, 150
   vascular, 111, 111*t*
Cavity, 36*t*
CBC (complete blood count), 135
CDT (Current Dental Terminology), 160
Cecum, 48*t*
Cellulitis, 36*t,* **200**
Central nervous system (CNS), 23,
   24*f,* 54
   assessments, 150*t*
Central venous access procedures,
   111, 111*t*
Cerebellum, 24, 56*t*
Cerebral cortex, 56*t*
Cerebrovascular accident (CVA),
   57*t,* 184
Cerebrovascular hemorrhage, 184
Cerebrovascular hypertension, 184
Cerebrovascular infarction, 184
Cerebrum, 24, 56*t*
Cerumen, 51*t*
   impacted, 52*t*
Cervical nerves, 25, 27*f*
Cervical vertebrae, 21, 22*f*
   surgery codes, 106*t*
Cervicitis, 43*t*
Cesarean section, 114
Chemistry, 134–135
Chemotherapy
   administration, 150–151
   complications, 178
Cheyne-Stokes respiration, 207
Chief complaint, 73, 73*f,* 78
Child abuse, 173
Childbirth, 114, 115*f; see also*
   Obstetrics; Pregnancy
   maternal complications, 196–200, 197*t*
   neonatal complications, 205
Children; *see also* Infants; Neonates;
   under Pediatric
   developmental milestones, 207
Chiropractic manipulative treatment
   (CMT), 151
Cholecystectomy, **65**
Cholecystitis, 49*t*
Choledocholithiasis, 195
Cholelithiasis, 49*t*

Chordae tendineae, 18, 18*f*
Chromatography, 134
Chronic cystic mastitis, 196
Chronic fatigue syndrome, 207
Chronic kidney disease (CKD),
   195–196
Chronic obstructive pulmonary disease
   (COPD), 37*t,* 185–186, 186*f*
Circulatory system; *see* Blood system;
   Cardiovascular system
Cirrhosis, **194**
CKD (chronic kidney disease), 195–196
Clavicle, 22, 22*f*
Clinical treatment planning, radiation
   therapy, 127–128, 128*t*
Clitoris, 17*f,* 18, 42*t*
CMT (chiropractic manipulative
   treatment), 151
CNS (central nervous system),
   23, 24*f,* 54
   assessments, 150*t*
Coagulation, 135
Coccygeal nerves, 25, 27*f*
Coccyx, 22, 22*f,* 53*t*
Cochlea, 51*t*
Code categories, CPT, 63*t,* 63–64
Code changes, 69
Code set rules (HIPAA), 187–188
Coding conventions, **6**
Coding examinations, 2–11
   anxiety about, 9–10
   CCS-P, 5–6, 8, 164, 255–258
   content, 5–6
   correlations to, 255–258
   CPC, 5–6, 8, 164, 255
   practice test, 218–235
   preparing for, 10
   questions on
      different kinds of, 7
      difficult, handling, 8
      multiple choice, 8–9, 10
   studying for, 2–5
   strategies, 6–9
   test-taking skills, 7–9
   time limits during, 3, 7–8, 10
Coding records, reading, 6
Colon, 48*t*
   diverticulum, 194
Colonoscopy, 112
Combining forms, 32–33
Community acquired conditions,
   neonatal, 205
Comorbidities, **79**
Compact bone, 21
Complete blood count (CBC), 135
Complexity, 79, 79*t,* 80
Comprehensive examination, 79
Comprehensive history, 78
Computed tomography (CT), 124
Concurrent, **69**, 74
Condition, finding codes by, 64
Conduction system, heart, 18–19, 19*f*
Confirmatory consultations, 82
Congenital anomalies, 203–204, 205
Congenital hydrocephalus, 203, 204*f*
Congestive heart failure, 46*t*
Conjunctiva, 50*t*
Conjunctivitis, **9,** 52*t*
Connective tissue diseases, 201*t,*
   201–203
Conscious sedation, 92, 94
   moderate, 151–152
Consultations, 82–83
   pathology, 135
   radiology, 127
Contact dermatitis, 200
Contact lenses, 147
Continuing intensive care services, 84

Contrast materials, administration of,
   124–125
Contusion, **74**
Conventions, **6**
Copayment, **210**
COPD (chronic obstructive pulmonary
   disease), 37*t,* 185–186, 186*f*
Cornea, 21, 21*f,* 50*t*
Coronal plane, 13, 13*f*
Coronary artery, 44*t*
Coronary artery bypass, vascular
   grafting for, 110
Corpus luteum, 42*t*
Correlate, **76**
Cortical, 39*t*
Counseling, 74
Counseling V codes, 171
Cowper's glands (bulbourethral
   glands), 16*f,* 17, 40*t*
CPT Assistant, 63
CPT Changes: An Insider's View, 63
CPT code(s)
   add-on, 67, 102–103, 107, 143
   anesthesia (*see* Anesthesia section)
   versus HCPCS Level II codes,
      157, 158
   indented, 65
   medicine (*see* Medicine section)
   modifiers, 67–68, 67*t*–68*t* (*see also*
      Modifier(s))
   pathology (*see* Pathology and
      Laboratory section)
   radiology (*see* Radiology section)
   surgery (*see* Surgery section)
   unlisted, 69, 102, 143
CPT Editorial Panel (AMA), 63
CPT Information Services, 63
CPT manual, 62–71
   Appendices, 69
      A, 69
      B, 69
      C, 77
      D, 67
      G, 151
      H, 153
   Evaluation and Management
      Section (*see* Evaluation and
      Management Services)
   guidelines, 65–67, 66*f*
   index, 64, 64*f*
   instructions for using, 64–65
   section numbers, 63*t,* 63–64
   terminology format, 65
CPT Principles of Coding, 63
Cranial, 13
Cranial bones, 21, 22*f*
Cranial nerves, 25, 26*f,* 54
Craniectomy, **25**
Cranioplasty, **116***t*
Critical care services, 83–84
Crohn's disease, 49*t,* 194
Cryptorchidism, 41*t*
CT (computed tomography), 124
Curettement, **104**
Current Dental Terminology (CDT), 160
Current Procedural Terminology, 158;
   see also CPT manual
Cushing syndrome, 58*t*
Custodial care services, 84
Cutaneous, 35*t*
CVA (cerebrovascular accident),
   57*t,* 184
Cystic mastitis, 196
Cystitis, 40*t*
Cystocele, 40*t,* 196, 197*f*
Cystoscope, 38, 38*f*
Cystoscopy, 113
Cystourethroscopy, 113

Cytopathology, 136
Cytotoxic, 46*t*

D

D codes, 158, 160
Daily planner, 3–5, 4*f,* 5*t*
Data quality and management, 210–212
Debridement, **15,** 209
Decision making, level of, 79, 79*t,* 80
Decubitus ulcer, **159,** 201
Definitive identification, 136
Dehydration, chemotherapy-
   induced, 178
Delivery services (childbirth), 114,
   115*f,* 197–199, 205
Deltoid muscle, 53*t*
Dementia, **84**
Dendrites, 23
Dental procedures, 160
Depilatory, 35*t*
Depolarization, 44*t*
Dermatitis, 36*t,* 200
Dermatology, 35*t*
Dermis, 13, 15*f*
Destruction, 104
Detailed examination, 78
Detailed history, 78
Developmental milestones, 207
Diabetes, gestational, 198
Diabetes mellitus, 58*t,* 179
   in pregnancy, 198
Diagnoses
   coding, 164 (*see also* ICD-9-CM
      codes)
   UHDDS reporting rules, 189
Diagnostic and Statistical Manual
   (DSM-IV-TR), 180, 181*t*
Diagnostic-related group (DRG), 212
Dialysis, **146**
Diaphysis, 21, 53*t*
Diastole, 45*t*
Digestive system, 19–20, 20*f*
   disorders, 49*t,* 193*t,* 193–195
   surgery codes, 112–113
   terminology review, 48, 48*t*–49*t*
Dilation, 43*t*
Dipstick, urinalysis, 134
Directional terms, 13, 13*f*
Discharge services, neonatal, 85
Disease; *see also specific disease or*
   system
   finding codes by, 64
Disease-oriented panels, 133, 133*f*
Dislocations, 107
Disseminated, **149**
Distal, 13
Diverticulitis, 49*t*
Diverticulum of colon, 194
DME (durable medical equipment),
   159, 160
Domiciliary, **81***t*
Domiciliary care services, 84
Donor codes, 171
Dorsal, 13
Dosimetry, **127**
Down syndrome, 204
Drainage, nervous system
   procedures, 116
DRG (diagnostic-related group), 212
Drug(s)
   adverse effects of, 173, 209–210
   overdose, 209
Drug abuse treatment services, 160
Drug administration routes,
   abbreviations for, 159*t*
Drug Enforcement Administration
   number, 188

Drug errors, 209
Drug table
  HCPCS, 159
  ICD-9-CM, 165, 173, 174*t*
Drug testing, 133–134
DSM-IV-TR *(Diagnostic and Statistical Manual)*, 180, 181*t*
Duodenal ulcer, 49*t*
Duodenitis, 193
Duodenum, 48*t*
  diseases of, 193
Durable medical equipment (DME), 159, 160
Dysdiadochokinesia, 207
Dysrhythmias, 109, 109*f*, 148

E

E codes
  HCPCS, 158, 160
  ICD-9-CM, 165, 171–173, 172*t*
Ears, 20–21, 118*f*
  disorders, 52*t*, 182, 182*t*
  otorhinolaryngological services, 147–148
  surgery codes, 117, 118*t*
  terminology review, 50, 51*t*
Echocardiography, 148
Eczema, 36*t*, 200
EDI (Electronic Data Interchange), 187–188
EEG (electroencephalography), 150*t*
Effacement, 43*t*
Ejaculatory duct, 16*f*, 17, 40*t*
Elastin, 35*t*
Electrical stimulation, acupuncture, 151
Electrodes, pacemaker, 109
Electroencephalography (EEG), 150*t*
Electromyography, 150*t*
Electronic Data Interchange (EDI), 187–188
Electronic medical evaluation, 151
Electrophysiological procedures, 109*f*, 109–110, 148, 148*t*
E&M Service; *see* Evaluation and Management Services
Embolus, 46*t*
  cerebral, **57***t*
  pulmonary, 38*t*
  versus thrombus, 44, 44*f*
Embryonic, 43*t*
Emergency department, evaluation and management services, 73, 76, 83
Emerging technology codes (Category III), 153–154
Emphysema, 37*t*, 186*f*, 187
Encephalitis, 57*t*
Encounter form, 210
End-stage renal disease (ESRD), 146, 195–196
Endocrine system, 25–26
  disorders, 58*t*, 179*t*, 179–180
  surgery codes, 115–117
  terminology review, 57, 57*t*–58*t*
Endometriosis, 43*t*
Endometrium, 43*t*
Endoscopy, 108
  digestive system, 112
  respiratory system, 107
  urinary system, 113
Endosteum, 53*t*
Endovascular repair, descending thoracic aorta, 110–111
Enforcement Rule (HIPAA), 188
Enterectomy, cadaver donor, 112
Enucleation, **137**
EOB (explanation of benefits), **210**
Epicardium, 45*t*
Epidermis, 13, 15*f*

Epididymis, 16*f*, 17, 40*t*
Epididymitis, 41*t*
Epidurography, 116
Epiglottis, 15, 15*f*, 37*t*
Epilepsy, 182
Epinephrine (adrenaline), **9**, 24
Epiphysis, 21, 53*t*
Epistaxis, 207
Epithelium, 35*t*
Erythrocyte, 47*t*
Esophagus, 15, 15*f*, 19, 20*f*, 37*t*, 48*t*
  disorders, 193
ESRD (end-stage renal disease), 146, 195–196
Essential hypertension, 175
Established patients, 73, 78, 146
Estradiol, 57*t*
Ethmoid sinuses, 51*t*
Etiology, unknown, 206
Etiology (note), **167***t*
Eupneic, 37*t*
Evaluation and Management Services, 72–90
  appropriate level, 80, 81*t*
  case management services, 85–86
  classification, 73–74
  clinical examples, 77
  consultations, 82–83
  critical care services, 83–84
  emergency department, 73, 76, 83
  extent of examination performed, 78–79
  extent of history, 77–78
  hospital inpatient services, 82
  hospital observation services, 81, 82
  immunizations, 86, 142, 143–144
  level of decision making, 79, 79*t*, 80
  levels of service, 74–75
  nursing facility services, 84–85
  office/outpatient services, 80
  past and social history, 75
  review of systems, 75
  selecting level of, instructions for, 77
  time factors, 76, 82
Evocative testing, **134**
Evoked potentials, 150*t*
Exacerbated, **83**
Exacerbation, respiratory disease, 185–187, 186*f*
Examination; *see* Coding examinations
Examination performed, extent of, 78–79
Exanthem, **176***t*
Excisions, **15**
  breast, 105
  intestinal, 112
  skin, 103
Excludes (note), 167*t*
Excretory, 39*t*
Exocrine glands, 25–26, 57*t*
Expanded examination, 78
Expanded history, 78
Explanation of benefits (EOB), **210**
Extension, 53*t*
External, 13
External causes of injury or poisoning (E codes), 171–173, 172*t*, 174*t*, 210
Eyes, 20–21, 21*f*
  disorders, 52*t*, 182, 182*t*
  ophthalmology, 146–147, 147*t*
  surgery codes, 117, 118*t*
  terminology review, 50, 50*t*–51*t*

F

Face-to-face time, 76
Facial bones, 21, 22*f*, 53*t*
Fallopian tubes (oviducts), 17*f*, 18, 43*t*

Family history, 74, 170
Federal Bureau of Investigation, terrorism identified by, 173
Female reproductive system, 17*f*, 17–18
  disorders, 43*t*–44*t*, 195*t*, 195–196, 197*f*
  surgery codes, 18, 114, 114*t*
  terminology review, 42, 42*t*–43*t*
Femoropopliteal vein grafting, 110
Femur, 22, 22*f*
Fetal alcohol syndrome, 206
Fetal conditions, 198, 204*t*, 204–206
Fetal growth retardation, 206
Fibrillation, 46*t*
Fibrocystic disease, 196
Fibroid tumor, 43*t*
Fibula, 22, 22*f*
Filtration, 39*t*
Fissures, 24, 36*t*
  anal, 194
Flexion, 53*t*
Floor time, 76
Fluoroscopy, 116, 126
Flush, infusion, 144, 150
Focusing, during study sessions, 6
Foley catheter, 113, 113*f*
Follicle, 35*t*
Follicle-stimulating hormone, 57*t*
Follow-up codes, 171
Foot bones, 22*f*, 23, 53*t*
Fractures, 52, 105, 105*t*, 106*f*, 107, 201, 202, 207
Fraud, health care, 187–188
Frontal lobes, 24, 56*t*
Frontal sinuses, 51*t*
Functional brain mapping, 150*t*
Furuncle, **6**, 36*t*

G

G codes, 158
Gallbladder, 19, 20*f*, **48**, 48*t*
  disorders, 49*t*
Ganglion cyst, 202
Gangrene, 36*t*
Gastritis, 193
Gastroenteritis, 49*t*
Gastrointestinal bleeding, 195
General anesthesia, 92, 94, 94*t*
General health panel, 133
Genetic counseling services, 150*t*
Genetic disorders, 203–204
Genital prolapse, 44*t*, 196, 197*f*
Genitourinary system; *see* Female reproductive system; Male reproductive system; Urinary system
Gestational diabetes, 198
Glands
  endocrine, 25–26, 57*t*
  exocrine, 25–26, 57*t*
Glaucoma, 52*t*, 182
Glomerulonephritis, 40*t*
Glomerulus, 39*t*
Glycogen, 58*t*
Glycoprotein, 47*t*
Goiter, 58*t*
Gonads, 40*t*, 41*t*
Goniometer, 151*f*
Gout, 55*t*
Granulocyte, 47*t*
Graves disease, 58*t*
Grouper program, 212
Guessing, during testing, 8
Guidelines
  CPT, 65–67, 66*f*
  ICD-9-CM coding, 168, 168*t*
Gyri, 24

H

H codes, 158, 160
Hair, 13, 15*f*
Hallux valgus, 202
Hand bones, 22, 22*f*, 53*t*
HCPCS Level I codes; *see* CPT code(s)
HCPCS Level II codes, 157–159
  assignment guidelines, 158–159
  versus CPT codes, 157, 158
  modifiers, 160–161, 161*t*
  section breakdowns, 158
  Table of Drugs, 159
Health and behavior assessment, 149
Health care fraud, 187–188
Health care setting, V codes use in, 170
Health insurance claims, 210–212, 211*f*
Health Insurance Portability and Accountability Act (HIPAA), 187–188
Health service, contact with, classification of, 169–171
Health status, factors influencing, classification of, 169–171
Hearing; *see* Ears
Heart
  conduction system, 18–19, 19*f*
  disorders, 46*t*, 148
  flow of blood through, 18
  procedure codes, 148
  structure, 18, 18*f*
  terminology review, 44, 44*t*–45*t*
Heart/lung transplantation, 111
Heart murmurs, 207
Heart muscle, 23
Heart valves, 18, 18*f*
Hematocrit, 135, 135*f*
Hematocytopenia, 47*t*
Hematology, 135
Hemiplegia, 182
Hemodialysis, 146, 147*f*
Hemoglobin, 47*t*
Hemophilia, 46*t*
Hemoptysis, 207
Hemorrhage
  cerebrovascular, 184
  gastrointestinal, 195
  nasal, 207
Hemothorax, 38*t*
Hepatic, 48*t*
Hepatic function panel, 133
Hepatitis, 194, 195
Hernias
  abdominal, 49*t*
  inguinal, **38**, 193
  repair of, 112
  types of, 193–194
  umbilical, 194
High-risk pregnancy, 197
High severity problem, 75
HIPAA (Health Insurance Portability and Accountability Act), 187–188
Hirsutism, 201
History, 74
  extent of, 77*t*, 77–78
  family, 74, 170
  past, 75
  personal, 170
    of neoplasm, 178
  of present illness, 74
  social, 75
History V codes, 170
HIV (human immunodeficiency virus) infections, 176, 177, 198
Hives, 201
Hodgkin's disease, 48*t*
Home services, 85
Hordeolum, 52*t*

Hormones, 25–26
  terminology review, 57, 57t–58t
Hospital, time factors, 76
Hospital discharge services, newborn, 85
Hospital inpatient services, 82
  pediatric critical care, 84
Hospital observation services, 81, 82
Human immunodeficiency virus (HIV)
  infections, 176, 177, 198
Humerus, 22, 22f
Hydration, **142**, 145
Hydrocele, 41t
Hydrocephalus, 57t, 203, 204f
Hymen, 43t
Hyoid bone, 21–22, 22f
Hypercalcemia, 58t
Hyperkeratotic, **105**
Hypertension, 183
  cerebrovascular, 184
  classification of, 175, 183
  diagnosis of, 183, 183f, 184
  renal, 40t, 183
Hypertension Table (ICD-9-CM), 175,
  176t, 183
Hypertensive heart disease, 46t
Hypertensive retinopathy, 184
Hypertrophy, **193**
Hypoglycemia, 58t
Hypospadias, 40t, 203
Hypothalamus, 58t
Hypothyroidism, 58t
Hypoxia, 47t
Hysterectomy, **43**, 43f

I

ICD-9-CM codes, 164–216
  conventions, 166–167, 167t
  guidelines, 168, 168t
  Hypertension Table, 175, 176t, 183
  Neoplasm Table, 173–174, 174t
  notes, 167, 167t, 175–187, 193–210
  supplementary classifications, 165,
    169–173
  Table of Drugs and Chemicals, 165,
    173, 174t
  Tabular List of Diseases, 165, 165t,
    173–175
  Tabular List of Procedures, 166, 166t
ICD-9-CM coding manual, 165t,
  165–166
Idiopathic, **176t**
Ileum, 48t
Ilium, 22, 22f, 53t
Ill-defined conditions, 206t, 206–207
Immune system
  disorders, 179t, 179–180
  terminology review, 46, 46t–47t
Immunity, 47t
Immunizations, 86, 142, 143–144, 144f
Immunoglobulin, **136**
Immunology, 136
Immunotherapy, complications of, 178
Impetigo, 36t
In utero surgery, 198
Includes (note), 167t
Inclusion terms, ICD-9-CM codes,
  167, 167t
Increased procedural services, 92–93
Incus, 51t
Indexes
  CPT manual, 64, 64f
  HCPCS code manual, 158
  ICD-9-CM manual, 165, 166, 168,
    169, 169t, 171, 173–175, 206
Indwelling catheter, access to, 144, 150
Infants; see also Neonates
  critical care services, 83–84
  developmental milestones, 207

Infarction
  cerebrovascular, 184
  myocardial, 184–185
Infectious diseases, 175–177, 176t–177t
Inferior, 13
Inferior vena cava, 18, 18f
Infiltration, **99**
Infusions, **134**, 144
  flushing, 144, 150
  intravenous, 95f, 151
    for hydration, 145
  supply codes, 144, 150
  time reporting, 144, 151
Inguinal canal, 40t
Inguinal hernia, **38**, 193
Inhalant solution, 159t
Injections, 144, 151
  cardiac procedures, 148
  contrast materials, 124–125
  intradermal, 95f
  intramuscular, 95f
  nervous system procedures, 116–117
  subcutaneous, 15
  supply codes, 144, 150
  vascular procedures, 111, 148
Injury, 207–210, 208t; see also
    specific injury
  caused by terrorism, 173
  external causes of, 171–173, 172t,
    174t, 210
  intentional, 173
  multiple, 207
  musculoskeletal, 201
Inpatient services
  hospital, 82
  pediatric critical care, 84
Insertion, 54t
Insomnia, 181
Instrumentation, spinal procedures, 106
Insulin, **20**, 179
Insulin pump malfunction, 179–180
Insurance claims, 210–212, 211f
Integumentary system, 13–15, 15f;
    see also Skin
  disorders, 36t, 200t, 200–201
  surgery codes, 15, 103t, 103–105
  terminology review, 34, 35t, 201
Intensive care services, pediatric, 84
Intentional injury, 173
Intentional overdose, 209
Intercostal, 37t
Intermediate care facilities, 84–85
Internal, 13
Interstitial cells, 40t
Intervertebral disc degeneration, 202
Interview, psychiatric, 145, 145t
Intestinal transplantation, 113
Intestines, 19, 20f, 48, 48t–49t
  disorders, 193–194
  surgery codes, 112
Intra-arterial, 151, 159t
Intra-articular injection, of contrast
  materials, 124–125
Intradermal injection, 95f
Intrahepatic, **65**
Intramuscular, 95f, 159t
Intraocular administration, 50t
Intraservice time, 76, 152; see also
    Time reporting
Intrathecal, 159t
Intrathecal injection, of contrast
  materials, 124–125
Intravascular injection, of contrast
  materials, 124–125
Intravascularly, **124**
Intravenous, 94t, **159t**
Intravenous (IV) start, 144, 150
Intravenous catheter, access to,
  144, 150

Intravenous infusion, 95f, 151
  for hydration, 145
Introitus, 114
Involuntary (smooth) muscle, 23, 54t
Iridectomy, **95**
Iris, 21, 21f, 50t
Ischemia, 46t
Ischium, 22, 22f
IV; see Intravenous

J

J codes, 158, 159
Jaundice, 206
Jaw diseases, 193
Jejunum, 49t
Joint injection, of contrast materials,
  124–125
Joint range of motion testing, 151f

K

K codes, 158
Keratin, 35t
Kidney(s), 16, 16f, 39t; see also under
    Renal
Kidney transplantation, 113
Kyphosis, 55t, 55f, 202–203

L

L codes, 158, 160
Labia majora, 17f, 18
Labia minora, 17f, 18
Laboratory testing; see Pathology and
    Laboratory section
Lacrimal glands, 21, 50t
Laminectomy, **93**
Laparoscopy, 112, 114
Large intestine, 19, 20f, **48**, 48t
Larynx (voice box), 15, 15f, 37t
Late effect **173**, 199
Lateral, 13
Leg bones, 22, 22f
Legally induced abortion, 199
Lens, 21, 21f
Lesions, 15
  skin, **103**, 104f
  skull base, 115–116, 116t
Leukemia, 48t
Leukocyte, 47t
Levels of service, 74–75
Lichen, 200, 201
Lidocaine, **3**
Life-work balance, 3
Lipocyte, 35t
Liver, 19, 20f; see also under
    Hepatic
  disorders, 194–195
Liver transplantation, 112
Lobar pneumonia, 38t
Local anesthesia, 94, 94t, 144, 150
Long bones, 21, 22f, 53t
Long-term care facilities, 84–85
Lordosis, 55t, 55f
Low severity problem, 75
Lower respiratory tract, 36
Lumbar nerves, 25, 27f
Lumbar vertebrae, 21, 22f
  surgery codes, 106f
Lung(s), 15f, 16; see also Respiratory
    system; under Pulmonary
Lung/heart transplantation, 111
Lung transplantation, 107
Lupus erythematosus, 200
  systemic, 55t, 201
Lymphadenectomy, **65**
Lymphadenitis, 48t
Lymphadenopathy, 48t

Lymphatic system
  disorders, 47t–48t
  radiological procedures, 126
  terminology review, 46, 46t–47t
Lymphocyte, 47t
Lymphoma, 48t

M

M codes, 158
Macula, 50t
Magnetic resonance (MR)
    arthrography, 124
Main term, finding codes by, 64
Major Diagnostic Categories
    (MDCs), 212
Malabsorption, 195
Maladaptive behavior, **145**
Male reproductive system,
    16f, 16–17
  disorders, 41t, 195t, 195–196
  surgery codes, 18, 114–115
  terminology review, 38, 40t–41t
Malignant hypertension, 175
Malignant lesions, 103, 104f
Malignant neoplasms, 174–175, 177f,
    177–178, 178t
Malleus, 51t
Managed health care, 210
Manifestation, **166**, 167t
Manual blood testing, 135, 135f
Mapping
  brain, 150t
  electrophysiologic, 148t
Mass, versus neoplasm, 175
Mastectomy, **69,** 105, **159**
Mastication, 49t
Mastitis, 43t
  chronic cystic, 196
Mastoid process, 51t
Maternal record, versus newborn
    record, 206
Maternity care, 114, 115f
Maxillary sinuses, 51t
MDCs (Major Diagnostic
    Categories), 212
Measurements, codes with, 158
Meconium aspiration syndrome, **206**
Medial, 13
Mediastinum, 37t
Medicaid, **160**
Medical decision making, level of,
    79, 79t, 80
Medical evaluation, on-line, 151
Medical genetics, 150t
Medical history; see History
Medical records, 189, 189f
  comprehending, 8
  maternal versus newborn, 206
Medical screening, 74
Medical supply codes, 159
Medical terminology, 31–59; see also
    specific term
  blood system, 46, 46t–47t
  cardiovascular system,
    44, 44t–46t, 184
  CPT manual format, 65
  digestive system, 48, 48t–49t
  endocrine system, 57, 57t–58t
  integumentary system, 34, 35t–36t
  lymphatic system, 46, 46t–47t
  musculoskeletal system,
    53, 53t–54t
  nervous system, 54, 56t–57t
  reproductive system
    female, 43, 43t–44t
    male, 38, 40t–41t
  respiratory system, 36, 36t–38t
  senses, 50, 50t–52t

Medical terminology—*Cont.*
  urinary system, 38, 39*t*–40*t*
  V codes, 169, 169*t*
  word components, 32–34
Medicare, 158, 189, 212
Medicinal substances; *see* Drug(s)
Medicine section (CPT), 141–156
  add-on codes, 143
  modifiers, 142, 143*t*, 146, 148
  notes, 141, 143–153
  separate procedures, 143
  special report, 142
  subsections, 142
  unlisted codes, 143
Medulla oblongata, 24, 56*t*
Melanin, 35*t*
Meniere's disease, 52*t*
Meninges, 56*t*, 183*f*
Meningitis, 57*t*, 182, 183*f*
Menses, 43*t*, **76**
Mental disorders, 145–146,
  180–181, 181*t*
Mental retardation, 181
Metabolic diseases, 179*t*, 179–180
Metabolism, **46**
Metacarpals, 22, 22*f*
Metastasis, 177, 177*f*, 178
Metatarsal bones, 53*t*
Microbiology, 136
Microorganisms, **46**, 136, 175–176
Microscopy
  blood testing using, 135
  urinalysis using, 134
Micturition, 39*t*
Midbrain, 24–25
Midsagittal plane, 13, 13*f*
Minimal problem, 74
Minimally invasive procedures, 142
Minor problem, 74–75
Misadventure, **172**
Mitral valve, 18, 18*f*, 45*t*
Moderate conscious sedation, 151–152
Moderate severity problem, 75
Modifier(s), 67–68, 67*t*–68*t*
  anesthesia, 92–93, 93*t*
  Category II codes, 153, 153*t*
  HCPCS Level II codes, 160–161, 161*t*
  medicine, 142, 143*t*, 146, 148
  pathology and laboratory,
    132*t*–133*t*, 136
  radiology, 123*t*, 123–124
  surgery, 99, 99*t*–101*t*, 101, 103, 106,
    107, 110, 113, 117
Modifier -51 exemption, 69, 105,
  107, 143
Morbidity, **75**
Moribund, **93***t*
Morphology, **136**
Mortality, **75**
Motion analysis, 150*t*
Motivation, 2
Mouth (oral cavity), 19, 20*f*, 193, 194*f*
MR (magnetic resonance)
  arthrography, 124
Mucosa, 51*t*
Multiple choice questions, 8–9, 10
Multiple gestation, 198
Multiple injury codes, 207
Multiple laboratory procedures,
  132, 136
Multiple physicians
  radiological procedures, 123
  surgical procedures, 117
Multiple surgical procedures
  anesthesia code, 92
  reporting, 101, 113
Muscle range of motion testing, 150*t*
Muscular dystrophy, 55*t*
Muscular system, 23, 23*f*

disorders, 54*t*–55*t*, 201*t*,
  201–203, 202*t*
  procedure codes, 149, 150*t*
  surgery codes, 23, 105–107
  terminology review, 53, 53*t*–54*t*
Myasthenia gravis, 55*t*
Mycology, 136
Myelin, 56*t*
Myocardial infarction, 184–185
Myocardium, 45*t*
Myofilaments, 54*t*
Myringotomy, **179**

N

Nails, 13, 34*f*
Nasolacrimal, 50*t*
Nasopharynx, 37*t*
National Provider Identifier
  (NPI), 188
Nature of presenting problem,
  74–75
Nausea, chemotherapy-induced, 178
NDR (Nurse's Drug Reference), 159
NEC (not elsewhere classifiable), 166
Neglect, 173
Neonatal care, 85
  critical, 83–84
  transfers, 205
Neonatal record, versus maternal
  record, 206
Neonatal sepsis, 206
Neonates, 43*t*, **83**
  congenital anomalies, 203–204, 205
  perinatal conditions, 204*t*, 204–206
  premature, 206
Neoplasm(s), **165**, 173, 177, 177*f*;
  see also Cancer
  subcategories, 177, 178*t*
Neoplasm Table (ICD-9-CM),
  173–174, 174*t*
Nephrectomy, 113
Nephroblastoma, 40*t*
Nephrolithiasis, 40*t*
Nephrolithotomy, 113
Nephron, **39***t*
Nerve cell terms, 23–24
Nerve conduction tests, 150*t*
Nerve receptors, **15**
  sensory, 20–21, 50
Nervous system, 23–25, 24*f*, 26*f*, 27*f*
  disorders, 57*t*, 181–182, 182*t*
  surgery codes, 25, 115–117, 116*t*
  terminology review, 54, 56*t*
Neuroglia, 23
Neurological deficits, 184
Neurology, 149, 150*t*
Neuromuscular procedures, 149, 150*t*
Neuron, 23, 56*t*
Neurophysiology, intraoperative, 150*t*
Neurostimulators, 150*t*
Neurotransmitter, 23, 54*t*, 56*t*
Nevus, 35*t*
New patients, 73, 78, 147
Newborns; *see* Neonates
Non-face-to-face time, 76
Noninvasive procedures, 142
Normocephalic, **149**
NOS (not otherwise specified),
  166, 206
Nose, 20–21
  otorhinolaryngological services,
    147–148
  terminology review, 50, 51*t*
Nosebleed, 207
Not elsewhere classifiable
  (NEC), 166
Not otherwise specified (NOS),
  166, 206

Notes
  CPT
    medicine, 141, 143–153
    pathology and laboratory,
      133–137
    radiology, 125–128
  ICD-9-CM, 167, 167*t*, 175–187,
    193–210
NPI (National Provider Identifier), 188
Numerical codes; *see* CPT code(s)
Numerical order, CPT codes, 64
Nurse anesthetist, 92
Nurse's Drug Reference (NDR), 159
Nursing facility services, 84–85
Nystagmus, **21**, 52*t*

O

Observation services, hospital, 81, 82
Observation V codes, 170
Obstetric panel, 133, 133*f*
Obstetrics, 43*t*, 196–200, 197*t*;
  see also Childbirth; Pregnancy
Occipital bone, 53*t*
Occipital lobes, 24, 56*t*
Ocular adnexa, surgery codes, 117, 118*t*
Oculomycosis, 52*t*
Office services, evaluation and
  management, 80
Oil glands, 13
Omit code (note), 167*t*
Oncology; *see* Cancer; Neoplasm(s)
  radiation (*see* Radiation oncology)
Onychomalacia, 36*t*
Oocyte, 43*t*
Oophoritis, 44*t*
Opacification, **148**
Open book tests, 6–7
Ophthalmologist, **9**
Ophthalmology, 146–147, 147*t*
Optic nerves, 21, 21*f*, 50*t*
Optometrist, 50*t*
Oral administration, 159*t*
Oral cavity (mouth), 19, 20*f*, 193, 194*f*
Orchiepididymitis, 41*t*
Organ-oriented panels, 133, 133*f*
Organ systems, 13, 14*f*; *see also*
  specific system
  extent of examination by, 79
  review of, 75
  surgery codes by, 98, 99, 102, 102*f*
Organ transplantation; *see*
  Transplantation
Organic sleep disorders, 181
Orthotic, **158**
Orthotic procedures, 160
Ossicles, 51*t*
Osteoarthritis, 55*t*, 202, 203*f*
Osteocarcinoma, 55*t*
Osteocyte, 53*t*
Osteomalacia, 55*t*, **202**
Osteomyelitis, 202
Osteopathy, 151
Osteopenia, 202
Osteoporosis, 202
Other (note), 167*t*
Other routes, 159*t*
Otitis media, 52*t*
Otorhinolaryngologic, **142**
Otorhinolaryngological services,
  special, 147–148
Otosclerosis, 52*t*
Outcome of delivery code, 198
Outpatient services
  evaluation and management, 80
  neonatal, 85
  obstetric, 197
  pediatric, 83, 84

Ovaries, 17, 17*f*, 26, 57
Overdose, 209
Oviducts (fallopian tubes), 17*f*, 18, 43*t*

P

P codes, 158
Pacemakers, 108–109
Paget's disease, 55*t*
Pancreas, 20, 20*f*, 57
Pancreatic islets, 26
Pancreatic transplantation, 112
Pancreatitis, 49*t*, 195
Panels, organ or disease-oriented,
  133, 133*f*
Pansinusitis, 38*t*
Papanicolaou smear screening, 136
Papilloma, **175**
Parasitic diseases, 175–177,
  176*t*–177*t*
Parasitology, 136
Parathyroid glands, 26, 57, 58*t*
Parietal bones, 53*t*
Parietal lobes, 24, 56*t*
Parietal pleura, 37*t*
Parkinson's disease, 57*t*
Past history, 75
Pathogen, 47*t*
Pathological fractures, 202
Pathology, **126**
  surgical, 136–137, 137*t*
Pathology and Laboratory section
  (CPT), 131–140
  modifiers, 132*t*–133*t*, 136
  notes, 133–137
  qualitative tests, **132**–133
  quantitative tests, **132**–133
  subsections, 132
Pathophysiology review, 31–59
Patient counseling, 74
PDR (Physician's Drug Reference), 159
Pectoralis major muscle, 54*t*
Pectus excavatum, 204
Pediatric critical care services, 83–84
Pediatric psychiatric services, 145
Pediculosis, 36*t*
Pelvic girdle, 22, 22*f*
Pelvic inflammatory disease (PID),
  44*t*, 196, 197*f*
Pelvis, 39*t*
Penis, 16*f*, 17
Percutaneous skeletal fixation, **105**
Performance Measures Advisory
  Group (PMAG), 152
Pericarditis, 46*t*
Perinatal period, conditions in,
  204*t*, 204–206
Perineum, 40*t*, 43*t*
  surgery codes, 114
Peripheral nervous system (PNS),
  23, 24*f*, 54
Peristalsis, 49*t*
Peritoneal dialysis, 146
Peritonitis, 49*t*, 194
Personal history, 170
  of neoplasm, 178
Personal strengths and weaknesses,
  identifying, 7
Peruse, **6**, 8
Petechia, 207
Phagocyte, 47*t*
Phalanges, 22, 22*f*
Pharynx (throat), 15, 15*f*, 19, 20*f*
  otorhinolaryngological services,
    147–148
PHI (Protected Health Information),
  187, 188*f*
Phimosis, 41*t*
Physical safeguards (HIPAA), 188

Physical status modifiers, anesthesia, 93, 93*t*
Physician services
  anesthesia, 92
  care plan oversight, 85
  surgery, 101
Physician's Drug Reference (PDR), 159
Physiology
  defined, 13
  overview, 13–26
PID (pelvic inflammatory disease), 44*t*, 196, 197*f*
Piloidal cyst, 200
Pineal gland, 58*t*
Pinna, 51*t*
Pituitary gland, 26, 57, 58*t*
Place of occurrence, for injuries or poisonings, 173
Placental disorders, 198
Planner, time, 3–5, 4*f*
Pleura, 16, 37*t*
Pleural effusion, 38*t*
PMAG (Performance Measures Advisory Group), 152
Pneumonectomy, cadaver donor, 107
Pneumonia, 38*t*, 187
Pneumothorax, 38*t*
PNS (peripheral nervous system), 23, 24*f*, 54
Poisoning, 207–210, 208*t*
  external causes of, 171–173, 172*t*, 174*t*, 210
Poliomyelitis, 57*t*
Polycythemia, 180
Polydactyly, 204
Polysomnography, **150***t*
Pons, 24
Popliteal artery, 45*t*
Posterior, 13
Postoperative, **67**
Postpartum care, 114, 198–199
Practice coding examination, 218–235
Pre-reading strategies, during study sessions, 6
Prefixes, 33, 33*t*
Pregnancy; *see also* Childbirth; Obstetrics
  complications of, 196–200, 197*t*
  high-risk, 197
Prematurity, 206
Prenatal care, 114, 197
Present illness, history of, 74
Presenting problem, nature of, 74–75
Presumptive identification, 136
Preventive medicine services, 85–86
Priapism, 41*t*
Principal diagnosis, 189, 210
  obstetrical cases, 196, 197–198
Privacy Rule (HIPAA), 187, 188*f*
Problem focused examination, 78
Problem focused history, 77
Procedural risk, 189
Procedure(s); *see also specific type of procedure*
  abnormal reactions to, 173
  anesthesia codes by, 95
  CPT manual descriptions, 65
  minimally invasive, 142
  surgery codes by, 102 (*see also* Surgical procedures)
  UHDDS reporting rules, 189
Proctor, following directions given by, 7, 10
Proctosigmoidoscopy, 112
Procurement, **110**
Professional component, of radiological procedure, 124
Progesterone, 58*t*

Prognosis, **69**
Prolapsed uterus, 44*t*, 196, 197*f*
Prolonged services, 85
Prophylactic, **142**
Prostate, 16*f*, 17, 41*t*
Prostatic hyperplasia, benign, 41*t*
Prostatitis, 41*t*
Prosthetic procedures, 160
Protected Health Information (PHI), 187, 188*f*
Prothrombin, 47*t*, **135**
Protocol, **7**
Proton beam treatment delivery, 128, 128*t*
Proximal, 13
Proximal convoluted tubule, 39*t*
Psoriasis, 200, 201
Psychiatric disorders, 145–146, 180–181, 181*t*
Psychiatry, 145*t*, 145–146
Psychogenic, **176***t*
Psychotherapy, **145**
Pubic bone, 22, 22*f*
Puerperium, **165**
  complications, 196–200, 197*t*
Pulmonary artery, 18, 18*f*
Pulmonary embolism, 38*t*
Pulmonary lobe, 37*t*
Pulmonary procedures, 149
Pulmonary semilunar valve, 18, 18*f*
Pulmonary vein, 18, 18*f*
Punctuation, ICD-9-CM codes, 166–167
Pupil, 21, 21*f*, 50*t*
Purkinje fibers, 19, 19*f*, 45*t*
Purpura, 180
Pustulent, **3**
Pyelonephritis, 40*t*
Pyloric sphincter, 49*t*
Pyloric stenosis, 203

Q

Q codes, 158
Qualifying circumstances, anesthesia, 93, 94*t*
Qualitative tests, **132**–133
  drug, 133–134
Quantitative tests, **132**–133

R

R codes, 158
Radiation oncology, 127–128
  clinical treatment planning, 127, 128*t*
  treatment management, 127–128
Radiology section (CPT), 122–130
  contrast materials, 124–125
  modifiers, 123*t*, 123–124
  notes, 125–128
  professional versus technical component, 124
  special report, 124
  supervision and interpretation, 123, 124, 148
Radiotherapy, complications, 178
Radius, 22, 22*f*
Range of motion testing, 150*t*, 151*f*
Reading
  coding records, 6
  medical records, 8
  test questions, 8
Receptors, **15**
  sensory, 20–21, 50
Recipient allotransplantation
  heart, 111
  intestinal, 112
  lung, 107
  renal, 113

Rectocele, 196, 197*f*
Rectum, 19, 20*f*
Reflex arc, 24
Reflex tests, 150*t*
Regional anesthesia, 92, 94, 94*t*
Regional enteritis, 194
Related procedures, 101
  versus separate procedures, 143
Renal disease, 146
  anemia in, 180
  chronic, 195–196
Renal disease services, 146
Renal failure, 183
Renal hypertension, 40*t*, 183
Repolarization, 45*t*
Reports
  radiology, 124
  versus results, 124, 132
Reproductive system; *see* Female reproductive system; Male reproductive system
Respiratory system, 15*f*, 15–16
  disorders, 37*t*–38*t*, 185*t*, 185–187
  procedure codes, 149
  surgery codes, 107–108
  terminology review, 36, 36*t*–37*t*
Rest home services, 84
Results, versus reports, 124, 132
Retained products of conception, 199–200
Retina, 21, 21*f*, 50*t*
Retinopathy, hypertensive, 184
Retroperitoneal, 39*t*
Review of systems, 75
Rheumatoid arthritis, 202
Ribs, 21–22, 22*f*
Roots, word, 32, 32*t*
Rosacea, 200
Routes of administration, abbreviations for, 159*t*
Routine examination V codes, 171
Rugae, 49*t*
Rule of nines, 209, 209*f*

S

S codes, 158
SA (sinoatrial) node, 18, 19*f*, 45*t*
Sacral nerves, 25, 27*f*
Sacrum, 22, 22*f*
Sagittal plane, 13, 13*f*
Salivary glands, 19, 20*f*
  disorders, 193
Salpinx, 43*t*
Same-day service, 74
Saphenous vein grafting, 110
Sarcoma, **174**
Scapula, 22, 22*f*
Schedule, daily, 3–5, 4*f*, 5*t*
Sclera, 21, 21*f*, 51*t*
Scleroderma, 36*t*
Scoliosis, 55*t*, 55*f*, 203
Screening, 74, 170
Scrotum, 16, 16*f*, 41*t*
Sebaceous cyst, 201
Sebaceous glands, 14, 35*t*
Secondary neoplasm, previously excised, 178
Secondary site of neoplasm, 177
Secretion, 39*t*
Security Rule (HIPAA), 188
Sedation, conscious, 92, 94, 151–152
See (note), 167*t*
See also (note), 167*t*
Seizures, 182, 206
Self-harm, 209–210
Self-limited problem, 74–75
Semen, 41*t*
Semilunar valves, 18, 18*f*

Seminal vesicles, 16*f*, 17, 41*t*
Seminiferous tubules, 41*t*
Senses, 20–21
  disorders, 52*t*, 181–182, 182*t*
  terminology review, 50, 50*t*–52*t*
Separate procedures, 101, 143
  versus related procedures, 143
Sepsis, neonatal, 206
Septicemia, 177, **206**
Sequela, **199**
Service, levels of, 74–75
Shoulder girdle, 22, 22*f*
Sialadenitis, **193**
Sight; *see* Eyes
Sigmoidoscopy, **112**
Signs, Symptoms, and Ill-Defined Conditions, 206*t*, 206–207
Sinoatrial (SA) node, 18, 19*f*, 45*t*
Sinus endoscopy, 107
SIRS (systemic inflammatory response syndrome), 177
Skeletal (voluntary) muscle, 23, 23*f*, 54*t*
Skeletal system, 21–23, 22*f*
  disorders, 54*t*–55*t*, 201*t*, 201–203, 202*t*
  surgery codes, 23, 105*t*, 105–107, 106*t*
  terminology review, 53, 53*t*
Skilled nursing facilities, 84–85
Skin; *see also* Integumentary system
  layers of, 13–15, 15*f*
Skin biopsy, 103
Skin lesions, 15, 103, 104*f*
Skull, 21, 22*f*, 53*t*
Skull base, surgery of, 115–116, 116*t*
Sleep disorders, 181
Sleep testing, 150*t*
Small intestine, 19, 20*f*, 49*t*
Smell; *see* Nose
Smooth (involuntary) muscle, 23, 54*t*
Social history, 75
Source documents, coding from, 210
Special report, 69
  anesthesia, 92
  medicine, 142
  radiology, 124
  surgery, 101–102
Specialized training, procedures requiring, 189
Specimen, 136
Spermatocyte, 41*t*
Sphygmomanometer, 183, 183*f*
Spinal cord, 25, 27*f*, 54, 183*f*
Spinal disorders, 55*t*, 55*f*, 202
Spinal instrumentation codes, 106
Spinal nerves, 25, 27*f*, 54
Spine (vertebral column), 21, 22*f*
  chiropractic regions, 151
  injection of contrast materials, 124
  surgery codes, 105–107, 106*t*
Spirometry, **149**
Splenomegaly, 48*t*
Spondylolisthesis, 203
Spondylosis, 202
Spongy bone, 21
ST segment elevation myocardial infarction (STEMI), 185
Stapes, 51*t*
Status asthmaticus, 187
STEMI (ST segment elevation myocardial infarction), 185
Stereotaxis, **25**
Sternocleidomastoid muscle, 54*t*
Sternum, 21–22, 22*f*, 37*t*
Stomach, 19, 20*f*
  disorders, 193
Strabismus, 52*t*
Strapping, 107
Stratum corneum, **13**

Strengths, personal, 7
Study habits, effective, 2–5
Study skills strategies, 6–9
Subcutaneous, 15, **103**, 159*t*
Subcutaneous catheter, access to, 144, 150
Subcutaneous layer, 15, 15*f*, 35*t*
Subcutaneous tissue diseases, 200*t*, 200–201
Subdural hematoma, 57*t*
Subsequent hospital care services, 84
Suffixes, 34, 34*t*
Sulci, 24
Superficial, 13
Superficial fascia, 15
Superior, 13
Superior vena cava, 18, 18*f*
Superlatives, **9**
Supplemental tracking codes (Category II), 152–153
Supplementary classifications, 165, 169–173
Supply codes, 142
  anesthesia, 92
  HCPCS Level II, 159
  injection/infusion, 144, 150
  surgery, 101
Suppression testing, 134
Supraventricular dysrhythmias, 109
Surgeons
  anesthesia by, 93
  multiple, 117
Surgery section (CPT), 98–121
  add-on codes, 102–103, 107
  auditory system, 117, 118*t*
  cardiovascular system, 19, 108*t*–109*t*, 108–111
  coding guidelines, 102*f*, 102–103
  digestive system, 112–113
  endocrine system, 115–117
  eye and ocular adnexa, 117, 118*t*
  integumentary system, 15, 103*t*, 103–105
  materials supplied by physician, 101
  modifiers, 99, 99*t*–101*t*, 101, 103, 106, 107, 110, 113, 117
  musculoskeletal system, 23, 105*t*, 105–107, 106*t*
  nervous system, 25, 115–117, 116*t*
  reproductive system, 18, 114*t*, 114–115
  respiratory system, 107–108
  separate procedures, 101
  special report, 101–102
  subsections, 99
  unlisted codes, 102
  urinary system, 16, 113–114
Surgical package, definition of, 99
Surgical pathology, 136–137, 137*t*
Surgical procedures
  abnormal reaction to, 173
  multiple
    anesthesia code, 92
    reporting, 101, 113
  UHDDS reporting rules, 189
Surgical supply codes, 159
Sweat glands, 13–14
Symbology, **6**
Sympathetic nervous system, 56*t*

Symptoms, 206*t*, 206–207
Synapse, 23
Synonyms, 65
Synovial joint, 53*t*
Synovitis, 202
Synthesize, **6**
Systemic, **75**
Systemic inflammatory response syndrome (SIRS), 177
Systemic lupus erythematosus, 55*t*, 201
Systolic, 45*t*

T

T codes, 158
Table of Drugs (HCPCS), 159
Table of Drugs and Chemicals (ICD-9-CM), 165, 173, 174*t*
Tabular List of Diseases (ICD-9-CM), 165, 165*t*, 173–175, 174*t*
Tabular List of Procedures (ICD-9-CM), 166, 166*t*
Tangential, **128**
Taste, 20–21, 50
Technical component, of radiological procedure, 124
Technical safeguards (HIPAA), 188
Temporal lobes, 24, 56*t*
Temporary codes (Category III), 153–154
Tendons, 23, 23*f*, 54*t*
Terminology; *see* Medical terminology
Terrorism, injury caused by, 173
Test; *see* Coding examinations
Testes, 16, 16*f*, 26, 41*t*, 57
Testicular carcinoma, 41*t*
Testicular torsion, 41*t*
Testosterone, 58*t*
Tetany, 58*t*
Thoracic aorta, endovascular repair of, 110–111
Thoracic nerves, 25, 27*f*
Thoracic vertebrae, 21, 22*f*
  surgery codes, 106*t*
Thoracotomy, **95**
Thorax, 37*t*
Throat (pharynx), 15, 15*f*, 19, 20*f*
  otorhinolaryngological services, 147–148
Thrombectomy, **19**
Thrombocyte, 47*t*
Thrombocytopenia, 180
Thrombophlebitis, 48*t*
Thrombus, 46*t*
  cerebral, 57*t*
  versus embolus, 44, 44*f*
Thymus, 26, 57, 58*t*
Thyroid gland, 26, 57, 58*t*
Tibia, 22, 22*f*
Time management
  for studying, 2–5
  for test preparation, 10
  during test-taking, 7–8, 10
Time reporting
  anesthesia codes, 92
  conscious sedation, 152
  critical care services, 83
  evaluation and management services, 76, 82

infusions, 144, 151
  psychotherapy, 146
Torticollis, 202
Touch, 20–21, 50
Toxic effects, 209–210
Toxoids, **142**
  administration (*see* Immunizations)
Trachea (windpipe), 15, 15*f*, 37*t*
Tracheostenosis, 38*t*
Tracheostomy, **159**
Tracking codes (Category II), 152–153
Transaction rules (HIPAA), 187–188
Transient, 206
Transient ischemic attack, 57*t*
Transplantation
  heart/lung, 111
  intestinal, 112
  liver, 112
  lung, 107
  pancreatic, 112
  renal, 113
Transverse plane, 13, 13*f*
Treatment management, radiation therapy, 127–128
Tricuspid valve, 45*t*
Trisomy, 21, 204
Tumor; *see* Cancer; Neoplasm(s)
Turbinates, 53*t*
Tympanic membrane, 51*t*

U

UHDDS (Uniform Hospital Data Discharge Set), 188–189
Ulcer
  decubitus, **159**, 201
  duodenal, 49*t*
Ulcerative colitis, 194
Ulna, 22, 22*f*, 53*t*
Ultrasound
  cardiac, 148
  diagnostic, 126*t*, 126–127
Umbilical hernia, 194
Uniform Hospital Data Discharge Set (UHDDS), 188–189
Unique Identifiers Rule (HIPAA), 188
Unit time, 76
Unknown etiology, 206
Unlisted codes, 69, 102, 143
Unspecified (note), 167*t*
Unspecified hypertension, 175
Unusual anesthesia, 93
Upper respiratory tract, 36
Upper respiratory tract infection, 38*t*
Uremia, 40*t*
Ureterolithiasis, 40*t*
Ureters, 16, 16*f*, 39*t*
Urethra, 16, 16*f*, 39*t*
Urethrocystitis, 40*t*
Urethroscopy, 113
Urinalysis, 134
Urinary bladder, 16, 16*f*, 38
Urinary meatus, 39*t*
Urinary system, 16, 16*f*; *see also* Kidney(s); *under* Renal
  disorders, 40*t*, 195*f*, 195–196
  surgery codes, 16, 113–114
  terminology review, 38, 39*t*
Urination, 39*t*

Urodynamics, **113**
Urticaria, 36*t*, 201
Use additional code (note), 167*t*, 205
Uterus (womb), 17*f*, 18, 43*t*
  prolapsed, 44*t*, 196, 197*f*

V

V codes
  HCPCS, 158
  ICD-9-CM, 165, 169*t*–170*t*, 169–171, 205
Vaccinations, 86, 142, 143–144, 144*f*
Vagina, 17*f*, 18
Vaginal delivery, 114, 115*f*
Varicose vein, 48*t*
Various routes, 159*t*
Vas deferens, 41*t*
Vascular procedures, **69**, 148
  injection, 111, 148
  radiological, 125*f*, 125–126
Vena cava, 18, 18*f*, 45*t*
Venography, 126
Venous grafting, for coronary artery bypass, 110
Ventral, 13
Ventricle, 18, 18*f*, 45*t*
Ventricular septal defect, 203
Verify codes, 65, 164
Vertebral column; *see* Spine
Vesicovaginal fistula, 44*t*
Vestibular function tests, 147–148
Viremia, 207
Virology, 136
Visceral, 49*t*
Vision; *see* Eyes
Visual cortex, 56*t*
Vitiligo, 201
Vitreous humor, 51*t*
Voice box (larynx), 15, 15*f*, 37*t*
Voluntary (skeletal) muscle, 23, 23*f*, 54*t*
Vomiting, chemotherapy-induced, 178
Vowel, combining, 32–33
Vulvectomy, 114, 114*t*

W

Weaknesses, personal, 7
Wheezing, 186
Windpipe (trachea), 15, 15*f*, 37*t*
With (note), 167*t*
Womb (uterus), 17*f*, 18, 43*t*
  prolapsed, 44*t*
Word beginnings, 33, 33*t*
Word endings, 34, 34*t*
Word roots, 32, 32*t*
Work-life balance, 3
Wound debridement, 209
Wound repair, 103*t*, 103–104
  multiple, 103
Written reports, radiology, 124
Wry neck, 202

Z

Zygomatic bones, 53*t*